Sponsored by the
International Life Sciences Institute

Caffeine

Perspectives from Recent Research

Edited by P. B. Dews

With 32 Figures and 36 Tables

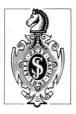

Springer-Verlag
Berlin Heidelberg New York Tokyo 1984

Dr. Peter B. Dews
181 Upland Road, Newtonville, MA 02160, USA

ILSI International Life Sciences Institute,
      1126 Sixteenth Street, N. W., Washington, DC 20036, USA

ISBN 3-540-13532-4 Springer-Verlag Berlin Heidelberg New York Tokyo
ISBN 0-387-13532-4 Springer-Verlag New York Heidelberg Berlin Tokyo

Library of Congress Cataloging in Publication Data. Caffeine : perspectives form recent research. "Sponsored by the International Life Sciences Institute"–Includes bibliographical references and index. 1. Caffeine–Physiological effect. 2. Caffeine–Metabolism. 3. Caffeine–Toxicology. I. Dews, Peter B., 1922 –. II. International Life Sciences Institute. [DNLM: 1. Caffeine–pharmacodynamics. 2. Caffeine–metabolism. QV 107 C129] QP801.C24C34 1984 615'.785 84–5602

Typesetting and binding: G. Appl, Wemding, printing: aprinta, Wemding
2123/3140-543210

Foreword

Before the late 1970s, interest in caffeine among both the general public and the scientific community was at a relatively low level for many years, even though it was recognized that caffeine was an almost universal component of the diet. The National Coffee Association was supporting a continuing program of research, some research was being conducted by a few of the largest companies selling coffee, and an occasional university researcher became interested in caffeine and conducted experiments, often on effects of caffeine in very high concentration in vitro on skeletal muscle fibres or on dividing cells. Since 1978, however, there has been a mighty upsurge in both public and scientific interest in caffeine. It is interesting to note that this was prompted not by discovery of hitherto unknown effects or hazards of caffeine, but by the actions of a regulatory agency, the Food & Drug Administration (FDA) of the U.S. Public Health Service.

The U.S. Congress passed new laws on foods and drugs in 1958. One of the provisions was for testing of food additives to assess risk to health. As it was clearly impracticable to require immediate testing of all additives already in use, a list was drawn up of some hundreds of additives that were generally recognized as safe (GRAS). When the law had been operating for some years, a presidential directive required the FDA to reexamine the evidence on risk of the substances on the GRAS list. The FDA commissioned a special committee on GRAS substances (SCOGS) to examine the evidence. Caffeine was on the GRAS list. In 1978, the SCOGS issued a draft of its commentary on caffeine, which immediately occasioned both public and industry interest. The soft drinks industry, because of their practice of adding caffeine to colas and other soft drinks, became particularly involved. Its main response, surely appropriate, took the form of initiation of support for scientific research on caffeine. The research program continues under the auspices of the International Life Sciences Institute (ILSI), a foundation developed primarily to permit companies to pool resources to support research programs of common interest. On caffeine, the ILSI has also supported a series of international workshops for exchange of information on caffeine between researchers, both supported and not supported by ILSI, and an interested technical audience, including individuals from regulatory agencies.

In 1981, the FDA published a proposed regulation on caffeine in the Federal Register and invited comments. Among the groups that commented was the ILSI, which collected a group of experts to review and address the various points raised by the FDA. The resulting report represented a rather comprehensive update of scientific information on caffeine by many of the leading experts in the fields covered. ILSI had been discussing the desirability of sponsoring a monograph on caffeine, and the work done for the report provided a good starting point. This volume is the result. While it shows clear signs of its origin, coverage has been expanded considerably beyond the original report by the addition of a number of authors to cover areas not addressed by the FDA. The book is by no means a primer, but it is intendend to be intelligible to the wide audience of people with technical interest in caffeine. It was suggested to authors that they start their update from the publication in 1976 of the comprehensive monograph by Eichler and collaborators (*Kaffee und Coffein,* Springer-Verlag, Berlin Heidelberg New York).

Preface

Caffeine is a regular component of the diet for most people. What happens to it when it has been ingested, and what are its consequences? In addressing these questions, the contributors to this monograph illustrate some of the strengths and weaknesses of contemporary dietary pharmacology, which studies the physiological, biochemical and behavioral consequences of dietary intake of substances. Never before has there been so much interest in dietary pharmacology. Millions of joggers and other athletes, as well as health zealots, spend much time and effort on selection of their diet, clearly on the premise that proper choice of diet can benefit them in an emphatic manner. In many top-ranking athletes the preoccupation approaches a fetish, strongly encouraged by coaches. Other classes of consumers are equally preoccupied with the possibility of being harmed by components of the diet, whether added deliberately or present as trace contaminants. "Organic" food stores prosper, and there are periodic "scares" about particular foods or classes of foods.

To an objective appraiser, it is likely that the great majority of effects in dietary pharmacology are subtle, making for problems in their detection and measurement. Subtle means hard to measure, but not necessarily trivial; people eat every day, and the effects of substances taken daily may, in the long run, have substantial effects. If a regimen including caffeine helps worker A do better than worker B by a 2.5% annual increment, then after 30 years A will be doing more than twice as well as B. Small margins in competitiveness can be cumulatively decisive.

We are accustomed to the analytical techniques of the chemist becoming progressively more sensitive, so that we can measure smaller and smaller amounts of components of the diet and of the body, from milligrams to micrograms to nanograms and even picograms. Pharmacologists and students of nutrition have taken avidly to modern analytical techniques and to other boons from the physical sciences in their studies of receptors and of the intimate molecular mechanisms of drugs and foods. In contrast, there has been no substantial increase in the sensitivity of methods of detecting physiological and behavioral effects, either beneficial or deleterious, in the past 20 years or so. Higher sensitivities in measuring subtle effects are needed, both for purely scientific purposes and to answer questions now being asked urgently by the public. Among the classical nutritional requirements for the maintenance of health are the inclusion of particular substances in the diet and a balanced intake of carbohydrates and fats. Beyond this, the influences of quantity, composition, and schedule of intake of foods on physiological and behavioral performance are largely unkown. Folklore abounds with stories ranging from the salutary effects of oysters to the "brain food" functions of fish. The superstition of many athletes has already been mentioned. In spite of the enduring public interest in diet, there has been little systematic scientific study until recent years, and many subtle effects may be unrecognized. These are not matters of life and death; but then, neither is music. It is to be hoped that the increase of interest in the subtle effects of caffeine, beneficial or deleterious, will be one more factor leading to increased work in dietary pharmacology.

On the basis of present information, some predictions about characteristics of dietary pharmacology may be ventured. First, to demonstrate an effect of a dietary component convincingly, it will be necessary to show a quantitative relation between intake and effect, corresponding to a dose-effect curve in classical pharmacology. But dose-effect curves in dietary pharmacology will often reach an asymptote at levels which are low relative to toxic levels, and so it will be easy to miss dependence of the effect on the size of the dose. Examples of asymptotes can be found in the fields of both nutrition and pharmacology. Take a subject deficient only in Vitamin A. Therapeutic effect is related to dose of vitamin A over a limited range. Once an optimum utilizable dose has been reached, additional, amounts have no clear incremental effect until, with doses which are orders of magnitude larger than the maximum therapeutic levels, toxic effects become manifest. Mechanistically, such effects may have little in common with the therapeutic effects. Among drugs, acetylsalicylic acid, in its therapeutic range, operates quantitatively in inhibiting synthetic pathways in the prostaglandin-prostacyclin systems. Once effectively complete inhibition has been achieved in any particular pathway, increasing doses have no substantial additional effect on that system until, again, toxic levels are reached. The mechanism of the toxic effects of acetylsalicylic acid, for example, on respiration is different from that of the effects of small doses on headache. It may be noted in passing that the irrelevance of actions at high dose levels poses decisive problems for conventional strategies of risk assessment. It should also be noted that the occurrence of asymptotes does not remove the necessity of demonstrating dose dependence; it just makes it harder to achieve.

A second feature of dietary pharmacology may be illustrated with the same two examples. Reasonable amounts of Vitamin A have no discernible effects in a nondeficient subject, and reasonable amounts of acetylsalicyclic acid have no discernible behavioral effects in subjects free from pain and fever. In both instances, many characteristic effects of the agent could not be detected and measured in samples of subjects – humans or experimental animals – chosen randomly from well cared for, normal populations.

Third, developments in dietary pharmacology are sure to blur further the dividing line between "foods" and "drugs". No one is about to reclassify penicillin or digoxin as a food, but what of, for example, minerals, amines, and amino acids, ubiquitous components of the diet that have undoubted conventional pharmacological effects?

Dietary pharmacology is well exemplified by caffeine. Caffeine can have subtle behavioral effects quantitatively related to dose at levels far below toxic levels. Increasing amounts do not then cause increases in most of the characteristic behavioral effects. Eventually, at toxic levels, the mechanisms have a dubious relationship to those of the characteristic effects at low doses. A variety of behavioral effects of caffeine that are relatively easily detected in fatigued, bored, or sleepy subjects may be essentially undetectable in alert, fresh subjects. Caffeine is a component of natural foods and is essentially completely metabolized in a way that is not characteristically qualitatively different from the general manner in which, for example, other purines in the diet are handled.

In this volume we start from the firm ground of metabolism and kinetics. We then consider consumption levels, always a crucial component in determining societal consequences of dietary practices. Physiological and behavioral effects are then assessed and information on molecular mechanism of action is examined. The next group of chapters reviews risk-assessment studies, which are useful without pretending to any "proof of safety." The volume concludes, deliberately, with a contribution to pure science, a designation which does not preclude possible practical importance.

Contents

Section II Intake

Section III Physiological and Behavioral Effects

Section V **Direct Assessments of Effects on Health**
Editor of Section V: W. R. Grice

XIV

XVI

List of Contributors

Dr. M.J. Arnaud, Nestle Products Technical Assistance Co. Ltd, Research Department, CH-1814 La Tour de Peilz, Switzerland

J.J. Barone, The Coca-Cola Company, External Technical Affairs Department, P.O. Drawer 1734, Atlanta, GA 30301, USA

Dr. M. Bonati, Istituto di Ricerche Farmacologiche, "Mario Negri", Via Eritrea 62, I-20157 Milano, Italy

Dr. R.W. von Borstel, Laboratory of Neuroendocrine Regulation, Department of Nutrition and Food Science, Massachusetts Institute of Technology, Cambridge, MA 02139, USA

Dr. H. D. Christensen, Department of Pharmacology, University of Oklahoma, Health Sciences Center, Oklahoma City, OK 73109, USA

Dr. J. D. B. Collins, Connaught Laboratories Ltd., Toronto, Ontario, Canada

Dr. P. W. Curatolo, New England Deaconess Hospital, Department of Surgery, 185 Pilgrim Road, Boston, MA 02115, USA

Dr. P. B. Dews, Vice-President, 181 Upland Road, Newtonville, MA 02160, USA

Dr. J. D. Fernstrom, Western Psychiatric Institute, 3811 O'Hara Street, Pittsburgh, PA 15213, USA

Dr. M. H. Fernstrom, Western Psychiatric Institute, 3811 O'Hara Street, Pittsburgh, PA 15213, USA

Dr. S. Garattini, Istituto di Ricerche Farmacologiche, "Mario Negri", Via Eritrea 62, I-20157 Milano, Italy

Dr. W. R. Gomes, University of Illinois, 315 Animal Sciences Laboratory, Urbana, IL 61801, USA

Dr. H. C. Grice, 71 Norice Drive, Nepean, Ontario, K2G 2X7, Canada

Dr. R. H. Haynes, York University, Department of Biology, Toronto, Ontario, M3J IP3, Canada

Dr. A. Leviton, Department of Neurology, The Children's Hospital, Medical Center, Boston, MA 02115, USA

Dr. A. H. Neims, Department of Pharmacology, University of Florida, Box J 267 JHMHC, Gainsville, Fl 32610, USA

Dr. H. Roberts, NSDA, 1101 16th NW, Washington DC 20036, USA

Dr. J. J. Roberts, Institute of Cancer Research, Royal Cancer Hospital, Molecular Pharmacology, F Block, Clifton Avenue, GB-Sutton, Surrey SM2 5PX, United Kingdom

Dr. D. Robertson, Division of Clinical Pharmacology, Vanderbilt University Medical School, Nashville, TN 37232, USA

Dr. W. J. Scott Jr., The Children's Hospital, Research Foundation, Cincinnati, OH 45229, USA

Dr. S. H. Snyder, Department of Pharmacology, John Hopkins University, Medical School, 725 North Wolfe St., Baltimore, MD 21205, USA

Dr. E. R. Spindel, Laboratory of Molecular Endocrinology, Massachusetts General Hospital, Boston, MA 02114, USA

Dr. J. G. Wilson, The Children's Hospital, Research Foundation, Cincinnati, OH 45229, USA

R. J. Wurtman, M. D., Laboratory of Neuroendocrine Regulation, Massachusetts Institute of Technology, Cambridge, MA 02139, USA

Section I
Metabolism and Kinetics

I Products of Metabolism of Caffeine

M. J. Arnaud

1 Discovery and Chemical Structure of Methylxanthines

The isolation of caffeine from green coffee beans was described in Germany in 1820 by Runge and confirmed the same year by von Giese. In France, Robiquet in 1823 and then Pelletier in 1826 independently discovered a white and volatile crystalline substance. The name "cofeina" appeared in 1823 in the "Dictionnaire des termes de médecine" and the word "caffein" or "coffein" was used by Fechner in 1826. The same year, Martius discovered a substance which he called "guaranin", and 1 year later a substance found in tea was named "thein" by Oudry. It was only in 1838 (Mulder; Jobst) and in 1840 (Martius; Berthemot and Dechastelus) that thein and guaranin respectively were shown to be identical with caffeine. In 1843 caffeine was found in maté prepared from *Ilex paraguayensis* (Stenhouse), and in 1865 in kola nuts (Daniell).

Theobromine was discovered in cocoa beans by Woskresensky in 1842, but it was only in 1888 that Kossel isolated theophylline from tea leaves and identified it as a dimethylxanthine. The third dimethylxanthine, paraxanthine, has been observed in plants very recently (Chou and Waller 1980) and was isolated for the first time from human urine by Salomon in 1883.

At that time, chemical identification of natural methylxanthines was closely linked with studies on purines in nucleic acids and uric acid discovered as early as 1776 (Scheele). Even today, the presence of methylated purine and pyrimidine in nucleic acids raises the question of the endogenous or exogenous origin of methylated xanthine and uric acid and more recently uracil derivatives identified in human urine (Burg 1975; Fink et al. 1964: De et al. 1980, 1981).

In 1861, using methyl iodide, Strecker converted theobromine to caffeine, leading to the important conclusion that theobromine was a dimethylxanthine and caffeine a trimethylxanthine. In 1875, Medicus described the structure of xanthine and caffeine correctly, but his formula of theobromine was incorrect with regard to the position of a methyl group. In 1882, Fischer demonstrated that theobromine was obtained by the methylation of xanthine. However, as the location of one of the oxy groups in the xanthine molecule was incorrect, the proposed formula for caffeine was also incorrect. In addition, the position of the methyl groups for theobromine was unchanged from the chemical structure proposed by Medicus (1875).

Finally, in 1895, Fischer and Ach achieved the complete synthesis of caffeine, but it was only 2 years later that after several years of experimental investigations, the formula for caffeine suggested by Medicus based on speculation by Fischer was

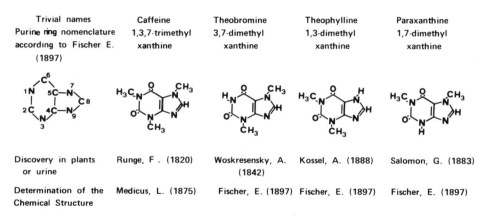

Trivial names	Caffeine	Theobromine	Theophylline	Paraxanthine
Purine ring nomenclature according to Fischer E. (1897)	1,3,7-trimethyl xanthine	3,7-dimethyl xanthine	1,3-dimethyl xanthine	1,7-dimethyl xanthine
Discovery in plants or urine	Runge, F. (1820)	Woskresensky, A. (1842)	Kossel, A. (1888)	Salomon, G. (1883)
Determination of the Chemical Structure	Medicus, L. (1875)	Fischer, E. (1897)	Fischer, E. (1897)	Fischer, E. (1897)

Fig. 1. Discovery and chemical identification of caffeine and dimethylxanthines

confirmed (Fischer 1897). The chemical structure of theobromine, theophylline, and paraxanthine was described. A monomethylxanthine already identified in human urine (Salomon 1885) called heteroxanthine and identified as 7-methylxanthine (Krüger and Salomon 1895/1896) was discovered in plants *(Beta vulgaris)* in 1904 by Bresler.

The chemical structures of caffeine and dimethylxanthines, named according to the numbering of the purine ring atoms proposed by Fischer (1897), are presented in Fig. 1.

The earliest known study on caffeine metabolism was carried out in 1850, before the chemical characterization of caffeine, by Lehmann, who failed to detect traces of caffeine in human urine following an oral dose. Albanese (1895) was the first to report that dogs and rabbits fed large doses of caffeine or theobromine excreted a monomethylxanthine, showing that ingested methylxanthines were demethylated. A few months later, Rost (1895) published data on the excretion of unchanged caffeine and theobromine in the cat, the dog, the rabbit, and man. In man, 0.5% and 19% of caffeine and theobromine doses respectively were recovered in urine, while the corresponding mean values were 16% and 15% in the rabbit, 4% and 22% in the dog, and 2.4% for caffeine in the cat. Most of the recent human studies (Cornish 1956; Arnaud and Welsch 1980a, 1981) have confirmed these percentages, which can be accepted as definitive.

In 1895 and 1896, Bondzynski and Gottlieb (1895a, b, 1896) isolated a monomethylxanthine in the rabbit corresponding to 20% of a daily dose of 2.5 g theobromine. This metabolite was later shown to be 7-methylxanthine.

Purine bases were isolated from normal human urine, and quantitative analysis of 10000 liters of normal human urine by Krüger and Salomon (1898, 1898/1899) showed the presence of 1,7-dimethylxanthine, 1-methylxanthine, 7-methylxanthine, and 7-methylguanine.

In 1899 and 1900, Krüger, in association with P. Schmidt and J. Schmidt, reported several studies performed with dogs, rabbits, and human subjects fed large doses of theobromine. They were the first to observe species difference in the metabolism of

4

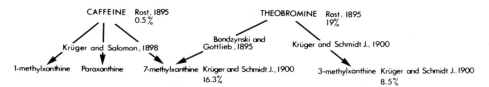

Fig. 2. Discovery of metabolic pathways in man and quantitative estimation of the metabolites before 1900 (expressed as % of the administered compound, caffeine or theobromine)

this dimethylxanthine, and in addition to 7-methylxanthine, they identified 3-methylxanthine, which amounted in man (Krüger and J. Schmidt 1900) to 8.5% of the dose of theobromine, a result in agreement with the most recent study (Arnaud and Welsch 1981). Oral administration of paraxanthine to rabbits showed the excretion of 8% unchanged paraxanthine, while 1-methylxanthine amounted to only 1% of the dose and 7-methylxanthine could not be detected (Krüger and P. Schmidt 1899).

In a study published in 1901, Krüger and J. Schmidt concluded that in man the methyl groups were decreasingly stable in the order 7, 1, 3, and that the methylated purines found in human urine were explained by the 3-methyl demethylation of the methylated purines present in food. The stability of the methyl groups of caffeine evaluated recently (Arnaud and Welsch 1981) by the quantitative analysis of metabolites excreted in human urine is in agreement with these conclusions made at the beginning of this century (Fig. 2).

2 Formation of Uric Acid Metabolites

The demonstration that caffeine was demethylated into dimethylxanthine and even monomethylxanthine raised the question of the subsequent formation of xanthine and uric acids as end-metabolic products. This problem was studied as early as 1868 by Leven, who found that coffee drinking did not increase the excretion of uric acid in man, while in 1896 and 1899 both tea and coffee drinking were shown in independent studies to increase uric acid excretion in urine (Hess and Schmoll 1896; Haig 1896). Finally, in 1900, Burian and Schur observed no modifications of uric acid excretion in urine after ingestion of caffeine.

Using a more accurate colorimetric method and a well-designed experimental protocol, whereby the subjects drank decaffeinated coffee for 3 days and caffeine was then added for the next 4 days at a dose of 200 mg/cup, corresponding to a total dose of 1 g caffeine/day, Benedict demonstrated in 1916 that ingested caffeine significantly increased the excretion of endogenous uric acids. These results were confirmed a few months later by Mendel and Wardell (1917) with subjects on a purine-free diet, who received coffee, tea, or caffeine. In 1926, Clark and de Lorimier observed that the concentration of uric acid in blood increased after caffeine administration, and increased excretion in urine was also found. This problem was studied in 1928 by Myers and Wardell after the administration of caffeine, theobromine, and theophylline in man, using several methods for the estimation of uric acid. The results obtained suggested the possibility that some products of caffeine me-

5

tabolism other than uric acid can react with the reagents. Although none of the methyluric acids had ever been found in the urine at that time, Myers and Wardell hypothesized that caffeine could be oxidized in the 8 position before it was completely demethylated. With standards of methyluric acids supplied by Biltz, they observed that 1-methyluric acid and 1,3-dimethyluric acid gave the same color development as uric acid, while 1,3,7-trimethyluric acid gave little color and 7-methyluric acid with 3,7-dimethyluric acid gave no color at all. In the light of the known instability of methyluric acids, they were able to show that color reaction can be obtained or not depending on the method employed, thus explaining the discrepancies reported in previous studies.

A study by Myers and Hanzal in 1929 suggested the formation of 3,7-dimethyluric acid from theobromine, and these authors succeeded in isolating crystals resembling those of 1,3-dimethyluric acid after administration of theophylline to Dalmatian dogs. They concluded that the methylated derivatives of uric acid were apparently quite stable in the animal organism.

Buchanan et al. (1945b) confirmed that after caffeine and theophylline administration in man, there was increased excretion of phosphotungstic-acid-reducing material, while theobromine did not show this effect. Using uricases (Buchanan et al. 1945a), they demonstrated that the observed increased excretion was not produced by true uric acid. They were the first to produce evidence that methylxanthines did not seem to be completely demethylated and then converted into uric acid. In addition, precipitation by ammoniacal silver suggested the presence of 1-methyluric acid after caffeine administration.

One year later, Myers and Hanzal (1946) reported the complete study of the metabolism of 1-methyl-, 3-methyl-, 1,3-dimethyl-, 1,7-dimethyl-, 3,7-dimethyl-, and 1,3,7-trimethyluric acids in the rat and the Dalmatian dog. They observed that theophylline seemed to be quantitatively oxidized to 1,3-dimethyluric acid and excreted in the urine of the dog, while caffeine appeared to be completely converted to methyluric acids. Although they recognized that the error in calculation was large, they concluded that trimethyluric acid was partially demethylated in the 7 position, 3-methyluric acid appeared to be completely demethylated into uric acid, 1,3-dimethyluric acid was excreted unchanged with some demethylation in the 3 position. It must be pointed out that in 1946 Myers and Hanzal changed their opinion on the metabolism of methyluric acids; they had reported previously (Myers and Hanzal 1929) that methylated derivatives of uric acid were quite stable in the animal organism. Metabolic pathways including demethylation of methyluric acids have often been presented, even recently (Khanna et al. 1972; Bonati et al. 1981; Tang-Liu et al. 1983), in spite of lack of proof and experiments showing that labeled 1,3,7-trimethyluric acid was not demethylated when given by tail vein injection to Sprague-Dawley rats (Arnaud and Welsch 1981). It is quite accepted today that methyluric acids are rapidly excreted in the urine and cannot be subjected to extensive further metabolism. However, there is no direct proof to support this statement for dimethyluric acids.

Increased excretion of uric acid was reported in the rat after oral administration of maximum tolerated doses of caffeine and theophylline. However, Martin was unaware in 1948 of the suggestion made by Myers and Wardell, 20 years earlier, that this increase could be due to methyluric acids, not uric acid.

6

3 Introduction of Chromatographic Techniques

With the introduction of paper chromatography, purines, pyrimidines, and methylxanthines were separated (Markham and Smith 1949) and only few micrograms were necessary for detection. Correlation between chemical structure and chromatographic behavior of some caffeine metabolites was reported using six different solvent systems.

In 1951, Weinfeld showed in a preliminary report that 1-methyluric acid and 1,3-dimethyluric acid, identified by paper chromatography, were excreted in rabbit urine after feeding with theophylline or caffeine.

Separation of purines and pyrimidines from biological material, particularly human urine, led Johnson (1952) to isolate the purine fractions by ammoniacal silver precipitation and to collect several well-defined fractions after chromatography on ion-exchange resin. In addition to uric acid, two fractions were eluted when caffeine was administered but only one fraction after theophylline administration. The first fraction was heterogeneous; by paper chromatography a spot corresponding to 7-methyluric acid was observed, and this compound was confirmed by absorption spectra. 1-methyluric acid was also present in this first fraction, while the second fraction was pure 1,7-dimethyluric acid. These methyluric acids disappeared from urine after 2 days abstinence from foods and beverages containing methylxanthines.

The administration of 750 mg theophylline divided into three equal doses over a 5-h period in a human subject fed a xanthine-free diet was followed by the isolation and characterization of 1,3-dimethyluric acid in the urine collected for 18 h after the last dose (Brodie et al. 1952). The isolation procedure began with chloroform extraction, followed by uric acid degradation with uricase and isobutyl alcohol extraction and then treatment with petroleum ether. In the aqueous phase, the authors observed the presence of a methyluric acid. Further separation by countercurrent showed that little if any 3-methyluric acid was present in the urine. After ion-exchange chromatography and crystallization of pooled fractions, solubility characteristics, ultraviolet absorption spectra at different pH values, and finally infrared spectra demonstrated the presence of 1,3-dimethyluric acid. Quantitative analyses were performed in two subjects. The excretion of theophylline and 1,3-dimethyluric acid was negligible after 18 h urine collection, and 7% and 12% of the theophylline dose was excreted unchanged, indicating extensive metabolism of theophylline in man. 1,3-dimethyluric acid amounted to 51% and 38% of the administered theophylline, and no excretion of 1-methyluric acid was observed. These results agree completely with those reported recently in nonsmoking adult men, using a high-pressure liquid chromatography (HPLC) method, where unchanged theophylline amounted to 12% ± 4% and 1,3-dimethyluric acid to 45% ± 7% (Arnaud and Welsch 1981; Arnaud et al. 1982), and also confirm previous observations on theophylline, caffeine, and theobromine (Morgan et al. 1922; Dixon 1926; Coombs 1927) that xanthine oxidase from milk was incapable of catalyzing the oxidation of theophylline in vitro.

In 1953, two important reports were published: "The Fate of Caffeine in Man and a Method for its Estimation in Biological Material" by Axelrod and Reichenthal, and "The Metabolism of Caffeine and Theophylline" by Weinfeld and Christman. These two groups stated that little was known concerning the fate of caffeine in the body although it was widely ingested in drugs and beverages.

Axelrod and Reichenthal (1953) confirmed the results of Rost in 1895, showing in three male subjects that only 0.5%–1.5% of a 500-mg intravenous dose of caffeine was excreted unchanged in the urine. Comparison of caffeine plasma levels after oral and intravenous administration demonstrated that absorption from the gastrointestinal tract was rapid and complete. In the dog, caffeine concentrations in the fluids of various tissues were equivalent to those in plasma. This observation in the cerebrospinal fluid suggested for the first time that caffeine freely crossed the blood-brain barrier. In the dog, caffeine was also almost entirely metabolized. Axelrod and Reichenthal reported caffeine plasma half-lives for both man and the dog, but the metabolites were not analyzed either in plasma or in urine.

In contrast, these analyses were the very aim of the study by Weinfeld and Christman (1953) who tried to identify by paper chromatography 1-methyl-, 3-methyl-, and 1,3-dimethyluric acids in the urine of man, rat, and rabbit after the administration of caffeine and theophylline. Their results confirmed that 1-methyluric acid is an important metabolite of caffeine in the human body, but 1,3-dimethyluric acid only appeared as a faint spot on chromatograms and they found no evidence for the presence of 3-methyluric acid. Recent work in man showed that 3-methyluric acid corresponds to only 0.1% of the administered dose of caffeine (Arnaud and Welsch 1981). After theophylline administration, Weinfeld and Christman confirmed with three different solvents that 1,3-dimethyluric acid and 1-methyluric acid were the principal chromogenic substances excreted in addition to uric acid in human urine. The quantitative importance of 1-methyluric acid as theophylline metabolite shown in this study confirmed the previous report by Buchanan et al. (1945b), but was not in agreement with the results of Brodie et al. (1952), who reported little 1-methyluric acid. After human theophylline administration, the quantitative excretion of metabolites, calculated with HPLC, showed that 1-methyluric acid amounted to 21% ± 5% of the dose, while 3-methyluric acid was a minor metabolite corresponding to 1.5% ± 1% (Arnaud and Welsch 1981). These results are thus in agreement with the estimations by Weinfeld and Christman (1953). In the rat, the increase in urinary chromogens after caffeine administration was very small when compared with the increase after administration of the same amount of theophylline. Chromatography of methyluric acids was not attempted for caffeine, but 1,3-dimethyluric and 1-methyluric acids were found after theophylline administration, so that theophylline metabolism appeared to be similar in man and the rat. In the rabbit, 13% of caffeine was excreted unchanged, and 1,3-dimethyluric acid was the most important methyluric acid identified after both theophylline and caffeine oral administration. 1-Methyluric acid as shown to be excreted during the second 24-h period after caffeine administration, but 3-methyluric acid could not be identified. In the discussion, the hypothesis of a slow demethylation of 1,3-dimethyluric acid into 1-methyluric acid was suggested, and although no significant demethylation of 1,3,7-trimethyluric acid (Arnaud and Welsch 1981), and 1-methyluric acid (Myers and Hanzal 1946) was reported, the possibility of 3-methyl demethylation of 1,3-dimethyluric acid and 3-methyluric acid has not yet been tested with radiolabeled compounds.

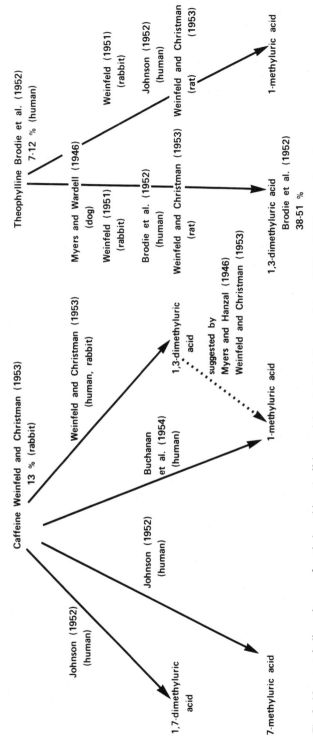

Fig. 3. New metabolic pathways of methylxanthines (caffeine and theophylline) discovered from 1900 to 1956 in animals and man

In 1954 and 1957, Weissmann et al. investigated individual variations of urinary purine excretion and identified xanthine in subjects on purine-free diets. The presence of 1-methylxanthine, 7-methylxanthine, and 1,7-dimethylxanthine after caffeine administration confirmed earlier observations made before 1900 (Fig. 3).

4 The Metabolic Studies by H. H. Cornish

The article most often referred to in work on human methylxanthine metabolism was published by Cornish and Christman in 1957. Their results concerned the identification and quantitative determination of methylxanthines and methyluric acids excreted by two volunteers after ingestion of theobromine, theophylline, and caffeine, and were obtained by Cornish and presented in 1956 at the University of Michigan as a doctoral dissertation. For caffeine and the dimethylxanthines ingested, 65%–75% of the 1-g oral dose was recovered in the urine as methylxanthines and methyluric acid. The chromatographic method used was ion-exchange resin to separate a uric acid fraction from a methylxanthine fraction. These fractions were then chromatographed on a filter paper by the ascending technique with standard compounds. Quantitative measurements were performed by light absorption on the eluate of the strips corresponding to the standards. Some identifications and quantitative determinations were performed by fractional precipitations as silver salts (7-methylxanthine, 3-methylxanthine, and theobromine, for example) at various pH values.

Although only two subjects were studied, this publication was the first to propose metabolic pathways for each methylxanthine, and confirmed previous quantitative data concerning urinary excretion, showing 11% and 12% of the dose of unchanged theobromine (confirming Rost 1895), 10% of unchanged theophylline (confirming Brodie et al. 1952), 35% of 1,3-dimethyluric acid produced from theophylline (confirming Brodie et al 1952), and 1% of unchanged caffeine (confirming Rost 1895).

7-Methylxanthine excreted after theobromine administration was observed by Krüger and P. Schmidt in 1899; their quantitative determination, corresponding to 16.3%, was low compared with the results of Cornish and Christman (1957), who reported 28% and 30% of the given dose, a result in agreement with the 33% ± 7% found recently (Arnaud and Welsch 1981). Cornish and Christman discovered 7-methyluric acid which amounted to 3% and 4% of the dose and observed important variations in the excretion of 3-methylxanthines, their values of 14% and 21% being higher than the 8.5% found by Krüger and P. Schmidt (1899) and the 11% ± 2% found by Arnaud and Welsch (1981).

After theophylline administration, 1-methyluric acid and 3-methylxanthine were quantified for the first time. The results of Cornish and Christman (1957) and Arnaud and Welsch (1981) are in agreement, with respectively 19% and 21% ± 5% for 1-methyluric acid and 13% and 7% ± 2% for 3-methylxanthine.

In the case of caffeine, metabolic pathways already identified by Krüger and Salomon in 1898 were quantified by Cornish and Christman (1957), who showed that paraxanthine amounted to 5% of the 1-g dose, compared to 6% and 5.8% found by Arnaud and Welsch (1980a, 1981) and Callahan et al. (1980, 1982) respectively. The results were also in agreement for 7-methylxanthine, with 6%, 6.4%, and 7.7% respectively for the three independent studies, and for 1-methylxanthine, with 19%, 12%, and 18% respectively, while 1-methyluric acid pathways observed by Buchanan et al. (1945b) were found in higher quantity by Cornish and Christman (1957); 27%, compared with 12% and 15% in the more recent studies. The 1,3-dimethyluric acid pathway discovered by Weinfeld and Christman (1953) was also higher; 9% compared to 2.6% and 1.8% respectively.

In 1964, Fink et al. discovered a new urinary pyrimidine, 5-acetylamino-6-amino-3-methyluracil. The aim of his study was the recovery from the urine of cancer patients of large amounts of 5-ribosyluracil for subsequent investigations, and the authors made only the statement that the excretion of this pyrimidine "may be" elevated by oral intake of caffeine, while theophylline and theobromine did not increase its excretion. Another explanation was the scission of the imidazole ring of endogenous methylated purines such as those found in nucleic acids, and 1-methylguanine was cited as an example. There have been no further metabolic studies to follow up this publication, except a recent and more accurate investigation (Arnaud and Welsch 1980a) of the relationship between caffeine intake and the urinary excretion of this uracil derivative.

Several metabolic studies were published by Schmidt, in collaboration with Huenisch on the detection of theobromine (1966), with Schoyerer for caffeine (1966), and with Kuehl for theophylline (1968) and their urinary metabolites. They confirmed that only 1% of a 300-mg dose of caffeine was excreted unchanged, 10% of a 300-mg dose of theobromine, and 11% of a 500-mg dose of theophylline. They did not quantify the metabolites extracted with chloroform, except 3-methylxanthine produced from theophylline, confirming the results of Cornish and Christman (1957). They were the first to detect theobromine after caffeine administration and 1-methylxanthine after administration of theophylline.

5 Use of Labeled Methylxanthines

In 1969, experiments performed on the pregnant rabbit, using [1-Me-^{14}C]caffeine administered orally at a dose of 3.5 mg were published for the first time (Fabro and Sieber). The results showed accumulation of radioactivity in the uterine secretion compared to the plasma and the transfer of caffeine to the preimplantation blastocyst, where theophylline, paraxanthine, and 1,3-dimethyluric acid were also detected, while 1-methylxanthine was only found in the plasma. In spite of the title "Metabolism of Xanthine Alkaloids in Man," Warren (1969) reported no new metabolic data except the simultaneous appearance in the blood of caffeine and paraxanthine after caffeine ingestion. Bülow and Larsson (1969) used tritium-labeled theophylline to study the oral absorption of theophylline preparations in man: aminophylline, choline theophyllinate, hydroxypropyltheophylline, and Brondaxin syrup. However, they only analyzed plasma theophylline concentrations and the cumulative excretion of radioactivity in the urine.

Most studies up to 1970 were devoted to man, the dog, and the rabbit; except for the experiments of Weinfeld and Christman (1953), caffeine metabolic pathways in rodents such as rats and mice were unkown.

In 1971, tissue distribution and urinary excretion of [^{3}H-^{14}C]caffeine and its metabolites were studied in the mouse by Burg and Werner (1972) and Burg and Stein (1972) respectively. 1,7-Dimethylxanthine was the major caffeine metabolite in tissue and was identified in the urine with 3-methylxanthine, 7-methylxanthine, 1,3-dimethyluric acid, and 1-methyluric acid. Quantitative determination was obtained only for unchanged caffeine, which accounted for 3%–6% of a 5–25 mg/kg body weight oral dose. A very important technical paper was published in 1972 by Cornish's group (Rao et al.); a direct mass spectrometric method was investigated for the identification of caffeine and 15 possible metabolites. The same group (Khanna et al. 1972) also published the first metabolic study of tritiated caffeine in the male Sprague-Dawley rat. Caffeine was injected intraperitoneally at a dose of 40 mg/kg and pooled urine samples were evaporated and extracted with chloroform-methanol (9:1 v/v). After thin-layer chromatography (TLC) of the extract, radioactive areas were eluted and counted. Thus, only 37% of the administered radioactivity was studied, in contrast with 64%–67% of total radioactivity recovered in the urine collected over a 24-h period. Mass spectrometry was used to identify paraxanthine, theobromine, theophylline, and caffeine. Theophylline corresponded to 1.2% of the radioactivity of the extract, theobromine to 5.1%, and paraxanthine to 8.8%. Traces of 1,3,7-trimethyluric acid and 3-methyluric acid were detected, and the most important observation was the discovery of two unknown metabolites corresponding to 11.4% (A) and 1.3% (B) of the radioactivity extracted. Metabolite A readily lost a molecule of water and appeared to be converted into caffeine under isolation conditions, while the spectra of metabolite B suggested the absence of an intact purine ring.

Inspite of the use of a very accurate method, the quantitative determination performed on only 37% of the ingested dose may lead to biased conclusions concerning the relative importance of metabolic pathways in the case of metabolites incompletely extracted and present both in the extract and in the aqueous phase (30% of the dose). It was thus premature to state that caffeine metabolism in the rat parallels that observed in man. Khanna et al. (1972) also proposed a metabolic pathway in the rat whereby metabolite A was tentatively identified as 1,3,7-trimethyldihydrouric acid, and speculated that this compound was the precursor of 1,3,7-trimethyluric acid. Although older literature stated that methylated uric acids were stable in the animal organism (Myers and Hanzal 1929) or partially demethylated in position 7 for 1,3,7-trimethyluric acid, giving 1,3-dimethyluric acid either excreted unchanged or with some 3-methyl demethylation (Myers and Hanzal 1946), Khanna et al. (1972) proposed that trimethyluric acid undergoes demethylation to form di- and monomethyluric acid (3-methyluric acid for example). One year later, the same group (Rao et al. 1973) published a short paper in which they assigned the structure of "1,3,7-trimethyldihydrouric acid" on the basis of mass spectra before and after derivatization. The solution analyzed contained 50% of the dihydrouric acid, 25% caffeine, and 25% of the open chain structure. They did not try to confirm this open chain structure with the standard synthesized 2 years before by Pfleiderer (1971). Metabolite B was identified as 3,6,8-trimethylallantoin, and Rao et al. (1973) hypothesized further oxidation into 1,6,8-trimethylallantoic acid, glyoxylic acid, methylurea, and 1,3-dimethylurea. These polar metabolites were suggested to represent most of the unextracted and unidentified metabolites present in the urine. It is quite

12

surprising to find in the introductions to several studies the statement that methyl-xanthine metabolism or the excretion of a particular compound has received little attention; the authors obviously did not refer to older literature. It was in fact the subject of several studies performed by Young et al. (1971), Mrochek et al. (1971), Butts et al. (1971), and Van Gennip et al. (1973) on 3-methylxanthine excretion in adults and children, this compound having been identified and quantitatively deter-mined in man by Krüger and P. Schmidt in 1899 (Fig. 4).

Burg et al. (1974) presented data on caffeine metabolism in the squirrel monkey. They identified the same metabolites as in other animals in tissues and urine, but observed a relatively prolonged half-life (11 h) compared with that in the rhesus monkey (2.4 h), which can be explained by a lower caffeine metabolic rate.

In 1975, the synthesis of [8-^{14}C]theophylline by Lohmann and Miech initiated the well-known work on theophylline metabolism in vivo and particularly in vitro. They confirmed the in vivo excretion of 1-methyluric acid and 1,3-dimethyluric acid in the rat. More important, they demonstrated in 1976, using tissue slices, that the-ophylline metabolism was localized only in the liver and that inhibition or induc-tion of metabolism was observed with chemicals known to act on microsomes. Little progress has been made in the understanding of enzymes involved in the me-tabolism of methylxanthines, in contrast to the intensive effort devoted since 1975 to metabolic investigations (pharmacokinetics, dose effects) and chemical identifi-cation of new metabolites.

A new sulfur-containing metabolite of caffeine, α-[7-(1,3-dimethylxanthi-nyl)]methyl methylsulfoxide, was identified in the urine of the horse, rabbit, rat, and mouse (Kamei et al. 1975). Two other metabolites, α-[7-(1,3-dimethylxanthi-nyl)]methyl methylsulfide and α-[7-(1,3-dimethylxanthinyl)]methyl methylsulfone, were also isolated from the urine of the mouse, and a metabolic pathway was pro-posed. The discovery of the methylsulfoxide was recently confirmed (Rafter and Nilsson 1981), and involvement of the intestinal microflora was suggested because the ratio of this metabolite in the urine of conventional and germ-free rats was 42 : 1. Using labeled caffeine and the sulfur-containing metabolite standards (provided by Kamei), it was impossible to detect any traces of these compounds (M. J. Arnaud, unpublished observations), which were easily separated by TLC (Arnaud 1976a), although caffeine methylsulfoxide amounted to 0.5% of the caffeine dose according to J. J. Rafter and 1%–1.8% of an intraperitoneal dose of caffeine according to K. Kamei (personal communications).

In 1976 and 1977, two short communications were published by Sved et al. and Sved and Wilson respectively. One demonstrated for the first time the appearance of theophylline in the plasma when 300 mg caffeine was ingested by subjects sub-mitted to a 9-day caffeine-free diet, the other dealt with the HPLC technique but presented results such as the half-life of ingested dimethylxanthines: 9½ h for both theophylline and theobromine and 5½ h for paraxanthine. They observed 3-methylxanthine and 7-methylxanthine in the plasma after the administration of each monomethylxanthine, but failed to detect 1-methylxanthine after its adminis-tration. They concluded from this observation that there is lack of absorption or fast elimination of 1-methylxanthine. Using [1-Me-^{14}C]- and [2-^{14}C]caffeine, the total ra-dioactivity in the urine, feces, and labeled CO_2 was measured in the rat (Arnaud 1976a). The results of fecal excretion (from 2% to 7% of the dose) and labeled CO_2

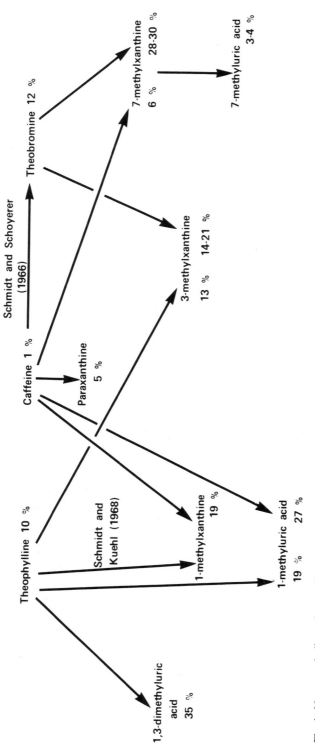

Fig. 4. New metabolic pathways discovered in man from 1956 to 1972 and quantitative estimation of the metabolites made by Cornish (1956) and Cornish and Christman (1957) after oral administration of caffeine, theobromine, and theophylline

14

produced by 1-methyl demethylation (15%) were reported for the first time. The analysis of total radioactivity excreted in the urine, using two-dimensional TLC followed by the visualization of labeled metabolites by autoradiography, showed a large number of unidentified derivatives. Quantification was made difficult for methylurates, which were not well chromatographed and can oxidize on silica plates. In this study, 1-methylxanthine, 3-methylxanthine, 7-methylxanthine, 1,3-dimethyluric acid, 1,7-dimethyluric acid, 3,7-diethyluric acid, methylurea, and dimethylurea were detected and quantified for the first time in the rat. It was also the first report on the presence of 7-methyluric acid and 1-methyluric acid in the rat, but these metabolites cannot be separated like 3-methyluric acid from other polar unknown compounds. Trimethyluric acid was oxidized on TLC into trimethylallantoin (compound 7), so that the true excretion of trimethylallantoin was not 14% but 7% and trimethyluric acid amounted to 11%. This study demonstrated that the results of Khanna et al. (1972) and Rao et al. (1973) underestimated the true excretion of water-soluble derivatives which were partially extracted with the solvent system used. This was the case for 1,3,7-trimethyluric acid, where 11% and only traces were recovered in the whole urine and in the extract respectively, trimethylallantoin (7% and 1.3%), and the compound called "1,3,7-trimethyldihydrouric acid" (20.4% and 11.4%). In contrast to the report of Rao et al. (1973), this last metabolite was reported to be stable and easy to isolate, so that it was for the first time also identified in human urine and characterized by chromatographic behavior and ultraviolet spectra of the isolated metabolite in human and rat urine.

From these analyses of whole urine, it can be concluded that the most important caffeine metabolites were identified in the rat, although several unknown minor metabolites were demonstrated by two-dimensional TLC autoradiography.

This study was followed by a short communication (Arnaud 1976 b) on the metabolism of "1,3,7-trimethyldihydrouric acid" isolated and purified from rat urine and administered orally to overnight-fasted rats. Between 75% and 90% of the dose was recovered in the urine and the excretion was approximately complete after the first 5 h following the administration. Urinalysis demonstrated that this metabolite was excreted unchanged and was not the intermediate in the formation of trimethylallantoin according to Khanna et al. (1972) and Rao et al. (1973). A new metabolic pathway was proposed with "1,3,7-trimethyldihydrouric acid" as end product of caffeine metabolism.

In 1977, Welch et al. and Aldridge et al. published two similar studies showing the effect of phenobarbital, 3-methylcholanthrene, benzo[a]pyrene, and polychlorinated biphenyls on the plasma clearance of caffeine administered orally or intravenously to rats. Although pharmacokinetics is not the subject of this chapter, it was interesting to learn from these studies that the metabolism of the dimethylxanthines formed from caffeine was stimulated similarly to that of caffeine. ^{14}C-labeled theophylline was intravenously administered to volunteers and a preliminary communication by Caldwell et al. (1978) reported no new metabolites, only the well-known 3-methylxanthine, 1,3-dimethyluric acid, and 1-methyluric acid. The recovery of radioactivity in the 24-h urine was 76%. This study did not resolve the divergent quantitative results obtained previously on theophylline metabolism. In 1976, theophylline metabolites were quantified by Jenne et al. in the 24-h urines of 15 patients using the HPLC technique; the excretion of unchanged theophylline,

1,3-dimethyluric acid, and 1-methyluric acid was in agreement with Cornish and Christman (1957) and more recent results also obtained with the HPLC technique (Arnaud and Welsch 1981). However, Jenne et al. (1976) found an excretion of 3-methylxanthine amounting to $36.2\% \pm 7.3\%$, compared to 13% and $7\% \pm 2\%$ respectively for the other two studies.

6 Metabolism of Theophylline in the Premature Infant

In 1978, several research groups in the United States and in France made a simultaneous discovery during the analysis of plasma theophylline concentrations of newborn children treated for apnea. Soyka and Neese (1978) reported in March, at the Annual Meeting of the American Society for Clinical Pharmacology and Therapeutics, the presence of caffeine in the plasma which could not be explained by blood perfusion or breast milk, and they suggested theophylline methylation into caffeine in the newborn infant. In December, Bory et al. published a letter in the Lancet describing how two premature infants showed an increase of both caffeine and theophylline in the plasma after the initiation of theophylline therapy. Transplacental and breast milk transfer of caffeine were excluded in both cases. They concluded that theophylline methylation into caffeine in the newborn can be explained by the immaturity of enzymes metabolizing theophylline through pathways known in the adult and by the well-known N-methylase activity already present in the human fetus. The appearance of caffeine was also observed by a third group in France (Boutroy 1978; Boutroy et al. 1979a), and a complete report comparing seven premature newborns with four adult volunteers was published by Bory et al. in 1979 in the *Journal of Pediatrics*. In the same issue, the methylation of theophylline to caffeine but also the formation of theophylline from caffeine was reported in 13 infants receiving methylxanthine therapy (Bada et al. 1979), while the clinical data of 38 premature infants were presented by Boutroy et al. (1979b).

The definitive experiment and demonstration was published by Aranda et al. (1979), who incubated liver explants of the aborted human fetus (12–20 weeks gestation) with theophylline and ^{3}H-labeled S-adenosylmethionine and found labeled caffeine and low amounts of 1,3-dimethyluric acid and 3-methylxanthine. From these in vitro experiments, it seemed that the predominant pathway of theophylline metabolism in the human fetus is methylation.

In vivo proof was provided later by Brazier et al. (1980a), who showed by gas chromatography–mass spectrometry (GC-MS) that two premature newborn infants receiving [1,3-^{15}N, 2-^{13}C]theophylline by nasogastric tube excreted theophylline, caffeine, theobromine, and paraxanthine labeled with stable isotopes in their urine. Brazier et al. (1980b) suggested that most of the theophylline was excreted unchanged and the methylation to caffeine seemed a minor biotransformation. They cited data, without references, on the three pathways of demethylation of caffeine in adults from which 17% paraxanthine seemed to be obtained, a figure three times higher than the values reported by Cornish and Christman (1957) and more recently by Arnaud and Welsch (1981) and Callahan et al. (1982). They did not find 3-methylxanthine in preterm infants and reported that 3-methylxanthine is quantitatively important in adult urine. This statement was not supported by a reference in the paper 1980a, while they found in paper 1980b that 35% of a dose of theophylline was excreted in the adult as 3-methylxanthine. From these papers, it is not possible to tell whether this figure was obtained experimentally or taken from the published data of Jenne et al. (1976).

Van Gennip et al. (1979) discussed the role of xanthine oxidase in the formation of 1-methyluric acid in the rat before and during loading with allopurinol and presented quantitative data on the urinary metabolites of theophylline in asthmatic children. Although the total amount of the metabolites recovered ranged from 40% to 79% of the administered dose, they confirmed the data of Cornish and Christman (1957) by showing that theophylline, 1-methyluric acid, and 3-methylxanthine were excreted in moderate amounts compared with 1,3-dimethyluric acid, and also observed 1-methylxanthine. Taking into account the low total recovery, these quantitative results for each metabolite are in complete agreement with recent data obtained by Arnaud and co-workers (Arnaud and Welsch 1981; Arnaud et al. 1982): respectively 8% and 12% of urinary metabolites for theophylline, 50% and 45% for 1,3-dimethyluric acid, 25.8% and 26% for 1-methyluric acid, 15% and 9% for 3-methylxanthine, and 0.3% and 4% for 1-methylxanthine. Figures of $2\% \pm 1\%$ were observed for 3-methyluric acid by Arnaud et al. (1982). Thus, in conclusion, these studies in children and adults are not in agreement with the excretion of 3-methylxanthine found by Jenne et al. (1976).

This discrepancy in 3-methylxanthine excretion was discussed in terms of variations of extraction recovery of the urinary metabolites by Muir et al. (1980). Also in 1980, Grygiel and Birkett published a study on the effect of age on the pattern of theophylline metabolism and found similar results in children and adults: respectively $23.5\% \pm 1\%$ and $20\% \pm 1\%$ of total metabolites recovered in urine for 1-methyluric acid, $16\% \pm 0.8\%$ and $13.5\% \pm 1\%$ for 3-methylxanthine, and $52.8\% \pm 2\%$ and $55.4\% \pm 2\%$ for 1,3-dimethyluric acid. They also observed traces of 1-methylxanthine. In premature neonates, these metabolites were not found with the exception of theophylline (98%), and only 2% of caffeine was detected. This last paper cannot confirm the quantitative results of Jenne et al. (1976) concerning 3-methylxanthine excretion. However, Staib et al. (1980) described the changes of metabolite pattern in urine observed in patients with acute hepatitis, liver cirrhosis, and cholestasis, compared with healthy subjects. Although their results exhibit wide variations, they were compared with and shown to be in agreement with those of Jenne et al. (1976) for 3-methylxanthine: 30–45% of the dose. In diseased patients, the excretion of theophylline was unchanged and lower amounts of 1,3-dimethyluric acid and 3-methylxanthine were found, compensated by an increased excretion of 1-methyluric acid.

Caffeine metabolism in the newborn child was studied using a chloroform-isopropanol extraction procedure to isolate the urinary metabolites and a HPLC system which separated caffeine and 13 metabolites (Aldridge et al. 1979). Caffeine was more than 85% of the identified metabolites in the newborn, but this percentage decreased to the adult value by the age of 7–9 months. This study demonstrated that the limited capacity for caffeine metabolism in the newborn and the slow urinary excretion of unchanged caffeine explained the 4-day plasma half-life which characterized these newborns. For convenience of presentation, the authors grouped the metabolites as dimethyl- and monomethylxanthines and uric acids, so that we learn only that trimethyluric acid, a minor metabolite, was reported for the first time in children and adult subjects. Quantitative data obtained in this study are difficult to correlate with other results because the percentage were calculated from the identified products in urine, a method which was explained by the constraints associated with the care of infants with recurrent apnea. However, a similar calculation was applied for the adult, and figures as high as 36% for paraxanthine/theophylline and 34% for 1-methyluric acid can be explained by the fact that ignoring unknown metabolites has the tendency to increase the percentages of the metabolites studied. In several reviews on methylxanthines in apnea of prematurity (Aranda and Turmen 1979; Aranda et al. 1980), the quantitative metabolism of theophylline has been described with reference to the papers of Cornish and Christman (1957) and Jenne et al. (1976). The problem of quantitative differences in 3-methylxanthine determination was not discussed, and only the results of Jenne et al. were in fact published.

Observation of the effect of deuterium substitution on the rate of caffeine metabolism in the rat showed that the demethylation of each methyl group occurs at comparable rates in vivo (Horning et al. 1979). These experiments demonstrated an important species difference between the rat, with equivalent first demethylation importance, and man, where 3-methyl demethylation was early described as the main metabolic pathway (Krüger and J. Schmidt 1901).

Another species difference in caffeine metabolism was shown by Aldridge et al. (1979) in the beagle. The metabolic effects of phenobarbital and β-naphthoflavone pretreatment were tested to evaluate the different cytochromes involved in caffeine metabolism. In the control dog, urinary metabolites indicating the predominance of 7-methyl demethylation and the quantitative excretion of 3-methylxanthine, 1,3-dimethyluric acid, 1-methyl uric acid, theobromine, caffeine, 1,3,7-trimethyluric acid, 7-methyluric acid, 1,7-dimethyluric acid, and 1-methylxanthine, while paraxanthine was not separated from theophylline, were reported for the first time. Phenobarbital pretreatment did not affect the metabolic pattern, while 1-methyluric acid and 1-methylxanthine excretion increased with β-naphthoflavone, with a corresponding decrease of 3-methylxanthine and dimethylxanthine metabolites.

In the rat, the effects of phenobarbital and 3-methylcholanthrene on theophylline metabolism were investigated by Williams et al. (1979), who used [8-^{14}C]theophylline and TLC to separate urinary metabolites, which were quantified by scraping the plates for counting the area corresponding to the metabolites. They found in control animals that 47.7% ± 1.4% of the injected radioactivity was excreted as unchanged theophylline, 14.9% ± 0.9% as 1,3-dimethyluric acid, and 6.6% ± 0.4% as 1-methyluric acid. More recently, in similar experiments using [8-^{14}C]theophylline, urinary metabolites were separated by HPLC and TLC followed by quantitative radioactivity analysis with flow cells or scanners (Arnaud et al. 1982). Divergent results were obtained, with 25.8% of the administered dose for unchanged theophylline (35% ± 3% of urine radioactivity), 25.1% for 1,3-dimethyluric acid (34% ± 32%), and 13.3% for 1-methyluric acid (18% ± 2%), and in addition 3-methylxanthine (3% ± 1%) and two unknown polar compounds (4.8% ± 0.6%) were found. These differences, particularly the higher excretion of unchanged theophylline reported by Williams et al., could be explained by a dose effect, a dose of 38 mg/kg being injected compared with the 4 mg/kg dose administered orally.

7 Metabolism of Labeled Theobromine and Identification of Uracil Derivatives

While caffeine and theophylline have been subjected to intensive human metabolic investigations, theobromine metabolism has not been studied since the pioneer work of Rost (1895), Krüger and P. Schmidt (1899), and more recently Cornish (1956). For the first time, [7-Me-^{14}C]theobromine was synthesized and its metabolism studied in the rat (Arnaud and Welsch 1979a). The demethylation of the 7-methyl group producing 3-methylxanthine and 3-methyluric acid was a minor pathway (6% ± 1% of the dose). Only 11% ± 1% of the dose was excreted in the feces, and the analysis of urine collected over a 24-h period after oral administration (84% ± 8%) showed the presence of unchanged theobromine (49% ± 4% of urine radioactivity), 7-methylxanthine (6% ± 1%), 3,7-dimethyluric acid (2.7% ± 0.2%), 7-methyluric acid (3.9% ± 0.5%), and traces of labeled dimethylallantoin and N-methylurea. After theobromine, the most important metabolite found in the urine (36% ± 4%) was unkown and identified as 4-amino-5[N-formylmethyl-amino]-3-methyluracil (purine ring nomenclature) or 6-amino-5[N-formylmethyl-amino]-1-methyluracil (pyrimidine ring nomenclature) using a synthetic standard provided by Pfleiderer (1971). In this study, the chemical structure of 1,3,7-tri-methyldihydrouric acid, the most important caffeine metabolite in the rat, was discussed and it was shown that this metabolite was in fact the 6-amino-5[N-formyl-methylamino]1,3-dimethyluracil. In this first theobromine metabolic study performed in the rat, the presence of 6-amino-5[N-formylmethylamino]1-methyluracil was also demonstrated in the urine of a human volunteer previously deprived of food containing methylxanthines and taking 1 g theobromine from defatted cocoa powder. This new metabolite and 3,7-dimethyluric acid were identified for the first time in the urine of both the rat and man.

The physiological properties and the metabolism of the third dimethylxanthine, paraxanthine, discovered in human urine by Salomon (1883) and detected as a metabolite of caffeine by Krüger and Salomon (1898), were completely unknown both in the animal and man. [1-M-^{14}C]paraxanthine was synthesized and administered to rats by tail vein injection (Arnaud and Welsch 1979b). The 1-methyl group was stable; only 2.3% ± 0.2% of the dose was recovered in expired CO_2. Fecal and urinary excretion amounted to 7% ± 1% and 85% ± 3% respectively. This metabolic study showed that 7-methylxanthine and 7-methyluric acid formation was a minor pathway in the rat. Most of the radioactivity in the urine (52% ± 3%) corresponded to unchanged paraxanthine, while the following metabolites were found in lower amounts: 1-methylxanthine, 11% ± 1%; 1-methyluric acid, 21% ± 3%; and 1,7-dimethyluric acid with a newly identified metabolite 6-amino-5[N-formylmeth-ylamino]-3-methyluracil, both corresponding to 15% ± 2%. These results in the rat can be compared with a similar study performed in man (Arnaud 1980). Paraxanthine demethylation was much more important in man and lower amounts of 1,7-dimethyluric acid and the new diaminouracil derivative were excreted in the human urine (Fig. 5).

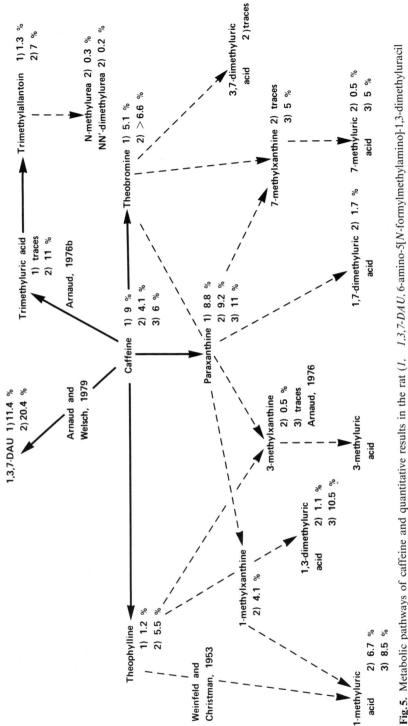

Fig. 5. Metabolic pathways of caffeine and quantitative results in the rat (*1,* Rao et al. 1973; *2,* Arnaud 1976a, b) and the mouse (*3,* Burg and Stein 1972). *1,3,7-DAU,* 6-amino-5[*N*-formylmethylamino]-1,3-dimethyluracil

In 1980, two studies were published on labeled caffeine breath tests. Desmond et al. (1980) injected [1-Me-^{14}C]caffeine into the tail vein of unanesthetized rats and demonstrated a dose-related impairment of caffeine elimination produced by cimetidine. They concluded that interactions such as the inhibition of the metabolism of warfarin, antipyrine, diazepam, aminopyrine, and caffeine by cimetidine may have widespread clinical implications. Breath tests were also performed in human volunteers after the oral administration of [1,3,7-Me-^{13}C]caffeine, a molecule labeled with stable isotopes (Arnaud et al. 1980). The ^{13}C content in expired CO_2 increased significantly by 15 min after caffeine ingestion, demonstrating that caffeine was immediately demethylated, the highest rate of demethylation being reached within 1 h after administration. The $^{13}CO_2$ enrichment remained stable until 5 h and then decreased continuously to reach a ^{13}C content close to the basal value 26 h after administration. With these experiments, the total demethylation process of caffeine in man was quantified and 21%–26% of total ^{13}C administered was recovered in expired CO_2 over 24 h. These figures also correspond to a mean rate of demethylation of each methyl group. This study showed that an oral load as low as 200 mg of [1,3,7-ME-^{13}C]caffeine was sufficient to perform this noninvasive and safe breath test and to study human liver functions linked with cytochrome P-448.

The first study on the human caffeine breath test was confirmed and extended in more recent investigations by Wietholtz et al. (1981), Arnaud (1981), and Kotake et al. (1982). Using specific methyl-labeled caffeine, the $^{14}CO_2$ exhalation curves were studied in the rat and also in healthy volunteers, cirrhotics, and smokers (Wietholtz et al. 1981). Compared to control animals, pretreatment with phenobarbital did not enhance demethylation of any labeled caffeine. In contrast, induction by 3-methylcholanthrene resulted in highly significant increases in peak $^{14}CO_2$ exhalation rates and areas under the exhalation rate-time curves. In the control animals a more pronounced and significant demethylation of the C-3 methyl group was demonstrated. These results indicated that demethylation of the three methyl groups was quantitatively more important in man than in the rat, and confirmed data showing that non-demethylated metabolites amounted to 42% in rat urine and only 5% in human urine (Arnaud 1981). The effects of liver disease on caffeine demethylation were demonstrated in patients with compensated liver cirrhosis, who exhibit $^{14}CO_2$ exhalation curves clearly different from those in normal volunteers, characterized by a slower rise and a lower specific activity. Variability in control subjects can be influenced by extraneous factors such as smoking. It was shown with 7-methyl- and 3-methyl-labeled caffeine that the average $^{14}CO_2$ exhalation rate was doubled in smokers (Wietholtz et al. 1981). Kotake et al. (1982) confirmed these results with ^{13}C- and ^{14}C-methyl-labeled caffeine in smokers and nonsmoking healthy volunteers. Their results on the quantitative demethylation of [1,3,7-Me-^{13}C]caffeine – 28.1% of the dose – was in agreement with previous data (Arnaud et al. 1980). They suggested that a saturation in the metabolism of caffeine occured in man at a dose between 3 and 5 mg/kg; $^{13}CO_2$ exhalation increased proportionately from 1 to 3 mg/kg and no further increase appeared when the dose reached 5 mg/kg. They found no convincing arguments to explain the disagreement between the saturation of caffeine N-demethylation observed during the first 2 h of the breath test and the absence of saturation on caffeine clearance reported at similar doses. They demonstrated that $80\% \pm 4\%$ of the labeled CO_2 expired during the first 2 h was derived from the 3 position, confirming the figure of 72% found from the analysis of urinary metabolites (Arnaud and Welsch 1981). Kotake et al. discussed the discrepancies between their results and the results of Aldridge et al. (1979) on urinary metabolites in man, although they did not take into consideration that their quantitative results on demethylation cannot be compared with the urinary profile of metabolites calculated not from the dose but from the identified metabolites. It is impossible for example, that in man 36% of the dose was recovered in the urine as paraxanthine and theophylline and 34% as 1-methyluric acid; 6.7%–7.7% and 11.7%–14.8% respectively, found independently by two laboratories (Arnaud and Welsch 1981; Callahan et al. 1982), seems more realistic.

Caldwell et al. (1980) showed the absence of any effect of an increased daily caffeine intake in theophylline metabolism in man. After intravenous infusion of labeled theophylline, they found 13% of the dose as unchanged theophylline in the 24-h urine, 17% as 3-methylxanthine, 33% as 1,3-dimethyluric acid, 14% as 1-methyluric acid and 2% as two minor unknown metabolites. These results did not confirm the data of Jenne et al. (1976), except if we consider the hypothese that 3-methylxanthine formation can be inhibited by the pool of methylxanthine normally present in subjects on their usual diet.

Caffeine metabolism by perfused rat liver and isolated microsomes was studied by Arnaud and Welsch (1980b). Only 3% of caffeine was transformed after 30 min microsome incubation, and theophylline, paraxanthine, 6-amino-5[N-formylmethylamino]-1,3-dimethyluracil, 1-methylxanthine, and trimethylallantoin were identified. The identification of the uracil derivative was the first demonstration that a microsomal enzyme was responsible for the hydration of the 8,9 double bond of caffeine followed by the opening of the imidazole ring. This biotransformation was recently confirmed in mouse liver microsomes and addition of cytosol or GSH was shown to increase the production of the uracil derivative of caffeine, with a concomitant decrease in trimethyluric acid formation (Ferrero and Neims 1983).

With perfused rat liver, caffeine was extensively metabolized, and after 3 h only 5% of caffeine remained unchanged in the perfusion liquid. 1-Methyl demethylation was followed by $^{14}CO_2$ formation which amounted to 12% of total radioactivity after 3 h. The metabolite pattern in the perfused liquid was similar to that produced by microsomes. After 3 h, 12.5% of the radioactivity was recovered in bile, with a preferential metabolite pattern containing trimethyluric acid (3.5%), trimethylallantoin (31%), and 1-methyluric acid with several unknown polar metabolites (40%) (Arnaud and Welsch 1980b).

Using [2-^{14}C]caffeine, Bonati et al. (1980) found an extremely low level (1.3%) of caffeine metabolism by rat liver microsome, with an equal production of theobromine, theophylline, and paraxanthine and twice the amount of 1,3,7-trimethyluric acid, but did not detect the uracil derivative of caffeine.

9 Perinatal Caffeine and Theophylline Metabolism

Postnatal caffeine metabolism was studied in 1980 in the beagle and in the rat.

Caffeine was administered intravenously to beagle puppies aged from 2 to 29 days (Aldridge and Neims 1980). In addition to caffeine, theophylline, paraxanthine, theobromine, and also 3-methylxanthine were assayed in whole blood. The peak concentration of theophylline in blood increased sixfold with increasing age, but the increase for paraxanthine and theobromine was much less pronounced. Caffeine and eleven of its metabolites were found in urine. In 2-day-old puppies the major caffeine metabolites excreted were 1-methyluric acid and 1,7-dimethyluric acid; by 22 days of age, 1-methyluric acid, 1,3-dimethyluric acid, and 3-methylxanthine. In addition, the molar percentage of the total identified compounds decreased significantly for paraxanthine, theophylline, theobromine, 3,7-dimethyluric acid, and 1,3,7-trimethyluric acid, whereas 7-methyluric acid, 1-methyluric acid, and 1-methylxanthine did not change. These results were consistent with an age-dependent increase in the rate of 7-N-demethylation of caffeine to yield theophylline. This observation was confirmed in 1981 by Tse and Szeto, who reported that in the 1-year-old beagle, theophylline and paraxanthine in plasma reached peak concentrations of 2.38 and 1.00 µg/ml respectively 8 h after oral administration of caffeine. A similar study performed on mongrel dogs, but using [1-Me-^{14}C]caffeine and presenting quantitative data expressed as percentages of the administered dose, was published in 1982 by Warszawski et al. The first important metabolites excreted by the 2-day-old dog were trimethyluric acid and 6-amino-5[N-formylmethylamino]-1,3-dimethyluracil, the latter identified for the first time in the dog. At any age, the pattern of caffeine metabolites varied considerably with the time after the dose, and major quantitative changes occurred in the 2- and 7-day-old dogs by 50 h after administration. Therefore, the quantification of urinary metabolites expressed as the molar percentage of the total identified compounds may lead to an erroneous proportion of caffeine metabolites in the puppies with longer caffeine half-life. This study confirmed that the excretion of 1,3-dimethyluric acid increased from 2 days to 5 weeks after birth, with a corresponding decrease in 1,7-dimethyluric acid excretion. The points in which the findings of Warszawski et al. (1982) differed from those of Aldridge and Neims (1980) were the presence of 6-amino-5[N-formylmethylamino]-1,3-dimethyluracil, which is a major metabolite in puppies (from 8% to 20% of the dose), the lower amounts of 1-methyluric acid, 1-methylxanthine, trimethyluric acid, and 1,7-dimethyluric acid and the higher amounts of paraxanthine in the 2-day-old dog. Trimethylallantoin and 6-amino-5[N-formylmethylamino]-3-methyluracil were identified, while unlabeled 3-methylxanthine, theobromine, and 3,7-dimethyluric acid were not quantified.

Arnaud and Bracco (1980) studied fetal and early postnatal [1-Me-^{14}C]caffeine metabolism in the rat. In the urine of newborn rats they found unchanged caffeine (10% of urine radioactivity), paraxanthine (11%), theophylline (16%), trimethyluric acid (10%), trimethylallantoin (3%), 6-amino-5[N-formylmethylamino]-1,3-dimethyluracil (22%), and unknown polar compounds with 1-methyluric acid (22%). The maturation of metabolic pathways in the rat seemed more rapid than in the human newborn. Tissue distribution and placental transfer of the uracil derivative of caffeine was demonstrated in the pregnant rat (Arnaud et al. 1983).

The metabolic pathway of theophylline in newborns, children, and adult volunteers was studied by Bonati et al. (1981). They confirmed the methylation of theophylline to caffeine in newborn infants, but did not observe this pathway in children and adults. The metabolites of theophylline excreted by newborns were 1-methyluric acid and 1,3-dimethyluric acid; 3-methylxanthine could not be found. In adults, 1-methylxanthine was not detected, and the quantitative results expressed as the percentage of urinary molar fraction of the identified metabolites were in agreement with the results of Cornish (1956) and Arnaud and Welsch (1980a). Tserng et al. (1981) studied theophylline metabolism in premature infants in the steady state of a multiple-dose regimen, and the metabolites identified and quantified were caffeine (9.6%), theophylline (50.4%), 3-methylxanthine (1.3%), 1,3-dimethyluric acid (27.7%), and 1-methyluric acid (9.3%). In addition they studied the plasma, finding caffeine (21.4%), theophylline (76.6%), 3-methylxanthine (0.7%), 1,3-dimethyluric acid (2.6%), and 1-methyluric acid (0.6%). These two studies on the neonate and premature infants are in agreement (Fig. 6).

In adult subjects, Tang-Liu and Riegelman (1981) tried to demonstrate the metabolism of theophylline to caffeine. In steady-state conditions, three different plasma theophylline concentrations were achieved and subsequent theophylline, caffeine, and paraxanthine plasma concentrations were determined. From their results, which showed that the caffeine concentration was 30 times lower than that of theophylline, they concluded that an average of 6% of a theophylline dose was methylated to caffeine. Such a pathway could be confirmed more easily by the administration of labeled theophylline (Caldwell et al. 1980) followed by the detection of labeled caffeine in the plasma, as it is obviously impossible to detect the urinary metabolites of caffeine produced after a single dose of theophylline. Although this methylation may explain the incomplete urinary recovery of theophylline and its metabolites – 90% according to Tang-Liu and Riegelman – they did not consider possible fecal excretion of theophylline, even after intravenous injection, and the limitations embodied in their assumptions in calculation were shown by their underestimation of the conversion of caffeine to paraxanthine – 20% compared with 72% (Arnaud and Welsch 1980a) and 80% (Kotake et al. 1982).

Caldwell et al. (1981) administered [8-^{14}C]caffeine to adult male chimpanzees, rhesus monkeys, and galagos and collected their urine and feces for 24 h. Although only 38%–56% of the dose was recovered in urine and less than 1% in feces, this study showed extensive metabolism of caffeine, less than 1% being excreted unchanged. The metabolites, separated into methylxanthines and methyluric acids, were shown to differ appreciably between the species, and trimethyluric acid was always a minor metabolite (3%–6%). Another study performed in the baboon with [1-Me-^{14}C]caffeine (Christensen et al. 1981) showed that caffeine was metabolized through 7-methyl demethylation into theophylline, which was the major urinary metabolite (25% of the administered dose), with 1,3-dimethyluric acid (10.5%), 1-methyluric acid (13.4%), paraxanthine (2.3%), 1-methylxanthine (2.5%), and 1,7-dimethyluric acid (1.2%), while unchanged caffeine amounted to 7.2% and trimethyluric acid to 2%. Christensen et al. reported that 6-amino-5[N-formylmethylamino]-1,3-dimethyluracil, the most important caffeine metabolite in the rat, amounted to only 2.8%. The excretion of this metabolite was studied quantitatively in the rat, monkey *(Macaca cynomolgus)* and man by Latini et al. (1981). They con-

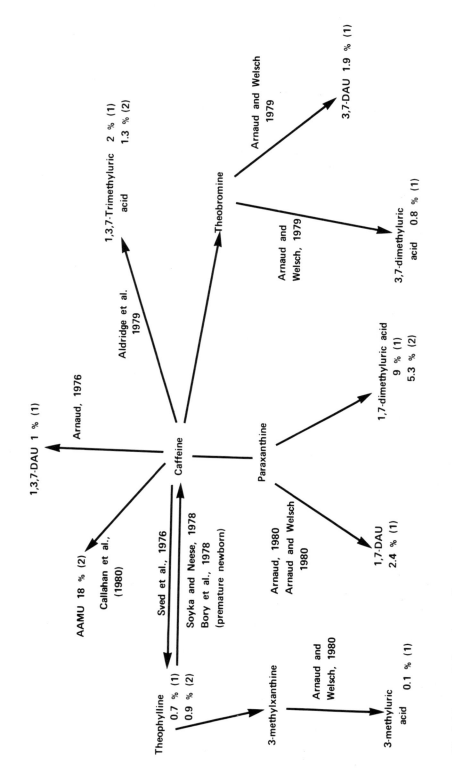

Fig. 6. New metabolic pathways discovered and quantitative estimation performed in man from 1972 to 1980. *1*, Arnaud and Welsch (1980a); *2*, Callahan et al. (1980). *1,3,7-DAU*, 6-amino-5[*N*-formylmethylamino]-1,3-di-methyluracil; *3,7-DAU*, 6-amino-5[*N*-formylmethylamino]-1-methyluracil; *1,7-DAU*, 6-amino-5 [*N*-formylmethylamino]-3-methyluracil; *AAMU*, 5-acetylamino-6-amino-3-methyluracil

firmed that this uracil derivative corresponded to only 1%–2% of the total urinary molar excretion in man (Arnaud and Welsch 1980a) and the monkey (Christensen et al. 1981), in contrast to the rat, where 30% was recovered (Arnaud 1976a). Discrepancies, perhaps explained by species differences in the case of monkeys, were observed in the study by Latini et al., where 50% of the urinary metabolites were identified as 1,3-dimethyluric acid (10.5% in the baboon) while 1-methyluric acid was not found both in the monkey (13.4% in the baboon) and the rat (6.7%) (Arnaud 1976a).

10 Quantitative Metabolic Pathways of Dimethylxanthines

After the discovery of 6-amino-5[N-formylmethylamino]-3-methyluracil (Fig. 7), a metabolite of paraxanthine in the rat (Arnaud and Welsch 1979b) and in man (Arnaud 1980; Arnaud and Welsch 1980a), it was identified in human urine by a group attempting to characterize urinary substances that could serve as potential tumor markers (De et al. 1980). This group (De et al. 1981) found two other uracil derivatives: 6-amino-5[N-formylmethylamino]-1-methyluracil, previously shown to be the main metabolite of theobromine in the rat (Arnaud and Welsch 1979a) and corresponding to 10% ± 4% of theobromine metabolites in man (Arnaud and Welsch 1980a, 1981), and 6-amino-5[N-formylamino]-3-methyluracil, which had never previously been reported and proved to be a metabolite of methylxanthines. In a short communication on theobromine metabolism in man, Klinge (1981) observed a recovery of only 60% of urinary metabolites after a 300-mg dose, but did not consider a previous animal and human study showing the presence of an uracil derivative of theobromine (Arnaud and Welsch 1979a). Only 10% was identified as 7-methylxanthine, compared with 28%–30% found by Cornish (1956). Arnaud and Welsch (1981), in a complete human study of theobromine, theophylline, and paraxanthine metabolism, found urinary excretion of 80%, 79.5%, and 70.3% of the dose respectively. A modified quantitative metabolic pathway of caffeine in man published to summarize this study is presented in Fig. 8.

In 1981 and 1982, Birkett et al. and Miners et al. respectively studied the metabolism of theophylline and theobromine. The total recovery of the administered dose in the urine was in disagreement with previously published data, but the quantification of urinary metabolite results agree with the results of Arnaud and Welsch (1980a, 1981). Birkett et al. (1981) reported theophylline and theobromine metabolic pathways where demethylation of 1,3-dimethyluric acid and 3,7-dimethyluric acid into 1-methyluric acid and 7-methyluric acid respectively were presented without experimental proof. One year later, a similar pathway was presented by Miners et al. (1982) for theobromine, but demethylation of 3,7-dimethyluric acid was no longer claimed, the authors stating that in a paper in press, they showed that dimethyluric acids appeared not to be demethylated. They introduced a tentative pathway for the formation of 6-amino-5[N-formylmethylamino]-1-methyluracil via the intermediate of 3,7-dimethyluric acid, a pathway the reverse of that proposed previously for trimethyluric acid formation through 6-amino-5[N-formylmethylamino]-1,3-dimethyluracil (formerly trimethyldihydrouric acid) (Rao et al. 1973). After administration of allopurinol, they demonstrated that the biotransformation of 1-methyl-

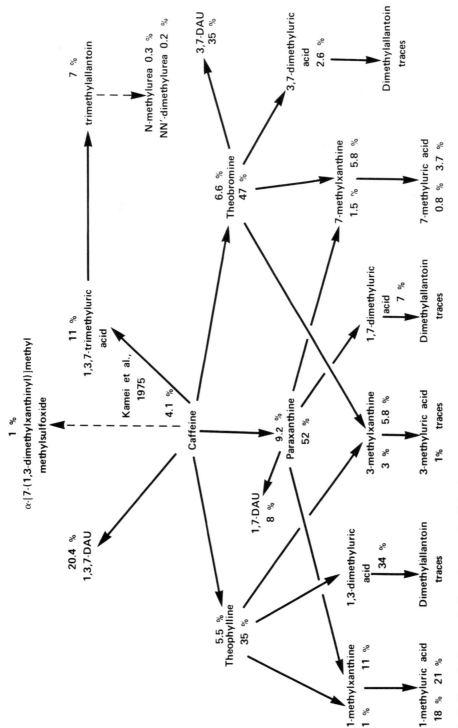

Fig. 7. Quantitative metabolic pathways of caffeine in the rat, determined from metabolic studies of caffeine (Arnaud 1976a), theobromine (Arnaud and Welsch 1979a), paraxanthine (Arnaud and Welsch 1979b) and theophylline (Arnaud et al. 1982). For abbreviations see legend to Fig. b

27

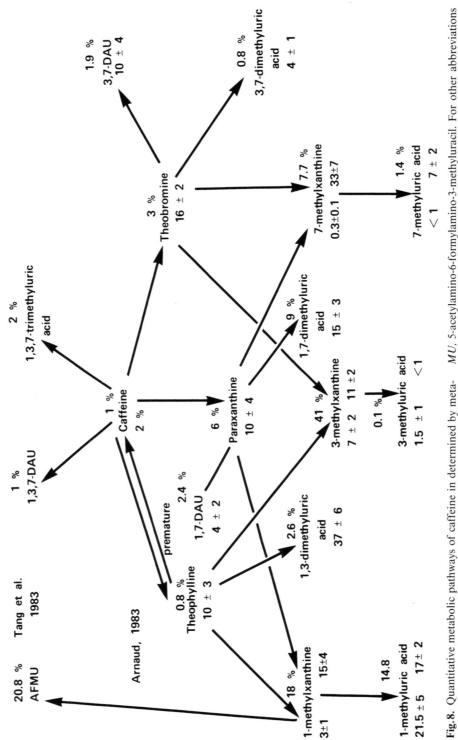

Fig. 8. Quantitative metabolic pathways of caffeine in determined by metabolic studies of each dimethylxanthine (Arnaud and Welsch 1981) and the studies of Callahan et al. (1982), Tang et al. (1983), and Arnaud (1983). *AF-* *MU*, 5-acetylamino-6-formylamino-3-methyluracil. For other abbreviations see legend to Fig. 6

28

xanthine and 7-methylxanthine into the corresponding methyluric acids were mediated by xanthine oxidase.

Arnaud and Gétaz (1982) studied theobromine metabolism in the newborn rat, and in addition to theobromine, identified 6-amino-5[N-formylmethylamino]-1-methyluracil, 3,7-dimethyluric acid, 3-methylxanthine, and 7-methylxanthine. Pregnancy was shown to impair theophylline metabolism in the rat (Arnaud et al. 1982). With [8-^{14}C]theophylline, fecal excretion was shown to amount to 18% ± 2% of the dose while 6% ± 1% was recovered in the expired CO_2 and 70% ± 7% in the urine. Unchanged theophylline amounted to 73% ± 6% of total urine radioactivity in the pregnant rat as compared to 35% ± 3% in the nonpregnant animal. This impairment of theophylline metabolism in late pregnancy was explained by the decreased formation of 1,3-dimethyluric acid, while the production of 1-methyluric acid was less affected.

Similar findings were recently obtained in the pregnant baboon with labeled theophylline and caffeine (Logan et al. 1983). Unchanged theophylline excreted in the urine increased from 48% to 74%, while 1,3-dimethyluric acid decreased from 30% to 12%. In the case of caffeine administration, unchanged caffeine and theophylline excreted in the urine increased from 5% to 22% and from 25% to 37% respectively, while 1,3-dimethyluric acid decreased from 20% to 10%.

Scalais et al. (1983) studied biotransformation of both theophylline and caffeine labeled with the stable isotope ^{15}N in neonates. The excreted metabolites of theophylline (expressed as the molar fraction of 15.6% of the dose recovered after 72 h) were unchanged theophylline (60%), caffeine (13%), and 1,3-dimethyluric acid (18%). Grygiel and Birkett (1980) and Birkett et al. (1981) found in premature neonates that caffeine constituted only about 2% of the theophylline dose, while 1,3-dimethyluric acid was not detected, in spite of a total recovery of the dose in the urine. For caffeine (Aranda et al. 1983), paraxanthine, theophylline, and theobromine were excreted at similar rates (1.3%–1.4% of dose in 72 h) and the results indicated that 3-N-demethylation with or without C-8 oxidation was a vital pathway of caffeine metabolism during early postnatal life.

Jager-Roman et al. (1982) did not measure the urinary metabolites of theophylline administered to preterm neonates, but identified caffeine, 7-methylxanthine, 1,3-dimethyluric acid, 1-methyluric acid, and occasionally theobromine in plasma. They observed that neonates of less than 35 weeks gestation did not show significant theophylline demethylation or oxidation during the first 2 weeks of life, which explained the reporting of the absence by some (Birkett et al. 1981) and the presence by others (Bonati et al. 1981; Tserng et al. 1981; Scalais et al. 1983) of theophylline metabolites in premature infants. Prenatal administration of corticosteroids induced theophylline metabolism, an increased appearance of theophylline metabolites in the plasma being demonstrated.

Using a sensitive HPLC assay for quantification of methylxanthines and methyluric acids in urine, Tang-Liu and Riegelman (1982) did not take into consideration the formation of uracil derivatives. In 1983, Tang Liu et al. studied caffeine metabolism in man, with no reference to the most recent papers, by Arnaud and Welsch (1980a, 1981) and Callahan et al. (1980, 1982). Particularly relevant would have been Callahan et al. (1982) where 80.9% of a dose of labeled caffeine was recovered in the urine and 95.9% of total urinary radioactivity was identified. The results of

Tang-Liu et al. (1983) are in agreement with these previous studies except that the amount of 1-methyluric acid found (21%) was high compared with the 11.7% and 14.8% found by Arnaud and Welsch (1981) and Callahan et al. (1982) respectively. For 1-methylxanthine, the 10% found by Tang-Liu et al. (1983) was in agreement with the 11.7% found by Arnaud and Welsch (1981), these values being lower than the 18.1% found by Callahan et al. (1982). Kinetics of plasma caffeine, theophylline, theobromine, and paraxanthine concentrations were in agreement with Arnaud and Welsch (1981). The metabolic pathway proposed was confusing and showed demethylation of trimethyluric acid into 1,3- and 1,7-dimethyluric acid and demethylation of the latter into 1-methyluric acid. Tang-Liu et al. suggested several hypotheses to explain the recovery of 70% of the dose in urinary metabolites. They did not know of the formation of uracil derivatives, although these had been reported in man as early as 1976 (Arnaud, a) and 1979 (Arnaud and Welsch, b) and the other routes of elimination proposed – the complete demethylation of xanthine or uric acid, the ring cleavage of methyluric acids to allantoins, the reduction of methylated uric acids to methylated dihydrouric acids – had already been shown to be absent (except allantoin formation in the rat). Finally, fecal excretion, where biliary metabolites could be included, was studied by Callahan et al. (1982), who found that no more than $2\% \pm 1.7\%$ was recovered, corresponding to 1,7-dimethyluric acid (44%), 1-methyluric acid (38%), 1,3-dimethyluric acid (14%), trimethyluric acid (6%), and caffeine (2%).

11 Identification of an Acetylated Uracil Metabolite in Man

In the complete and accurate study conducted by Callahan et al. (1982), one of the major human metabolites corresponded to 5-acetylamino-6-amino-3-methyluracil and exhibited a great interindividual variability in its excretion, ranging from 7% to 35% of the administered dose (mean $14.7\% \pm 6.4\%$). Another radiolabeled polar metabolite called A_2 was detected ($3\% \pm 1\%$), and this unidentified compound was shown to be unstable in methanol solution left at room temperature, transforming to 5-acetylamino-6-amino-3-methyluracil. Although this metabolite has long been known to be both a component of human urine and associated with caffeine (Fink et al. 1964; Young 1970; Kelley and Wyngaarden 1970; Butts et al. 1971; Pinkard et al. 1972), Callahan et al. were the first to establish caffeine as its primary source. However, faced with the instability of its precursor A_2, one may wonder whether or not 5-acetylamino-6-amino-3-methyluracil was not an artefact of isolation and chromatographic procedure. Recently, Tang et al. (1983) confirmed this hypothesis and isolated and identified 5-acetylamino-6-formylamino-3-methyluracil as a major metabolite of caffeine in man. This newly discovered ring-opened metabolite of caffeine was analyzed in urine and the results suggested that acetylation polymorphism was involved in its formation in man (Grant et al. 1983).

The identification of this metabolite was recently confirmed after its isolation from the urine of a volunteer fed 1-methylxanthine (Arnaud and Welsch 1981) by comparison with an authentic standard of 5-acetylamino-6-formylamino-3-methyluracil synthesized by G. Philippossian (cited in Callahan et al. 1982). The mechanism of formation of this acetylated uracil is unknown, and we noticed that its uri-

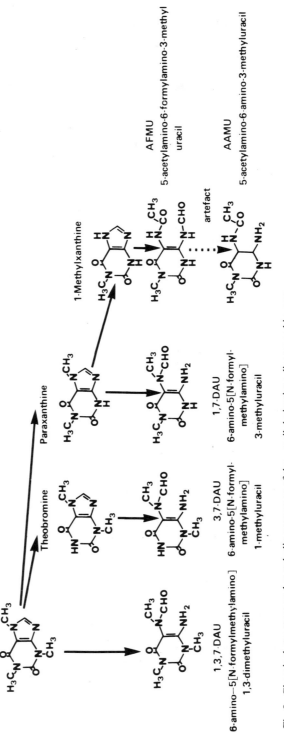

Fig. 9. Chemical structure and metabolic precursor of the uracil derivatives discovered in man

31

nary excretion was more rapid and quantitatively more important after oral paraxanthine administration than after 1-methylxanthine administration. Thus, this first identification as a 1-methylxanthine metabolite could be explained by an incomplete clearance of caffeine due to a protocol with too short a period of xanthine-free diet. Another problem of 1-methylxanthine oral administration in man is the very efficient transformation of 1-methylxanthine into 1-methyluric acid by xanthine oxidase (unpublished results). This observation may explain why 1-methylxanthine produced from paraxanthine is not metabolized in the same way as 1-methylxanthine administered orally or produced from theophylline. A short review of the identified uracil metabolites in man has been presented (Arnaud 1983), and Fig. 9 shows the chemical structure of these metabolites.

With this last discovery, one may consider that all the caffeine metabolites corresponding to more than 1% of the dose are now identified, and a comprehensive metabolic pathway (Fig. 8) has been established which may only be subjected to minor modifications in the future. However, further studies may be aimed at elucidating the enzymatic formation of uracil derivatives, the exact role of xanthine oxidase, the inhibition/induction of caffeine metabolism by exogenous or endogenous compounds or by disease states, diet, smoking, or genetic and environmental factors, and finally, experiments must be initiated showing clear evidence whether (Monks et al. 1981) or not (Rovei et al. 1982) dose effects can be produced by saturation of metabolic pathways.

Acknowledgement. The author is grateful to Professor F. H. Kemper of the University of Münster, West Germany, for providing reprints of the German literature.

References

Albanese M (1895) Über das Verhalten des Caffeïns und des Theobromins im Organismus. Arch Exp Pathol Pharmakol 35: 449–466

Aldridge A, Neims AH (1979) The effect of phenobarbital and β-naphtolflavone on the elimination kinetics and metabolite pattern of caffeine in the beagle dog. Drug Metab Dispos 7: 378–382

Aldridge A, Neims AH (1980) Relationship between the clearance of caffeine and its 7-N-demethylation in developing beagle puppies. Biochem Pharmacol 29: 1909–1914

Aldridge A, Parsons WD, Neims AH (1977) Stimulation of caffeine metabolism in the rat by 3-methylcholanthrene. Life Sci 21: 967–974

Aldridge A, Aranda JV, Neims AH (1979) Caffeine metabolism in the newborn. Clin Pharmacol Ther 25: 447–453

Aranda JV, Turmen T (1979) Methylxanthines in apnea of prematurity. Clin Perinatol 6: 87–108

Aranda JV, Louridas TA, Vitullo BB, Thom P, Aldridge A, Haber R (1979) Metabolism of theophylline to caffeine in human fetal liver. Science 206: 1319–1321

Aranda JV, Turmen T, Sasyniuk BI (1980) Pharmacokinetics of diuretics and methylxanthines in the neonate. Eur J Clin Pharmacol 18: 55–63

Aranda JV, Beharry K, Kinlough L (1983) Development of caffeine biotransformation in humans (Abstr). Pediatr Res 17: 353

Arnaud MJ (1976a) Identification kinetic and quantitative study of [2-^{14}C] and [1-Me^{14}C] caffeine metabolites in rat's urine by chromatographic separations. Biochem Med 16: 67–76

Arnaud MJ (1976b) Metabolism of 1,3,7-trimethyldihydrouric acid in the rat: new metabolic pathway of caffeine. Experientia 32: 1238–1240

Arnaud MJ (1980) Second international caffeine workshop. Nutr Rev 38: 197

Arnaud MJ (1981) Third international caffeine workshop. Nutr Rev 39: 183

Arnaud MJ (1983) Formation de dérivés de l'uracile au cours du métabolisme de la caféine. Med 5: 375–376

Arnaud MJ, Bracco I (1980) Fetal and early postnatal caffeine metabolism in the rat. World Conf Clin Pharm Ther, London, Abstract 0556

Arnaud MJ, Gétaz F (1982) Postnatal establishment of a bloodbrain barrier for theobromine in the rat. Experienta 38: 752

Arnaud MJ, Welsch C (1979 a) Metabolic pathway of theobromine in the rat and identification of two new metabolites in human urine. J Agric Food Chem 27: 524–527

Arnaud MJ, Welsch C (1979 b) Metabolism of [1-Me¹⁴C]paraxanthine in the rat: identification of a new metabolite. Experientia 35: 34

Arnaud MJ, Welsch C (1980 a) Caffeine metabolism in human subjetcs. In: IXth international colloquium in the sicence and technology of coffee, vol 1. Association Scientifique Internationale du Café, Paris, 1981, pp 385–396

Arnaud MJ, Welsch C (1980 b) Comparison of caffeine metabolism by perfused rat liver and isolated microsomes. In: Estabrook RW, Gelboni HV, Gilette JR, O'Brien PJ (eds) Microsomes, drug oxidations, and chemical carcinogenesis, Academic, New York, pp 813–816

Arnaud MJ, Welsch C (1981) Theophylline and caffeine metabolism in man. In: Rietbrock N, Woodcook BG, Staib AH (eds) Methods in clinical pharmacology, vol 3. Vieweg, Braunschweig Wiesbaden, pp 135–148

Arnaud MJ, Thélin-Dorner A, Ravussin E, Acheson KJ (1980) Study of the demethylation of [1,3,7-Me¹³C]caffeine in man using respiratory exchange measurement. Biomed Mass Spectrom 7: 521–524

Arnaud MJ, Bracco I, Welsch C (1982) Metabolism and distribution of labeled theophylline in the pregnant rat. Impairment of theophylline metabolism by pregnancy and absence of blood-brain-barrier in the fetus. Pediatr Res 16: 167–171

Arnaud MJ, Bracco I, Sauvageat JL, Clerc MF (1983) Placental transfer of the major caffeine metabolite in the rat using 6-amino-5[N-formylmethylamino]1,3[Me¹⁴C]-dimethyluracil administered orally or intravenously to the pregnant rat. Toxicol Lett 16: 271–279

Axelrod J, Reichenthal J (1953) The fate of caffeine in man and a method for its estimation in biological material. J Pharmacol Exp Ther 107: 519–523

Bada HS, Khanna NN, Somani SM, Tin AA (1979) Interconversion of theophylline and caffeine in newborn infants. J Pediatr 94: 993–995

Benedict SR (1916) Uric acid in its relation to metabolism. J Lab Clin Med 2: 1–15

Berthemot, Dechastelus (1840) Chemische Untersuchung des Guarana. Liebigs Ann Chem 36: 90–93

Birkett DJ, Grygiel JJ, Miners JO (1981) Metabolic disposition of the methylxanthines in man. In: Rietbrock N, Woodcock BG, Staib AH, (eds) Methods in clinical pharmacology, vol 3. Vieweg, Braunschweig Wiesbaden, pp 149–158

Bonati M, Latini R, Marzi E, Cantoni R, Belvedere G (1980) [2-¹⁴C] caffeine metabolism in control and 3-methylcholanthrene induced rat liver microsome by high pressure liquid chromatography. Toxicol Lett 7: 1–7

Bonati M, Latini R, Marra G, Assael BM, Parini R (1981) Theophylline metabolism during the first month of life and development. Pediatr Res 15: 304–308

Bondzynski S, Gottlieb R (1895 a) Über Methylxanthin, ein Stoffwechselprodukt des Theobromins und Caffeïns. Ber Chem Ges 28: 1113–1118

Bondzynski S, Gottlieb R (1895 b) Über Methylxanthin, ein Stoffwechselprodukt des Theobromins und Caffeïns. Arch Exp Pathol Pharmakol 25: 45–55

Bondzynski S, Gottlieb R (1896) Über die Constitution des nach Coffeïn und Theobromin im Harne auftretenden Methylxanthins. Arch Exp Pathol Pharmakol 37: 385–388

Bory C, Baltassat P, Porthault M, Bethenod M, Frederich A, Aranda JV (1978) Biotransformation of theophylline to caffeine in premature newborn. Lancet 1204–1205

Bory C, Baltassat P, Porthault M, Bethenod M, Frederich A, Aranda JV (1979) Metabolism of theophylline to caffeine in premature newborn infants. J Pediatr 94: 988–993

Boutroy M-J (1978) Etude de la pharmacologie de la 1,3-dimethylxanthine chez le prématuré. Master's Thesis, University of Nancy

Boutroy M-J, Vert P, Monin P, Royer RJ, Royer-Morrot M-J (1979 a) Methylation of theophylline to caffeine in premature infants. Lancet 830

Boutroy M-J, Vert P, Royer RJ, Monin P, Royer-Morrot M-J (1979b) Caffeine, metabolite of theophylline during the treatment of apnea in premature infant. J Pediatr 94: 996–998

Brazier JL, Ribon B, Desage M, Salle B (1980a) Study of theophylline metabolism in premature human newborns using stable isotope labelling. Biomed Mass Spectrom 7: 189–192

Brazier JL, Salle BL, Ribon B, Renaud H, Desage M (1980b) Metabolism of theophylline labeled with stable isotopes in the premature newborn infant. Colloq Inst Natl Sante Rech Med (Pharmacol Dev) 89: 309–316

Bresler HW (1904) Über die Bestimmung der Nucleinbasen im Safte von Beta vulgaris. Hoppe Seylers Z Physiol Chem 4: 535–541

Brodie BB, Axelrod J, Reichenthal J (1952) Metabolism of theophylline (1,3-dimethylxanthine) in man. J Biol Chem 194: 215–222

Buchanan OH, Block WD, Christman AA (1945a) The metabolism of the methylated purines. I. The enzymatic determination of urinary uric acid. J Biol Chem 157: 181–187

Buchanan OH, Christman AA, Block WD (1945b) The metabolism of the methylated purines. II. Uric acid excretion following the ingestion of caffeine, theophylline and theobromine. J Biol Chem 157: 189–201

Bülow KB, Larsson H (1969) Absorption of orally administered tritium labelled theophylline preparations. Pharmacol Clin 1: 156–160

Burg AW (1975) Physiological disposition of caffeine. Drug Metab Rev 4: 199–228

Burg AW, Stein ME (1972) Urinary excretion of caffeine and its metabolites in the mouse. Biochem Pharmacol 21: 909–922

Burg AW, Werner E (1972) Tissue distribution of caffeine and its metabolites in the mouse. Biochem Pharmacol 21: 923–936

Burg AW, Burrows R, Kensler CJ (1974) Unusual metabolism of caffeine in the squirrel monkey. Toxicol Appl Pharmacol 28: 162–166

Burian R, Schur H (1900) Über die Stellung der Purinkörper im menschlichen Stoffwechsel. Arch Gesamte Physiol 80: 241–343

Butts WC, Mrochek JE, Young DS (1971) Influence of certain components of a chemically defined diet on urinary excretion of ultraviolet-absorbing compounds. Clin Chem 17: 956–957

Caldwell J, Monks TJ, Smith RL (1978) A comparison of the metabolism and pharmacokinetics of intravenously administered theophylline and aminophylline in man. Br J Pharmacol 63: 369P–370P

Caldwell J, Lawrie CA, Monks TJ (1980) The effect of increased caffeine intake on the metabolism and pharmacokinetics of theophylline in man. Br J Pharmacol 70: 111P–112P

Caldwell J, O'Gorman J, Adamson RH (1981) The metabolism of caffeine in three non-human primate species. In: Rietbrock N, Woodcock GB, Staib AH (eds) Methods in clinical pharmacology, vol 3. Vieweg, Braunschweig Wiesbaden, pp 181–185

Callahan MM, Robertson RS, Branfman AR, McComish M, Yesair DW (1980) In: IXth international colloquium on the science and technology of coffee, vol 1. Association Scientifique International du Café, Paris, 1981, pp 371–384

Callahan MM, Robertson RS, Arnaud MJ, Branfman AR, McComish MF, Yesair DW (1982) Human metabolism of [1-methyl-^{14}C] and [2-^{14}C] caffeine after oral administration. Drug Metab Dispos 10: 417–423

Chou C-H, Waller GR (1980) Possible allelopathic constituents of coffea arabica. J Chem Ecol 6: 643–654

Christensen HD, Manion CV, Kling OR (1981) Caffeine kinetics during late pregnancy. In: Soyka LF, Redmond G (eds) Drug metabolism in the immature human. Raven, New York, pp 163–181

Clark GW, de Lorimier AA (1926) The effects of caffeine and theobromine upon the formation and excretion of uric acid. Am J Physiol 77: 491–502

Coombs HI (1927) Studies on xanthine oxidase. IX. The specificity of the system. Biochem J 21: 1259–1265

Cornish HH (1956) A study of the metabolism of theobromine, theophylline and caffeine. University Microfilms, Ann Arbor/Mich, publ no 21, p 165

Cornish HH, Christman AA (1957) A study of the metabolism of theobromine, theophylline and caffeine in man. J Biol Chem 228: 315–323

Daniell WF (1865) On the kola-nut of tropical West Africa (The gurunut of Soudan). Pharm J 6: 450–457

34

De NC, Mittelman A, Jenkins EE, Crain PF, McCloskey JA, Chheda GB (1980) Isolation of a new modified uracil derivative from huma urine. J Carbohydrates Nucleosides Nucleotides 7: 113–129

De NC, Mittelman A, Dutta SP, Edmonds CG, Jenkins EE, McCloskey JA, Blakley CR, Vestal ML, Chheda GB (1981) Isolation and characterization of two new modified uracil derivates from human urine. J Carbohydrates Nucleosides Nucleotides 8: 363–389

Desmond PV, Patwardhan R, Parker R, Schenker S, Speeg KV Jr (1980) Effect of cimetidine and other antihistaminics on the elimination of aminopyrine, phenacetin and caffeine. Life Sci 26: 1261–1268

Dictionnaire des termes de médecine, chirurgie, art vétérinaire, pharmacie, histoire naturelle, botanique, physique, chimie, etc. (1823), Paris, p 109

Dixon M (1926) Studies on xanthine oxidase. VII. The specificity of the system. Biochem J 20: 703–718

Fabro S, Sieber SM (1969) Caffeine and nicotine penetrate the preimplantation blastocyst. Nature 223: 410–411

Fechner MGT (1826) Repertorium der organischen Chemie. Leipzig

Ferrero JL, Neims AH (1983) Biotransformation of caffeine by mouse liver microsomes: GSH or cytosol causes a shift in products from 1,3,7-trimethyluric acid to 6-amino-5[N-formylmethylamino]1,3-dimethyluracil (Abstr 5871). Fed Proc 42: 1293

Fink K, Adams WS, Pfleiderer W (1964) A new urinary pyrimidine, 5-acetylamino-6-amino-3-methyluracil. Its isolation, identification and synthesis. J Biol Chem 239: 4250–4256

Fischer E (1882) Über Caffeïn, Theobromin, Xanthin und Guanin. Liebigs Ann Chem 215: 253–320

Fischer E (1897) Über die Constitution des Caffeïns, Xanthins, Hypoxanthins und verwandter Basen. Ber Dtsch Chem Ges 30: 549–559

Fischer E, Ach L (1895) Synthese des Caffeïns. Ber Dtsch Chem Ges 28: 3135–3143

Grant DM, Tang BK, Kalow W (1983) Polymorphic N-acetylation of a caffeine metabolite. Clin Pharmacol Ther 33: 335–359

Grygiel JJ, Birkett DH (1980) Effect of age on patterns of theophylline metabolism. Clin Pharmacol Ther 28: 456–462

Haig A (1896) Uric acid as a factor in causation of diseases. London

Hess N, Schmoll E (1896) Über die Beziehungen der Eiweiß- und Paranucleinsubstanzen der Nahrung zur Alloxurkörperausscheidung im Harn. Arch Exp Pathol Pharmakol 37: 243–253

Horning MG, Nowlin J, Thenot JP, Bouwsma OJ (1979) Effect of deuterium substitution on the rate of caffeine metabolism. In: Stable Isotopes, Proceedings of 3rd International Conference, 1978, pp 379–384

Jager-Roman E, Doyle PE, Thomas D, Baird-Lambert J, Cvejic M, Buchanan N (1982) Increased theophylline metabolism on premature infants after prenatal betamethasone administration. Dev Pharmacol Ther 5: 127–135

Jenne JW, Nagasawa HT, Thompson RD (1976) Relationship of urinary metabolites of theophylline to serum theophylline levels. Clin Pharmacol Ther 19: 375–381

Jobst C (1838) Thein identisch mit Caffein. Ann Chem Pharm 25: 63–66

Johnson EA (1952) The occurence of substituted uric acids in human urine. Biochem J 51: 133–138

Kamei K, Matsuda M, Momose A (1975) New sulfur-containing metabolites of caffeine. Chem Pharm Bull (Tokyo) 23: 683–685

Kelley WN, Wyngaarden JB (1970) Effect of dietary purine restriction, allopurinol, and oxipurinol on urinary excretion of ultraviolet-absorbing compounds. Clin Chem 16: 707–713

Khanna KL, Rao GS, Cornish HH (1972) Metabolism of caffeine-^{3}H in the rat. Toxicol Appl Pharmacol 23: 720–730

Klinge WE (1981) Method for the separation and quantification of methylated hydroxypurines found in urine of man and its application to the study of human metabolism of methylxanthines. Biochem Soc Trans 9: 120–121

Kossel A (1888) Über eine neue Base aus dem Pflanzenreich. Ber Dtsch Chem Ges 21: 2164–2167

Kotake AN, Schoeller DA, Lambert GH, Baker AL, Schaffer DD, Josephs H (1982) The caffeine CO_2 breath test: dose response and route of N-demethylation in smokers and nonsmokers. Clin. Pharmacol Ther 32: 261–269

Krüger M (1899a) Über den Abbau des Caffeïns im Organismus des Hundes. Ber Chem Ges 32: 2818–2824

Krüger M (1899b) Über den Abbau des Caffeïns im Organismus des Kaninchens. Ber Chem Ges 32: 3336–3337

Krüger M, Salomon G (1895/1896) Die Constitution des Heteroxanthins und seine physiologischen Wirkungen. Z Physiol Chem 21: 169–185

Krüger M, Salomon G (1898) Die Alloxurbasen des Harnes. Z Physiol Chem 24: 364–394

Krüger M, Salomon G (1898/1899) Die Alloxurbasen des Harnes. Z Physiol Chem 26: 350–380

Krüger M, Schmidt J (1900) Das Verhalten von Theobromin im Organismus des Menschen. Arch Exp Pathol Pharmakol 45: 259–261

Krüger M, Schmidt J (1901) Der Einfluß des Caffeïns und Theobromins auf die Ausscheidung der Purinkörper im Harne. Z Physiol Chem 32: 104–110

Krüger M, Schmidt P (1899) Über das Verhalten von Theobromin, Paraxanthin und 3-Methylxanthin im Organismus. Ber Chem Ges 32: 2677–2682

Latini R, Bonati M, Marzi E, Garattini S (1981) Urinary excretion of an uracilic metabolite from caffeine by rat, monkey and man. Toxicol Lett 7: 267–272

Lehmann CG (1850) Lehrbuch der physiologischen Chemie, 2nd edn. Leipzig, p 367

Leven (1868) Action physiologique et médicamenteuse de la caféine. Arch Physiol Norm Pathol 1: 179–189

Logan L, Kling OR, Christensen HD (1983) Xanthine metabolism in pregnant baboons (Abstr 5870). Fed Proc 42

Lohmann SM, Miech RP (1975) Synthesis and purification of 8-^{14}C-theophylline. J Labelled Compd 11: 515–519

Lohmann SM, Miech RP (1976) Theophylline metabolism by the rat liver microsomal system. J Pharmacol Exp Ther 196: 213–225

Markham R, Smith JD (1949) Chromatographic studies of nucleic acids. 1. A technique for the identification and estimation of purine and pyrimidine bases, nucleosides and related substances. Biochem J 45: 294–298

Martin GJ (1948) The effect of various agents on the excretion of uric acid and allantoin. Exp Med Surg 6: 24–27

Martius T (1826) Das Guaranin; ein neuer Pflanzenbildungstheil. Arch Gesamte Nat 7: 266–271

Martius T (1840) Über die Zusammensetzung des Guaranins. Ann Chem 36: 93–95

Medicus L (1875) Zur Constitution der Harnsäuregruppe. Liebigs Ann Chem 175: 230–251

Mendel LB, Wardell EL (1917) Effect of ingestion of coffee, tea and caffeine on the excretion of uric acid in man. JAMA 68: 1805–1807

Miners JO, Attwood J, Birkett DJ (1982) Theobromine metabolism in man. Drug Metab Dispos 10: 692–675

Monks TJ, Lawrie CA, Caldwell J (1981) The effect of increased caffeine intake on the metabolism and pharmacokinetics of theophylline in man. Biopharm Drug Dispos 2: 31–37

Morgan EJ, Stewart CP, Hopkins FG (1922) Anaerobic and aerobic oxidation of xanthine and hypoxanthine by tissues and by milk. Proc R Soc Lond [Biol] 94: 109–131

Mrocheck JE, Butts WC, Rainey WT Jr, Burtis CA (1971) Separation and identification of urinary constituents by use of multiple-analytical techniques. Clin Chem 17: 72–77

Muir KT, Jonkman JHG, Tang DS, Kunitani M, Riegelman S (1980) Simultaneous determination of theophylline and its major metabolites in urine by reverse-phase ion-pair HPLC. J Chromatogr 221: 85–95

Mulder CJ (1838) Chemische Untersuchung des chinesischen und des javanischen Thees. Arch Pharm 65: 68–84

Myer VC, Hanzal RF (1929) A study of methyl uric acids. Am J Physiol 90: 458–459

Myers VC, Hanzal RF (1946) The metabolism of methylxanthines and their related methyluric acids. J Biol Chem 162: 309–323

Myers VC, Wardell EL (1928) The influence of the ingestion of methylxanthine on the excretion of uric acid. J Biol Chem 77: 697–722

Oudry V (1827) Thein, eine organische Salzbase im Thee (Thea chinesis). Mag Pharm 19: 49–50

Pelletier MJ (1826) Note sur la caféine. J Pharm 12: 229–233

Pfleiderer W (1971) Synthese und Eigenschaften von 5,6,7,8-Tetrahydroluminazinen und ihren 5-Acetyl-Derivaten. Liebigs Ann Chem 747: 111–222

Pinkard KJ, Cooper IA, Motteram R, Turner CN (1972) Purine and pyrimidine excretion in Hodgkin's disease. J Natl Cancer Inst 49: 27–38

36

Rafter JJ, Nilsson L (1981) Involvement of the intestinal microflora in the formation of sulfur-containing metabolites of caffeine. Xenobiotica 11: 771–778

Rao GS, Khanna KL, Cornish HH (1972) Mass spectrometric identification of methylxanthines and methyluric acids, the possible metabolites of caffeine. J Pharm Sci 61: 1822–1825

Rao GS, Khanna KL, Cornish HH (1973) Identification of two new metabolites of caffeine in the rat urine. Experientia 19: 953–955

Robiquet (1823) Café. In: Dictionnaire technologique, vol 4. Thomine et Fortic, Paris

Rost E (1895) Über die Ausscheidung des Coffeïns und Theobromins im Harn. Arch Exp Pathol Pharmakol 36: 56–71

Rovei V, Chanoine F, Strolin-Benedetti M (1982) Pharmacokinetics of theophylline: a dose-range study. Br J Clin Pharmacol 14: 769–778

Runge F (1820) Phytochemische Entdeckungen. Berlin, p 204

Salomon G (1883) Über das Paraxanthin, einen neuen Bestandtheil des normalen menschlichen Harns. Ber Dtsch Chem Ges 16: 195–200

Salomon G (1885) Über Paraxanthin und Heteroxanthin. Ber Dtsch Chem Ges 18: 3406–3410

Scalais E, Papageorgiou A, Aranda JV (1983) Biotransformation of theophylline during the first six weeks of life (Abstr 409). Pediatr Res 17

Scheele KW (1776) Calculi urinarii. Opuscula 2: 73–79

Schmidt G, Huenisch E (1966) Detection of theobromine and its metabolites in urine. Dtsch Z Gesamte Gerichtl Med 57: 393–401

Schmidt G, Kuehl H (1968) Detection of theophylline and its metabolites in human urine. Wiss Z Martin Luther Univ Halle Wittenberg Math Naturwiss Reihe 17: 553–559

Schmidt G, Schoyerer R (1966) Detection of caffeine and its metabolites in the urine. Dtsch Z Gesamte Gerichtl Med 57: 402–409

Soyka LF, Neese AL (1978) Perinatal exposure to methylxanthines: Possible effects of pregnancy outcome (Abstr). Clin Pharmacol Ther 23: 130

Staib AH, Schuppan D, Lissner R, Zilly W, V Bomhard G, Richter E (1980) Pharmacokinetics and metabolism of theophylline in patients with liver diseases. Int J Clin Pharmacol Ther Toxicol 18: 500–502

Stenhouse J (1843) Über Thein und seine Darstellung. Liebigs Ann Chem 45: 366–372

Strecker A (1861) Untersuchungen über die chemischen Beziehungen zwischen Guanin, Xanthin, Theobromin, Caffeïn und Kreatinin. Liebigs Ann Chem 118: 151–177

Sved S, Wilson DL (1977) Simultaneous assay of the methylxanthine metabolites of caffeine in plasma by high performance liquide chromatography. Res Commun Chem Pathol Pharmacol 17: 319–331

Sved S, Hossie RD, McGilveray IJ (1976) The human metabolism of caffeine to theophylline. Res Commun Chem Pathol Pharmacol 13: 185–192

Tang BK, Grant DM, Kalow W (1983) Isolation and identification of 5-acetylamino-6-formylamino-3-methyluracil as a major metabolite of caffeine in man. Drug Metab Dispos 11: 218–220

Tang-Liu DD-S, Riegelman S (1981) Metabolism of theophylline to caffeine in adults. Res Commun Chem Pathol Pharmacol 34: 371–380

Tang-Liu DD-S, Riegelman S (1982) An automated HPLC assay for simultaneous quantitation of methylated xanthines and uric acids in urine. J Chromatogr Sci 20: 155–159

Tang-Liu DD-S, Williams RL, Riegelman S (1983) Disposition of caffeine and its metabolites in man. J Pharmacol Exp Ther 224: 180–185

Tse FLS, Szeto DW (1981) Reversed-phase high performance liquid chromatographic determination of caffeine and its N-demethylated metabolites in dog plasma. J Chromatogr 226: 231–236

Tserng K-Y, King C, Takieddine FN (1981) Theophylline metabolism in premature infants. Clin Pharmacol Ther 29: 594–600

Van Gennip AH, de Bree PK, van der Heiden C, Wadman SK, Haverkamp J, Vliegenthart JFG (1973) Urinary excretion of 3-methylxanthine and related compounds in children. Clin Chem Acta 45: 119–127

Van Gennip AH, Grift J, van Bree-Blom EJ, Ketting D, Wadman SK (1979) Urinary excretion of methylated purines in man and in the rat after the administration of theophylline. J Chromatogr 163: 351–362

Von Giese F (1820) Vermischte Notizen. 1. Kaffeestoff und Salzgehalt des Quassia Extrakts. Allg Nord Ann Chem Freunde Naturkd Arzneiwiss 4: 240–241

Warren RN (1969) Metabolism of xanthine alkaloids in man. J Chromatogr 40: 468–469

Warszawski D, Ben-Zvi Z, Gorodischer R, Arnaud MJ, Bracco I (1982) Urinary metabolites of caffeine in young dogs. Drug Metab Dispos 10: 424–428

Weinfeld H (1951) Metabolism of methylxanthines. Fed Proc 10: 267

Weinfeld H, Christman A (1953) The metabolism of caffeine and theophylline. J Biol Chem 200: 345–355

Weissmann B, Bromberg PA, Gutman AB (1954) Chromatographic investigation of purines in normal human urine. Proc Soc Exp Biol Med 87: 257–260

Weissmann B, Bromberg PA, Gutman AB (1957) The purine bases of human urine. II. Semiquantitative estimation and isotope incorporation. J Biol Chem 224: 423–434

Welch RM, Hsu SY, DeAngelis RL (1977) Effect of Aroclor 1254, phenobarbitol and polycyclic aromatic hydrocarbons on the plasma clearance of caffeine in the rat. Clin Pharmacol Ther 22: 791–798

Wietholtz H, Voegelin M, Arnaud MJ, Bircher J, Preisig R (1981) Assessment of the cytochrome P-448 dependent liver enzyme system by a caffeine breath test. Eur J Clin Pharmacol 21: 53–59

Williams JF, Lowitt S, Szentivanyi A (1979) Effect of phenobarbital and 3-methylcholanthrene pretreatment on the plasma half-life and urinary excretion profile of theophylline and its metabolites in rats. Biochem Pharmacol 28: 2935–2940

Woskresensky A (1842) Über das Theobromin. Liebigs Ann Chem 41: 125–127

Young DS (1970) Effect of a chemically defined diet on urinary excretion of minerals and aromatic compounds. Clin Chem 16: 681–686

Young DS, Epley JA, Goldman P (1971) Influence of a chemically-defined diet on the composition of serum and urine. Clin Chem 17: 765–773

II Measurement of Caffeine and Its Metabolites in Biological Fluids

H. D. Christensen and A. H. Neims

Methods for the detection and quantification of caffeine in biological material have paralleled the development of analytical technology in general. Early in this century, the analysis of caffeine depended on its purification and a classical approach to chemical identification (Salant and Rieger 1912). Subsequently, ultraviolet spectrophotometry was introduced in the 1940s (Ishler et al. 1948; Fisher et al. 1949), paper chromatography in the 1950s (Cornish and Christman 1957), gas chromatography in the 1960s (Grab and Reinstein 1968), and liquid chromatography and radioimmunoassay in the 1970s (Cook et al. 1976). These advancements not only tended to add sensitivity, ease, and specificity, but also increased the feasibility of measuring metabolites as well as caffeine itself. Tobias (1982) has recently reviewed several methods for the assay of caffeine in critical detail. We present an overview of the various procedures, selected methodological details, and a brief discussion of the advantages and disadvantages of the various options. Because caffeine is not measured routinely in clinical laboratories, there is no recommended or selected method of clinical chemistry.

1 Ultraviolet Spectrophotometry

The ultraviolet spectrophotometric procedure developed by Axelrod and Reichenthal (1953) received wide experimental application. In this method, caffeine is extracted into benzene from a biological matrix saturated with sodium chloride at pH 7–8. Benzene was chosen as solvent because of its relative selectivity for extraction of caffeine in comparison to potential interfering compounds such as the metabolites of caffeine under the conditions defined above. Caffeine is then back-extracted into 5 N HCl and measured direclty by its absorbance at 273 nm. Slight modifications of the procedure have been described, and a comparison of it to a differential absorbance method is available (Routh et al. 1969). Despite several potential interferences, results obtained with the spectrophotometric procedure have in large measure been confirmed with the use of more modern analytic methods. The latter methods offer convenience, improved specificity, the capacity to measure caffeine's metabolites, and increased sensitivity. Most of the newer procedures can be used to measure caffeine in small samples at concentrations less than 0.1 µg/ml, and the limit can often be extended to 0.01 µg/ml without resorting to extraction of a large specimen.

2 Liquid Chromatography

Liquid chromatography is the analytical method used by most investigators for the measurement of caffeine and its metabolites at this time. Caffeine itself is assayed with such ease that several procedures seem adequate. In the English literature alone there are more than 60 reports of liquid chromatographic procedures for the measurement of theophylline and caffeine (Christensen and Neims, to be published). The various methods differ with regard to chromatographic conditions and mode of sample preparation (direct injection, protein precipitation, extraction and/or ultrafiltration). We employ a procedure in which the sample is prepared by protein precipitation. This is accomplished by mixing the sample with an equal volume of 30% acetonitrile: 1% glacial acetic acid. Chromatographic conditions consist of

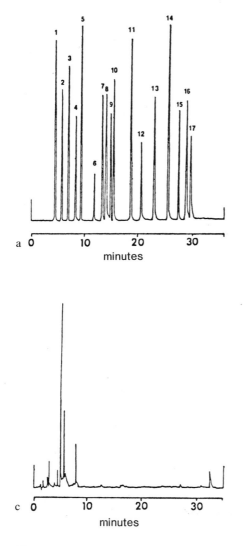

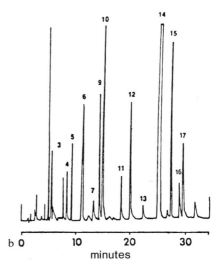

Fig. 1 a–c. Liquid chromatographic separation of methylated xanthines (MX) and uric acids (MU). **a** Chromatogram of a spiked standard mixture: *1*, xanthine; *2*, uric acid; *3*, 3-MU; *4*, 7-MX; *5*, 3-MX; *6*, 1-MX; *7*, 3,7-MX; *8*, 3,7-MU; *9*, 7-MU; *10*, 1-MU; *11*, 1,3-MU; *12*, 1,7-MX; *13*, 1,3-MX; *15*, 1,7-MU; *16*, 1,3,7-MU; *17*, 1,3,7-MX; each at 15 µg/ml. *14*, internal standard (β-hydroxyethyltheophylline). **b** Chromatogram of a volunteer's urine collected after concomitant administration of theophylline and caffeine. For significance of numbers, see Fig. 1 a. **c** Chromatogram of a volunteer's urine after 3 days abstinence from food and beverages containing methylxanthines. [Adapted with permission from Tang-Liu and Riegelmann (1982)]

1. a mobile phase of 15% acetonitrile: 0.5% glacial acetic acid,
2. a 10-μm Ultrasil-ODS column,
3. a flow rate of 2.5 ml/min, and
4. detection by absorbance at 280 nm.

Under these conditions caffeine has a retention time of about 4 min. Although the precision of liquid chromatographic procedures is usually decreased by solvent extraction in comparison to direct injection, coefficients of variation become equivalent after procedures become routine. Most investigators use reverse-phase columns, but normal-phase columns can be used in the assay of caffeine (Van der Meer and Haas 1980).

Even in the most straightforward procedures, seemingly trivial modifications can be important. The concentration of organic solvent used for precipitation of protein can influence the solubility of compounds under study or be of potential interference. Also, in sample preparation, initial acidification, can alter recoveries particularly when 8-chlorotheophylline serves as internal standard (Peat et al. 1977). The caffeine dose form (Blanchard et al. 1981), as well as preservatives and anticoagulants can also affect the suitability of particular assays. As usual, quality control is required to obtain reliable results.

Caffeine can be measured by liquid chromatography in plasma/serum, urine, saliva, milk, cerebrospinal fluid, semen, amniotic fluid, aqueous humor, and a variety of tissue affusates, perfusates, and extracts (Sved and Wilson 1977; Christensen and Whitsett 1979; Aldridge et al. 1979; Tin et al. 1979; Foenander et al. 1980; Christensen and Isernhagen 1981; Beach et al. 1982; Klassen and Stravric 1983).

Table 1. Extraction efficiency and retention time of the methylxanthines (MX) and methyluric acids (MU)

	3-MU	7-MX	3-MX	1-MX	3,7-MX	3,7-MU	7-MU
Extraction efficiency (%)[a]							
Mean	80.3	78.1	96.8	95.5	96.2	76.7	81.3
CV (%)	10.1	9.3	5.4	5.6	4.3	10.3	7.7
Retention time (min)[b]							
Mean	6.85	7.91	8.90	11.56	13.33	14.00	14.84
CV (%)	0.31	0.20	0.50	0.39	0.21	0.40	0.22
	1-MU	1,3-MU	1,7-MX	1,3-MX	1,7-MU	1,3,7-MU	1,3,7-MX
Extraction efficiency (%)[a]							
Mean	92.1	98.9	97.7	100.1	87.5	91.8	101.5
CV (%)	9.9	3.2	4.4	3.2	4.8	3.7	6.5
Retention time (min)[b]							
Mean	15.41	18.35	20.14	22.61	27.19	28.55	29.60
CV (%)	0.23	0.29	0.37	0.37	0.33	0.34	0.40

Adapted with permission from Tang-Liu and Riegelman (1982)
[a] $n = 7$ [b] $n = 26$

Liquid chromatography is particularly useful for studies in which caffeine and its metabolites are to be measured. In these circumstances, methods are more complicated and the time of analysis must be greater than in the multitude of procedures that can be used when only caffeine is to be analyzed. Tang-Liu and Riegelman (1982) have described a method for simultaneous analysis of methylated xanthines and uric acids (Table 1, Fig. 1). The sample, internal standard (β-hydroxyethyltheophylline), 0.1 M tetrabutylammonium hydrogen sulfate, and 0.01 M sodium carbonate buffer, pH 11.0, were admixed and agitated for 30 s before and after addition of about 1 g ammonium sulfate. This mixture was then extracted with ethyl acetate : chloroform : isopropanol (45 : 45 : 10). The organic layer was removed, evaporated to dryness under nitrogen and reconstituted in an aqueous solution of 50 mM tetrabutylammonium hydrogen sulfate and 10 mM sodium acetate, pH 4.9. The chromatographic conditions used solvent programming; solvent A was the aforementioned reconstitution solution, and Solvent B was Solvent A mixed with an equal volume fo 50% methanol pH adjusted to 4.8 with glacial acetic acid. The eluant flowed at 1.25–1.5 ml/min with the following changes in Solvent B: 0% for 7.5 min, 0%–15% in 7.5 min, 15%–30% in 10 min, 30%–32% in 8 min, 32%–45% in 5 min, and 45%–0% in 3 min. A precolumn (Lichrosorb RP-2, 4 cm $\times$ 2.1 mm, 10 μm) and analytical column (5 μm Ultrasphere ODS) were water-jacketed at 25 °C. The column effluent was monitored at 280 nM. The 15 methylated xanthines and uric acids were resolved in 30 min (Table 1, Fig. 1). The retention of methylated uracil metabolites and possible interference by these metabolites were not reported. Another approach used by various groups of investigators, especially with the substituted diaminouracils in mind, involved the use of two different sets of chromatographic conditions (Callahan et al. 1982, 1983; Arnaud 1980; Grant et al. 1983). Since the metabolic profile of caffeine is extensive only in urine, adequate sample size has not been a difficulty. The elucidation of the metabolic pathways has been assisted by the availability of both methyl and ring-labeled xanthines. More detailed discussion of the identification and measurement of the various diaminouracil metabolites of caffeine can be found in the chapter by Arnaud in this volume (p. 19).

3 Thin-Layer Chromatography

Thin-layer chromatography, especially in conjunction with the use of radiolabeled caffeine, is also utilized widely in studies of the biotransformation of caffeine. The two-dimensional method described by Arnaud (1976) resolves the various metabolites of caffeine. In this procedure, a silica gel plate (Merck F_{254}, 0.25 mm thickness) is developed first with chloroform : methanol (4 : 1, v/v) and then with chloroform : acetone : n-butanol : concentrated ammonium hydroxide (3 : 3 : 4 : 1, v/v). One-dimensional chromatography with chloroform : aceton : n-butanol : concentrated ammonium sulfate (3 : 3 : 2 : 0.5, v/v) will separate the five primary or initial metabolites of caffeine (theophylline, theobromine, paraxanthine, 1,3,7-trimethyluric acid, and 6-amino-5-[N-formylmethylamino]-1,3-diaminouracil); such separations are particuarly convenient and useful in experiments involving in vitro metabolism of caffeine in the presence of subcellular fractions because of the limited secondary metabolism of the metabolites (Ferrero and Neims 1983). Caffeine and its metabolites can be assayed by radioscanner and/or autoradiography, scraping or cutting, and scintillation counting.

A few potential problems exist in the utilization of radiolabeled caffeine. The first is simple and obvious, yet important. Caffeine that is labeled in the 1-, 3-, or 7-N-methyl substituent will yield nonradioactive metabolites if that methyl group is removed in the process of biotransformation. Indeed, the release of label as a one-carbon fragment forms the basis fo the CO_2 breath tests discussed below. Ring-labeled caffeine is available, and excellent metabolite recoveries have been obtained using such compounds (Callahan et al. 1982). The second potential problem is more subtle. If a compound such as caffeine is metabolized by multiple alternative and competitive pathways, the route of metabolism may be shifted by the isotope effect of deuterium labeling. Horning et al. (1976) showed in the rat that replacement of the 1-CH_3 substituent with a 1-CD_3 group favored the formation of theophylline instead of theobromine; replacement of the 7-CH_3 substituent with a 7-CD_3 group switched the pathway toward paraxanthine. The use of ^{14}C or ^{13}C rather than deuterium in the labeled xanthines would not be expected to cause an appreciable isotope effect in this context, and such compounds have been of great value in studies of caffeine. The combination of various methodologies can be particularly useful, as illustrated by the papers of Branfman et al. (1983) and Tang et al. (1983) for the identification of uracil metabolites.

A rather novel thin-layer chromatographic procedure for measurement of caffeine and/or theophylline has been developed by Riechert (1978); the method has been used to monitor newborn infants treated with methylxanthines for apnea. Serum, saliva, or urine (5–10 µl) is applied directly onto a wet ethanol spot on the plate (Kieselgel 60 F_{254} DC-Fertig Platten). The chromatogram is developed with ethylacetate:methanol:25% ammonia (80:20:10), and ultraviolet absorbance is measured with a dual-wavelength thin-layer chromatogram scanner (CS-910, Shimadzu, Kyoto, Japan) in reflection mode with a sample wavelength of 273 nm and a reference wavelength of 315 nm. The detection limit is about 1 µg/ml.

4 Immunoassays

The caffeine radioimmunoassay developed by Cook et al. (1976) has been used in several kinetic studies. Antiserum was prepared by immunizing rabbits with 7-[5-carboxypentyl]-1,3-dimethylxanthine–bovine serum albumin conjugate. Both good antibody titer and good selectivity (cross-reaction with theophylline, 7%; paraxanthine, 0.3%; theobromine, 0.6%, 1,3,7-trimethyluric acid, 0.9%; other metabolites, less than 0.05%) were obtained. The radioligand used initially was 7-[2,3-$^3H_2$]propyl-1,3-dimethylxanthine, but [8-^3H]caffeine was substituted when it became available. The procedure involved 2 h incubation followed by separation of bound and unbound ligand with dextran-coated charcoal. Analysis of plasma samples containing more than 20 ng/ml caffeine required only 20 µl or less plasma.

In contrast to the situation with theophylline, there has been no development of an enzyme-multiplied immunoassay technique (EMIT) assay for caffeine. A sub-

43

strate-labeled fluorescent immunoassay (SLFIA) using antisera that extensively cross-reacted with theophylline has been investigated (Briggs et al., to be published). Results comparable to radioimmunoassay and liquid chromatography were obtained as long as no significant amounts of theophylline were present.

5 Gas Chromatography–Mass Spectrometry

The resolution of caffeine by gas chromatography was described in 1960 (Llyod et al. 1960), but a procedure for use with a biological matrix did not appear until 1968 (Grab and Reinstein 1968). In this procedure, 3% OV17 on a Chromosorb W 100–120 mesh AW/DMCS H.P. 6-ft column was used with a flame-ionization detector. Operating temperature was oven 200 °C injection port 260 °C and detector 260 °C. Plasma pH was adjusted to 11.5–12.0 with 2.5 N sodium hydroxide during sample preparation, and caffeine was extracted with chloroform. Hexobarbital was used as an internal standard.

None of the clinical laboratories in the American College of Pathologists therapeutic drug monitoring survey currently use gas chromatography for the assay of theophylline, and we suspect that few laboratories use it as a primary method for studies of the kinetics of caffeine (Milton and Antonioli 1979; Cohen et al. 1978; Bradbrook et al. 1979; Bonati et al. 1979). The procedure remains useful, however, especially when linked to mass spectrometry, in the identification of metabolites of caffeine (Merriman et al. 1978; Tserng 1983; Midha et al. 1977). In the procedure used by Horning et al. (1976), caffeine and metabolites were extracted using ammonium carbonate–ethyl acetate as a salt–solvent pair. For the quantitative studies, 7-trideuteromethyl-1,3-dimethylxanthine and 1,3,7-tri-trideuteromethylxanthine were used as internal standards. Samples were ethylated with diazoethane before analysis. Quantification was accomplished by selected ion detection using a Finnegan mass spectrometer quipped with a chemical ionization (CI) source. Glass coil columns (270 mm × 2 mm) were packed with 1% SE-30 or 3% PZ-176 on 80–100 mesh Gas Chrom Q. Nitrogen was used as the carrier gas and chemical ionization was carried out with a mixture of equal amounts of N_2 and N_2^+ obtained by adjusting the voltage of the CI source.

6 Carbon Dioxide Breath Test

As noted above, N-demethylation of caffeine releases one-carbon fragments; the rate of this process can be ascertained by measurement of the rate of appearance of isotope, ^{13}C or ^{14}C, in exhaled CO_2 by mass spectrometry or liquid scintillation counting respectively (Arnaud et al. 1980; Kotake et al. 1982; Wietholtz et al. 1981). Specific labeling of the various methyl groups can be used to distinguish rates of 1-N-, 3-N-, and 7-N-demethylation. The procedure offers interesting opportunities for the study of special groups (e.g., man, newborn animals). Nonetheless, care must be taken to distinguish primary demethylation of caffeine (e.g., 3-N-demethylation to yield paraxanthine) from secondary demethylation of one of caffeine's metabolites (e.g., 7.N-demethylation of paraxanthine to yield 1-methylxanthine).

44

One must also realize that in some species metabolic processes that do not involve *N*-demethylation (e. g., production of 1,3,7-trimethyluric acid and of 6-amino-5[*N*-formylmethylamino]-1,3-dimethyluracil) are predominant initial steps.

7 Conclusions

We would like to emphasize four points in summary

1. Several methods for analysis of caffeine and its metabolites are now available; each has advantages and disadvantages. For any given experimental objective, an appropriately selective and sensitive procedure probably exists.
2. It is important to periodically assess reliability, since seemingly trivial changes in methodology have had significant consequences.
3. Periodic monitoring of caffeine is probably indicated in human studies to attempt to control for compliance.
4. The rather elegant methods now available have allowed rapid acquisition of kinetic data and metabolic profiles in several species and in several subgroups of the human population. We anticipate that mechanistic generalizations are forthcoming.

References

Aldridge A, Aranda JV, Neims AH, (1979) Caffeine metabolism in the newborn. Clin Pharmacol Ther 25: 447–453
Arnaud MJ (1976) Identification, kinetic and quantitative study of [2-^{14}C] and [1-Me-^{14}C] caffeine metabolites in rat's urine by chromatographic separations. Biochem Med 16: 67–76
Arnaud MJ (1980) Caffeine metabolism in human subjects. In: IXth Colloquium on the science and technology of coffee, vol 1. Association Scientifique Internationale du Café, Paris, pp 385–396
Arnaud MJ, Thelin-Doerner A, Ravussin R, Acheson KJ (1980) Study of the demethylation of [1,3,7-Me-^{13}C] caffeine in man using respiratory exchange measurement. Biomed Mass Spectrom 7: 521–524
Axelrod J, Reichenthal J (1953) The fate of caffeine in man and a method for its estimation in biological material. J Pharmacol Exp Ther 107: 519–523
Beach CA, Bianchine JR, Gerber N (1982) Excretion of caffeine in semen of men: comparison with concentrations in blood. Proc West Pharmacol Soc 25: 377–380
Blanchard J, Mohammadi JD, Trang JM (1981) Elimination of a potential interference in assay for plasma caffeine. Clin Chem 27: 637–639
Bonati M, Castelli D, Latini R, Garattini S (1979) Comparison of gas-liquid chromatography with nitrogen-phosphorus selective detection and high-performance liquid chromatographic methods for caffeine determination in plasma and tissues. J Chromatogr 164: 109–113
Bradbrook ID, James CA, Morrison PJ, Rogers HJ (1979) Comparison of thin-layer and gas chromatographic assays for caffeine in plasma. J Chromatogr 163: 118–122
Branfman AR, McComish MF, Bruni RJ, Callahan MM, Robertson R, Yesair DW (1983) Characterization of diaminouracil metabolites of caffeine in human urine. Drug Metab Dispos 11: 206–210
Briggs GM, Christensen HD, Benovic JL (to be published) Substrate labeled fluorescence immunoassay (SLFIA) for caffeine
Callahan MM, Robertson RS, Arnaud MJ, Branfman AR, McComish MF, Yesair DW (1982) Human metabolism of [1-methyl-^{14}C]- and [2-^{14}C] caffeine after oral administration. Drug Metab Dispos 10: 417–423

Callahan MM, Robertson RS, Branfman AR, McCormish MF, Yesair DW (1983) Comparison of caffeine metabolism in three non-smoking populations after oral administration of radiolabeled caffeine. Drug Metab Dispos 11: 211–217

Christensen HD, Isernhagen R (1981) The application of the radial compression separation system for biological materials. In: Hawk GL (ed) Biological/biomedical applications of liquid chromatography III. Dekker, New York, pp 71–93

Christensen HD, Neims AH (to be published) Antiasthmatics. In: Wong SH (ed) Therapeutic drug monitoring and toxicology by liquid chromatography. Dekker, New York

Christensen HD, Whitsett TL (1979) Measurement of xanthines by means of high pressure liquid chromatography. In: Hawk GL (ed) Biological/biomedical applications of liquid chromatography. Dekker, New York, pp 507–537

Cohen JL, Cheng C, Henry JP, Chan YL (1978) GLC determination of caffeine in plasma using alkali flame detection. J Pharm Sci 67: 1093–1095

Cook CE, Tallent CR, Amerson EW, Myers MW, Kepler JA, Taylor GF, Christensen HD (1976) Caffeine in plasma and saliva by a radioimmunoassay procedure. J Pharmacol Exp Ther 199: 679–686

Cornish HH, Christman AA (1957) A study of the metabolism of theobromine, theophylline and caffeine in man. J Biol Chem 228: 315–323

Ferrero JL, Neims AH (1983) Metabolism of caffeine by mouse liver microsomes; GSH or cytosol causes a shift in products from 1,3,7-trimethylurate to substituted diaminouracil. Life Sci 33: 1173–1178

Fisher RS, Algeri EJ, Walker JT (1949) The determination and the urinary excretion of caffeine in animals. J Biol Chem 179: 71–79

Foenander T, Birkett DJ, Miners JO, Wing LMH (1980) The simultaneous determination of theophylline, theobromide and caffeine in plasma by high performance liquid chromatography. Clin Biochem 13: 132–134

Grab FL, Reinstein JA (1968) Determination of caffeine in plasma by gas chromatography. J Pharm Sci 57: 1703–1706

Grant DM, Tang BK, Kalow W (1983) Variability in caffeine metabolism. Clin Pharmacol Ther 33: 591–602

Horning MG, Haegele KD, Sommer KR, Nowlin J, Stafford M, Thenot J-P (1976) Metabolic switching of drug pathways as a consequence of deuterium substitution. In: Klein ER, Klein PD (eds) Proceedings of the 2nd international conference on stable isotopes in chemical biology and medicine. National Technical Information Service, US Dept Commerce, Springfield/VA, pp 41–54

Ishler NH, Finucane TP, Borker E (1948) Rapid spectrometric determination of caffeine. Anal Chem 20: 1162–1166

Klassen R, Stavric B (1983) HPLC separation of theophylline, paraxanthine, theobromine, caffeine and other caffeine metabolites in biological fluids. J Liquid Chromatogr 6: 895–906

Kotake AN, Schoeller DA, Lambert GH, Baker AL, Schaffer DD, Josephs H (1982) The caffeine CO_2 breath test: dose response and route of N-demethylation in smokers and nonsmokers. Clin Pharmacol Ther 32: 262–269

Lloyd HA, Fales HM, Highet PF, van den Heuvel WJA, Wildman WC (1960) Separation of alkaloids by gas chromatography. J Am Chem Soc 82: 3791

Merriman RL, Swanson A, Anders M-W, Sladek NE (1978) Microdetermination of caffeine in blood by gas chromatography-mass spectrometry. J Chromatogr 146: 85–90

Midha KK, Sved S, Hossie RD, McGilveray IJ (1977) High performance liquid chromatographic and mass spectrometric identification of dimethylxanthine metabolites of caffeine in human plasma. Biomed Mass Spectrom 4: 172–177

Milton H, Antonioli J (1979) Caffeine determination in rat plasma. A comparative study of micromethods. J Chromatogr 162: 223–228

Peat MA, Jennison TA, Chinn DM (1977) Analysis fo theophylline in serum and whole blood samples by high pressure liquid chromatography. J Anal Toxicol 1: 204–207

Riechert M (1978) Micro-method for the determination of caffeine and theophylline allowing direct application of biological fluids to thin-layer chromatography plates. J Chromatogr 146: 175–180

Routh JI, Shane NA, Arredondo EG, Paul WD (1969) Determination of caffeine in serum and urine. Clin Chem 15: 661–668

Salant W, Rieger JB (1912) The elimination of caffeine: an experimental study on herbivora and carnivora. Bull Bur Chem 157: 1–23

Sved S, Wilson DL (1977) Simultaneous assay of the methylxanthine metabolites of caffeine in plasma by high performance liquid chromatography. Res Commun Chem Pathol Pharmacol 17: 319–331

Tang BK, Grant DM, Kalow W (1983) Isolation and identification of 5-acetylamino-6-formylamino-3-methyluracil as a major metabolite of caffeine in man. Drug Metab Dispos 11: 218–220

Tang-Liu DD-S, Riegelman S (1982) An automated HPLC assay for simultaneous quantitation of methylated xanthines and uric acids in urine. J Chromatogr Sci 20: 155–159

Tin AA, Somani SM, Bada HS, Khanna NN (1979) Caffeine, theophylline and theobromine determinations in serum, saliva and spinal fluid. J Anal Toxicol 3: 26–29

Tobias DY (1982) Current methods of caffeine determination: review of the literature, 1975–1980. FDA By Lines 3: 129–156

Tserng KY (1983) Gas chromatographic-mass spectrometric quantitation of theophylline and its metabolites in biological fluids. J Pharm Sci 72: 526–529

Van der Meer C, Haas RE (1980) Determination of caffeine in serum by straight-phase high-performance liquid chromatography. J Chromatogr 182: 121–124

Wietholtz H, Voegelin M, Arnaud MJ, Bircher J, Preisig R (1981) Assessment of the cytochrome P-448 dependent liver enzyme system by a caffeine breath test. Eur J Clin Pharmacol 21: 53–59

III Interspecies Comparison of Caffeine Disposition

M. Bonati and S. Garattini

1 Absorption

In line with its physiochemical characteristics (undissociated weak electrolyte at physiological pH, pK_a 1 and 14, partition coefficient 0.85 (Gaspari et al. 1983; Bonati et al. 1982a), caffeine is rapidly and completely absorbed from the gastrointestinal tract after oral administration (Axelrod and Reichenthal 1953; Bonati et al. 1982b, Blanchard and Sawers 1983a). In animals and man no significant first-pass effect occurs after oral caffeine (Aldridge et al. 1977). Although different absorption rates have been estimated for different species, mean values of the rate constant of absorption (k_{abs}) range from 4 to $6\,h^{-1}$; plasma peal levels are reached within 30–120 min of dosing in animals and man (Latini et al. 1978; Garattini et al. 1979; Bonati et al. 1982b). Lower k_{abs} values were reported after ingestion of caffeine in a soft drink than after coffee and caffeine aqueous solutions (Marks and Kelly 1973; Bonati et al. 1982b), suggesting that the characteristics (volume, pH, composition) of sources in which caffeine is dissyolved may influence its absorption rate. A tendency for the absorption rate to rise with increasing doses of caffeine was described (Garattini et al. 1980b; Bonati et al. 1982b). The absorption rate was lower after intramusuclar than oral dosing, indicating that solubility at site of administration may be another variable to consider (Sant'Ambrogio et al. 1964).

2 Plasma Protein Binding

In vivo and in vitro studies have shown that caffeine is poorly bound (10%–30%) to plasma albumin over a wide range of concentrations (1–100 µg/ml), ages, and species examined (Eichman et al. 1962; Desmond et al. 1980; Axelrod and Reichenthal 1953; M. Bonati and S. Garattini, unpublished results). These findings are confirmed by saliva/plasma and CSF/plasma concentration ratios (Parsons and Neims 1978; Cook et al. 1976; Somani et al. 1980).

3 Distribution

Once in the body, caffeine is rapidly distributed, and no specific binding to tissues has been observed. A mean volume of distribution of 0.8 liters/kg for different species has been reported (Bonati et al. 1983), leading to the conclusion that caffeine does distribute into total body fluids. This is in agreement with findings showing that caffeine moves rapidly into and out of cells (blood/plasma ratio equal to unity; Garattini et al. 1979) and tissues (Bianchi 1962).

Animal and human studies have shown that no physiological "barriers" limit the passage of caffeine through tissues, so that easy and rapid equilibrium is reached between mother and fetus and between blood and all tissues, brain and testes included (Burg 1975). Generally caffeine enters and leaves tissues by simple diffusion, although a partial carrier-mediated blood-brain barrier has recently been reported (McCall et al. 1982). Neither brain/blood ratios, calculated between the peak levels (after oral administration), nor the AUC, showed any significant differences between rat and mouse or at different dose levels (1,10, and 100 mg/kg), suggesting that the wide interspecies difference in caffeine disposition (see below) depends more on clearance than on distribution, at least for the mouse and rat (Garattini et al. 1980a).

4 Clearance

Caffeine is efficiently eliminated by animals and humans through liver biotransformation to several metabolites, dimethylxanthines (theophylline, paraxanthine, theobromine), which can be further demethylated to the respective monomethylxanthines. Xanthines can also be substrates for oxidation to the respective urate and/or hydration to the respective diaminouracil compounds (see the chapter by Arnaud, pp 19, 30).

4.1 Renal Clearance

Five percent of the administered dose of caffeine is eliminated unchanged in urine by all investigated species except the guinea pig (comparable for age, weight, and physiopathological status). Urinary excretion of caffeine is not affected by urinary pH or plasma concentrations (Bonati et al. 1982b), whereas it is linearly related to urine flow rate (Blanchard and Sawers, 1983b). After glomerular filtration it is rapidly and passively reabsorbed. Agreement was found between renal and body clearance ratios (around 1.5% in rat, beagle, and man) and the fraction of caffeine excreted unchanged in urine (Garattini et al. 1980a; Aldridge and Neims 1979; Bonati et al. 1982b; Neims and von Borstel, 1983).

4.2 Metabolic Clearance

In various species, caffeine is usually eliminated by apparent first-order kinetics, described by a one-compartment open model system, over different ranges of doses (see this chapter Sect. 6).

Despite the ample kinetic information reported in literature concerning caffeine disposition in different species, only a few systematic studies can be used to com-

Table 1. Average kinetic parameters for caffeine after administrations for which first-order kinetics is applicable

Parameter	Man	Monkey	Dog	Rabbit	Rat	Mouse
Dose (mg/kg)	10	10	20	10	2.5	10
k_{el} (h^{-1})	0.13	0.13	0.17	0.60	0.82	0.70
Half-life (h)	5.2	5.4	4.0	1.1	0.88	0.99
aVd (liters/kg)	0.66	0.99	0.78	1.00	0.92	0.84
Cl (liters/h/kg)	0.09	0.13	0.13	0.60	0.75	0.59

References: Bonati et al. (1982b), Garattini et al. (1979, 1980a, b, 1982) Aldridge and Neims (1979) k_{el}, apparent first-order elimination rate constant; aVd, apparent volume of distribution = aVd = f · D/(AUC · k_{el}) Cl, body clearance = aVd · k_{el}

Table 2. Average bloodstream AUC $_{0-24 h}$ values (mg/liter/min) for caffeine and its metabolites after normalization to 1 mg/kg of the doses reported in Table 1

Compound	Man	Monkey	Dog	Rabbit	Mouse
Caffeine	941	464	486	100	102
Theophylline	79	648	342[a]	24	3
Paraxanthine	393	41		173	20
Theobromine	83	74	100	11	47

References: see Table 1
[a] In the dog, theophylline and paraxanthine were measured together (see Sect. 4.3)

pare caffeine kinetics in different species (Aldrige and Neims 1979; Bonati et al. 1983). Kinetic parameters for the six most thoroughly investigated species are summarized in Table 1.

After administration of caffeine a few of its less polar metabolites can be measured in the bloodstream. The AUC values can be used as the basis for comparison between species, taking into account the circulating metabolites also produced (Table 2). Paraxanthine is the primary caffeine metabolite found in the bloodstream of man and the rabbit, theophylline in the monkey, and theobromine in the mouse. Since in the rat caffeine disposition is dose-dependent at around 5 mg/kg (Latini et al. 1978; Aldridge et al. 1977; see below), these data are not included. No dose-AUC relation exists, and at lower doses bloodstream kinetics of caffeine metabolites cannot be accurately described. At doses over 10 mg/kg in the rat, theophylline and theobromine producion are of the same order, while paraxanthine formation is lower (Garattini et al. 1980a). A similar metabolic profile was reported in relation to brain concentrations in the rat and mouse (Garattini et al. 1979).

Thus from Tables 1 and 2 different statements can be deduced concerning interspecies similarity according to whether kinetic or metabolic profiles are taken into account; man and monkey have the same clearance and half-life, but different metabolic profiles in blood (Garattini et al. 1980b).

Table 3. Comparative urinary excretion of caffeine metabolites in seven animal species (% of administered dose)

Compound	Man	Monkey	Dog	Rabbit	Rat	Mouse	Guinea pig
1,3,7-TMX	1.1	1.6	2.8	1.5	2.9	5.1	14.9
3,7-DMX	2.5	1.3	4.9	2.7	7.1	–	12.4
1,3-DMX	2.3	27.6	8.1[a]	–	4.4	5.0	6.8
1,7-DMX	5.4	1.4		13.7	8.6	10.4	13.6
1-MX	13.1	–	1.0	10.8	3.0	4.2	2.1
3-MX	2.5	7.6	21.2	–	1.5	2.3	3.1
7-MX	6.6	–	–	–	–	4.1	–
1,3,7-TMU	1.2	1.0	2.6	1.9	5.8	15.0	–
1,3-DMU	2.7	44.0	13.0	–	2.1	15.0	–
3,7-DMU	0.8	–	–	6.5	–	–	–
1,7-DMU	8.2	–	1.9	3.0	1.8	6.4	–
1-MU	24.1	2.0	8.2	–	3.6	9.7	–
3-MU	0.1	–	–	–	–	7.8	–
7-MU	–	–	2.3	–	–	2.1	–
1,3,7-TAU	1.1	0.4	–	2.1	19.5	–	8.1
3,7-DAU	1.9	–	–	–	3.0	–	–
1,7-DAU	2.4	–	–	–	–	–	–
7-A-3-MAU	17.8	–	–	–	–	–	–
Recovery	94.1	76.9	66.0	42.2	63.3	87.1	52.9

References: Bonati et al. (1982b), Garattini et al. (1979, 1980a, b, 1982), Aldridge and Neims (1979), Arnaud (1976a), Burg and Stein (1972), Grant et al. (1983b)
[a] In the dog, 1,3-DMX and 1,7-DMX were measured together (see Sect 4.3)

4.3 Urinary Metabolism

Since there are interspecies differences in caffeine metabolite production and the different physiochemical characteristics if each metabolite contribute to their faster (than the parent drug) urinary excretion, metabolite profiles in urine tend to be more species-specific than in blood or tissue. Table 3 shows comparative urinary patterns of caffeine metabolites (the averages of published values when more than one set was available). Even a swift analysis shows that the pattern is qualitatively and quantitatively different for the various species.

In adult humans most of the administered caffeine undergoes 3-N-demethylation to paraxanthine the primary metabolite found in the blood). The major metabolites excreted in urine are 1-methyluric acid 5-acetylamino-6-amino-3-methyluracil, and 1-methylxanthine. The acetylated diaminouracil derivative was recovered exclusively in human urine (Callahan et al. 1982; Grant et al. 1983 a,b; Tang et al. 1983).

Caffeine is biotransformed in the monkey *(Macaca cynomolgus)* by 7-demethylation. Theophylline (the primary metabolite in the blood) and 1,3-dimethyluric acid account for almost the whole metabolic excretion of the compound (Latini et al., 1981). Comparison of caffeine disposition in three different monkey strains revealed different profiles in each (Caldwell et al. 1981).

Regarding initial 7-N-demethylation, the metabolic pattern in the beagle resembles the *Macaca* profile, but they cannot be compared in detail because paraxanthine and theophylline were measured together. The beagle is the only species in which 3-methylxanthine was measured in serum after caffeine administration (Aldridge and Neims 1979). As in man, paraxanthine is the major metabolite measured in the bloodstream and urine of rabbits, though the complete urinary and kinetic profiles are quite different (Garattini et al. 1979, 1980 a,b). The urinary metabolic pattern in the rat (CD-COBS) is diffuse, involving all the primary routes of caffeine degradation (Arnaud 1976 a; Latini et al. 1981). A few minor metabolites, such as trimethylallantoin, were detected in this species alone, in which the main significant metabolite is 6-amino-5-[N-formylmethylamino]-1,3-dimethyluracil (Arnaud 1976 b; Latini et al. 1981).

In the mouse as in the rat, initial degradation of caffeine seems flexible (Burg and Stein 1972; Garattini et al. 1980 a,b). 1-, 3-, and 7-demethylation and 8-oxidation pathways seem equally involved (confirming bloodstream data). Unlike in other species investigated, in mouse and beagle urine, no 6-amino-5-[N-formylmethylamino]-1,3-dimethyluracil was detected.

The guinea pig seems to differ significantly from other species (Garattini et al. 1982). Unchanged caffeine accounts for 3–10 times more (15% of administered dose), and the three dimethylxanthines comprise an additional 35%. A larger amount of 6-amino-5-[N-formylmethylamino]-1,3-dimethyluracil was also measured. Thus, unlike the other species investigated, the guinea pig seems to have substantial difficulty in metabolizing caffeine and its primary metabolites.

5 Kinetics of Primary Metabolites of Caffeine

In order to better understand the disposition of caffeine it is important to know not only the biotransformation of the parent drug and each further metabolite after administration of the compound itself (as reported by Arnaud, this volume p 5), but also their kinetic parameters, because the values calculated might be different from the constants calculated after administration of parent drug (Gibaldi and Perrier 1975).

Despite the long and ample study of xanthine compounds, systematic comparable data are available only for rats given 5 mg/kg i. v. of each compound (Table 4) Garattini et al. 1982). Major differences were found in the kinetic profile of 1,3,7-trimethyluric acid, whose total body clearance and apparent volume of distribution were up to 10 times those of other primary metabolites. Values of the same order were found for other metabolites, but the half-lives for theophylline, theobromine, and 1,3,7-trimethyluric acid were double those of caffeine, paraxanthine, and 6-amino-5-[N-formylmethylamino]-1,3-dimethyluracil.

6 Nonlinear Kinetics

Plasma and brain concentrations of caffeine given at different doses to rats indicated a limited capacity to absorb and metabolize the drug (Garattini et al. 1979, 1980 a,b, 1982; Latini et al. 1978). Ratios between doses were much lower than be-

Table 4. Average kinetic parameters for caffeine and its primary metabolites after 5 mg/kg i.v. doses of each compound in male Sprague-Dawley rats

1,3,7-TMU ↖   ↗ 1,3,7-TAU

            1,3,7-TMX
                ↓

1,3-DMX ↙   3,7-DMX   ↘ 1,7-DMX

Parameter	1,3,7-TMX	1,3-DMX	3,7-DMX	1,7-DMX	1,3,7-TAU	1,3,7-TMU
β (h^{-1})	0.46	0.22	0.24	0.55	0.42	0.18
Half-life (h)	1.52	3.13	2.90	1.25	1.63	3.75
Cl (liters/h/kg)	0.38	0.20	0.23	0.39	0.40	2.04
aVd (liters/kg)	0.78	0.88	0.94	0.70	0.94	12.14

β, apparent first-order elimination rate constant obtained from the terminal slope of a semilogarithmic plot of drug concentration in blood vs time. For other abbreviations, see Table 1.

tween AUC in plasma and in brain because of a disproportionate increase in the dose-concentration relationship (46- instead of 10-fold from 1 to 10 mg/kg doses). After oral administration, peak level and k_{abs} also rose faster than the dose (Garattini et al. 1979; Latini et al. 1978). Thus the rat's metabolic capacity is saturable at relatively low doses (around 5 mg/kg). The consequences of saturation kinetics in rats are that exposure to caffeine increases disproportionately after either single or repeated dosing, and metabolic profiles can change with dose (Garattini et al. 1979, 1980a,b, 1982).

Since data were available after increasing doses in the same subject (man) and in the same species (rat, rabbit, monkey, mouse), Bonati et al. (1983) undertook an interspecies comparison of caffeine pharmacokinetics at increasing doses. Using AUC-dose relationships for a one-compartment model with Michaelis-Menten metabolism (Wagner 1973; Chau 1976), the nonlinear kinetic elimination of caffeine was investigated in all five species (Fig. 1). For rabbits and rats the AUC increases proportionally more than the dose.

For rats, rabbits, and mice, the in vivo apparent K_m and V_{max} values (Table 5) could be estimated. Similar values were reported for the rat by Aldridge et al. (1977) using another approach. These findings have important consequences in extrapolation of toxicological data across species. Ratios between animals and man must be calculated for rats and rabbits on the basis of the caffeine AUC, and not on the dose (Garattini et al. 1982), and account must be taken of the fact that first-order kinetics prevails in man [at least up to 10 mg/kg, the highest administrable dose (Bonati et al. 1982b)], monkey, and mouse (up to around 100 mg/kg).

7 Chronic Treatment in the Rat

Comparing results after acute administration with those after daily caffeine doses and those after the addition of 0.14% of the compound to drinking water over a period of 10 days, findings concerning caffeine disposition in blood and brain were similar, suggesting no accumulation of the drug even after high doses. Food intake did not affect caffeine disposition during chronic treatment (Garattini et al. 1979).

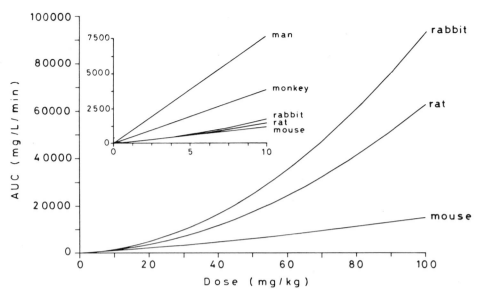

Fig. 1. AUC-dose relationship after caffeine administration in five species

Table 5. Estimates of K_m and V_{max} in three animal species after 1–100 mg/kg caffeine

Species	K_m (μg/ml)	F_{max} (μg/ml/ min)
Rat	8.74	0.159
Rabbit	7.13	0.096
Mouse	85.24	0.153

References

Aldridge A, Neims AH (1979) The effects of phenobarbital and β-naphthoflavone on the elimination kinetics and metabolite pattern of caffeine in the beagle dog. Drug Metab Dispos 7: 378–382

Aldridge A, Parsons WD, Neims AH (1977) Stimulation of caffeine metabolism in the rat by 3-methylcholanthrene. Life Sci 21: 967–974

Arnaud MJ (1976a) Identification, kinetic and quantitative study of [2-^{14}C] and [1-Me-^{14}C]caffeine metabolites in rat's urine by chromatographic separations. Biochem Med 16: 67–76

Arnaud MJ (1976b) Metabolism of 1,3,7-trimethyldihydrouric acid in the rat: new metabolic pathway of caffeine. Epxerientia 32: 1238–1240

Axelrod J, Reichenthal J (1953) The fate of caffeine in man and a method for its estimation in biological material. J Pharmacol Exp Ther 107: 519–523

Bianchi CP (1962) Kinetics of radiocaffeine uptake and release in frog sartorius. J Pharmacol Exp Ther 138: 41–47

Blanchard J, Sawers SJA (1983a) The absolute bioavailability of caffeine in man. Eur J Clin Pharmacol 24: 93–98

Blanchard J, Sawers SJA (1938b) Relationship between urine flow rate and renal clearance of caffeine in man. J Clin Pharmacol 23: 134–138

Bonati M, Kanto J, Tognoni G (1982a) Clinical pharmacokinetics of cerebrospinal fluid. Clin Pharmacokinet 7: 312–335

Bonati M, Latini R, Galetti F, Young JF, Tognoni G, Garattini S (1982b) Caffeine disposition after oral doses. Clin Pharmacol Ther 32: 98–106

Bonati M, Latini R, Young JF, Garattini S (1983) Interspecies Comparison of caffeine pharmacokinetics in man, monkey, rabbit, rat and mouse. In: Proceeding of Second World Conference in Clinical Pharmacology and Therapeutics, July 31–August 5, Washington, D.C.

Burg AW (1975) Physiological disposition of caffeine. Drug Metab Rev 4: 199–228

Burg AW, Stein M (1972) Urinary excretion of caffeine and its metabolites in the mouse. Biochem Pharmacol 21: 909–922

Caldwell J, O'Gorman J, Adamson RH (1981) Urinary metabolites of caffeine in the chimpanzee, rhesus monkey and galago (Abstr). Pharmacologist 23: 212

Callahan MM, Robertson RS, Arnaud MJ, Branfman AR, McComish MF, Yesair DW (1982) Human metabolism of [1-methyl-^{14}C]- and [2-^{14}C]caffeine after oral administration. Drug Metab. Dispos 10: 417–423

Chau NP (1976) Area-dose relationships in nonlinear models. J Pharmacokinet Biopharm 4: 537–551

Cook CE, Tallent CR, Amerson EW, Myers MW, Kepler JA, Taylor GF, Christensen HD (1976) Caffeine in plasma and saliva by a radioimmunoassay procedure. J Pharmacol Exp Ther 199: 679–686

Desmond PV, Patwardhan R, Parker R, Schenker S, Speeg KV Jr (1980) Effect of cimetidine and other antihistamines on the elimination of aminopyrine, phenacetin and caffeine. Life Sci 26: 1261–1268

Eichman ML, Guttman DE, Van Winkle C, Guth EP (1962) Interactions of xanthine molecules with bovine serum albumin. J Pharm Sci 51: 66–71

Garattini S, Bonati M, Latini R (1979) Studies on the kinetics and metabolism of caffeine. In: Proceedings of First International Caffeine Committee Workshop. November 8–10, 1978, Keauhou-Kona, Hawaii

Garattini S, Bonati M, Latini R (1980a) Caffeine kinetics. In: Proceedings of Second International Caffeine Committee Workshop. October 22–24, 1979, Monaco

Garattini S, Bonati M, Latini R, Galetti F (1980b) Caffeine kinetics and metabolism. In: Proceedings of Third International Caffeine Committee Workshop. October 27–28, 1980, Hunt Valley, Maryland

Garattini S, Bonati M, Latini R (1982) Caffeine kinetics and metabolism in several animal species. In: Proceedings of Fourth International Caffeine Committee Workshop. October 17–21, 1982, Athens

Gaspari F, Celardo A, Bonati M (1983) Apparent dissociation constants of some possible uracil metabolites of methylxanthines. Anal Lett 16: 167–180

Gibaldi M, Perrier, D (1975) Pharmacokinetics. Dekker, New York

Grant DM, Tang BK, Kalow W (1983a) Polymorphic N-acetylation of caffeine metabolite. Clin Pharmacol Ther 33: 355–359

Grant DM, Tang BK, Kalow W (1983b) Variability in caffeine metabolism. Clin Pharmacol Ther 33: 591–602

Latini R, Bonati M, Castelli D, Garattini S (1978) Dose-dependent kinetics of caffeine in rats. Toxicol Lett 2: 267–270

Latini R, Bonati M, Marzi E Garattini S (1981) Urinary excretion of an uracilic metabolite from caffeine by rat, monkey and man. Toxicol Lett 7: 267–272

Marks V, Kelly JF (1973) Absorption of caffeine from tea, coffee, and Coca Cola. Lancet 1: 827

McCall AL, Millington WR, Wurtman RJ (1982) Blood-brain barrier transport of caffeine: dose-related restriction of adenine transport. Life Sci 31: 2709–2715

Neims AH, von Borstel RW (1983). Caffeine: Its metabolism and biochemical mechanisms of action. In: Wurtman RJ, Wurtman JJ (eds) Nutrition and the brain, vol 6. Raven, New York

Parsons WD, Neims AH (1978) Effect of smoking on caffeine clearance. Clin Pharmacol Ther 24: 40–45

Sant'Ambrogio G, Mognoni P, Ventrella L (1964) Plasma levels of caffeine after oral, intramuscular and intravenous administration. Arch Int Pharmacodyn Ther 150: 259–263

Somani SM, Khanna NN, Bada SB (1980) Caffeine and theophylline: serum/CSF correlation in premature infants. J Pediatr 96: 1091–1093

Tang BK, Grant DM, Kalow W (1983) Isolation and identification of 5-acetylamino-6-formylamino-3-methyluracil as a major metabolite of caffeine in man. Drug Metab Dispos (in press)

Wagner JG (1973) Properties of the Michaelis-Menten equation and its integrated form which are useful in pharmacokinetics. J Pharmacokinet Biopharm 1: 103–121

Section II
Intake

IV Human Consumption of Caffeine*

J. J. Barone and H. Roberts

1 Introduction

Caffeine from natural sources has been consumed and enjoyed by people through-out the world for centuries, dating back to perhaps as early as the Paleolithic period. The widespread natural occurrence of caffeine in a variety of plants undoubtedly played a major role in the long-standing popularity of caffeine-containing products, especially beverages. More than 60 plant species throughout the world have been identified as containing caffeine. Caffeine-containing beverages made form native plants in South America, such as guarana, yoco, and mate, have been traced back to antiquity (Rall 1980). Similarly, North American natives made use of the caffeine-containing cassina.

The earliest written mention of coffee was in the tenth century, but coffee may have been cultivated in Ethiopia, where it is indigenous, as early as 575 A.D. Coffee was first used as a food, the berries being eaten whole or crushed and mixed with fat. Later, fermented juice from the berries was used to make a kind of wine. When coffee as a hot beverage came into use about 1000 A.D. the Arabians gave it their poetic name for wine, *gahwah*. Through the Turkish equivalent, *kahveh,* it finally became *café* in French and *Kaffee* in German. Coffee did not reach Europe until the seventeenth century, but then its use spread rapidly (Roden 1977). Today over half of the U.S. population drinks coffee and the coffee break has become an American institution.

The oldest caffeine-containing beverage, according to historical records, is tea. Tradition attributes the first written mention of tea to the legendary Chinese emperor Shen Nung in 2737 B.C. However, the first more reliable reference is the listing of tea in a Chinese dictionary of about 350 A.D. Despite its long-standing popularity in the Orient, tea did not reach Europe until Dutch traders introduced it in about 1600 (Ukers 1935).

Cocoa and other caffeine-containing chocolate products also have a long history. A sweetened chocolate drink was served by the Aztec emperor Montezuma to the Spanish conquerors in 1519, and soon thereafter chocolate drinks became a Spanish favorite. A way of making milk chocolate bars was invented in Switzerland in

---

* This chapter is based on a paper presented during the IFT Toxicology and Safety Evaluation Division Program "Caffeine – Biological Effects" at the 43rd Annual Meeting of the Institute of Food Technologists, New Orleans, Louisiana, June 19–22, 1983.

59

1876, and chocolate and chocolate-containing products enjoy current popularity in a wide variety of forms.

The major ingredient use of caffeine, as a flavor component in cola-type soft drinks, originated around the turn of the century (e. g., Dr Pepper in 1885, Coca-Cola in 1886, Pepsi-Cola in 1896, and Royal Crown Cola in 1912). According to the Food and Drug Administration (FDA), caffeine is also used, to a much lesser extent, as a flavoring agent in baked goods, dairy desserts, puddings and fillings, and candy (FDA 1980a).

Since its original chemical isolation in 1820, caffeine has been used therapeutically in infant apnea, as a bronchial and cardiac stimulant, in acne and other skin disorders, and in migraine headaches. Caffeine also occurs in a variety of over-the-counter (OTC) products used as analgesics, diuretics, weight control aids, allergy relief preparations, and alertness compounds.

In general, the human response to a given substance, whether therapeutic or adverse, depends not only on the substance itself but also on its concentration in body tissues or organs. That concentration is, in turn, dependent in the case of a therapeutic agent on the dose administered or in the case of a dietary constituent on the levels and time distribution of intake. The dependence of response on the intake involved is especially important in the case of caffeine, as is abundantly evident from the other chapters of this monograph. It is, therefore, of critical importance to examine the individual sources of human caffeine intake and the resulting patterns of consumption.

2 Sources and Levels

A wide variety of caffeine content values appears in the popular and scientific literature, especially with reference to coffee. As Burg (1975) has noted, many of the caffeine content values appearing in the literature are undocumented and different values can arise from miscitation of previous literature, differences in the analytical methods employed for determining caffeine content, or the use of different reference volumes (e. g., "cup" size). Plant variety and growing conditions can also affect the caffeine content of the natural product, and with coffee and tea, the method of preparation can significantly affect the caffeine content of the beverages as consumed.

2.1 Coffee

In general, brewed coffee has the highest and most variable caffeine content among those dietary items containing caffeine. Caffeine levels ranging from 0.8% to 1.8% in freshly ground roasted coffee beans were reported by Kaplan et al. (1974). Caffeine levels in coffee also depend on the product form (e. g., ground roasted vs instant), the method of brewing (e. g. percolator vs drip), the amount of coffee used, and the brewing time.

Table 1. Caffeine content of food products

Product	Volume or weight	Caffeine content (mg)		Reference
		Range	Average	
Roasted and ground coffee (percolated)[a]	5 oz	64–124	83	Burg (1975)
	5 oz	–	74	Gilbert (1981)
Instant coffee	5 oz	40–108	59	Burg (1975)
	5 oz	–	66	Gilbert (1981)
	5 oz	–	66	FDA (1980b)
Roasted and ground coffee (decaffeinated)	5 oz	2– 5	3	Burg (1975)
	5 oz	–	2	Gilbert (1981)
Instant coffee (decaffeinated)	5 oz	2– 8	3	Burg (1975)
Roasted and ground coffee (drip)[a]	5 oz	–	112	Gilbert (1981)
Instant coffee (percolated and drip)	5 oz	29–176	–	Gilbert (1981)
Tea	5 oz	8– 91	27	Gilbert (1981)
Bagged tea	5 oz	–	42	Burg (1975)
	5 oz	28– 44	–	FDA (1980b)
Leaf tea	5 oz	30– 48	41	Burg (1975)
Instant tea	5 oz	24– 31	28	Burg (1975)
Cocoa – African	5 oz	–	6	Burg (1975)
– South American	5 oz	–	42	Burg (1975)
Cocoa	5 oz	–	5	FDA (1980b)
	5 oz	less than 40	–	Gilbert (1981)
	5 oz	2– 7	4	Zoumas et al. (1980)
Chocolate bar	30 g	–	20	Gilbert (1981)
Milk chocolate	1 oz	–	6	FDA (1980b)
	1 oz	1– 15	6	Zoumas et al. (1980)
Sweet chocolate	1 oz	5– 35	20	Zoumas et al. (1980)
Chocolate milk	8 oz	2– 7	5	Zoumas et al. (1980)
Baking chocolate	1 oz	–	35	FDA (1980b)
	1 oz	18–118	60	Zoumas et al. (1980)
Soft drinks				
Regular colas	6 oz	15– 23	–	NSDA (1982)
Decaffeinated colas	6 oz	trace	–	NSDA (1982)
Diet colas	6 oz	1– 29	–	NSDA (1982)
Decaffeinated diet colas	6 oz	0–trace	–	NSDA (1982)
Orange, lemon-lime, root beer, tonic, ginger ale, club soda	6 oz	0	–	NSDA (1982)
Others	6 oz	22– 27	–	NSDA (1982)

[a] The FDA cites a range of 75–155 mg caffeine per cup of coffee, noting that percolated coffee is in the lower part of this range and drip coffee in the upper

In order to address the differing values reported in the literature, Burg (1975) assembled standardized data on over 2000 caffeine analyses of coffee. Average values were 83, 59, and 3 mg of caffeine per cup of percolated, instant, and decaffeinated coffee respectively, as shown in Table 1. Based on these data, Burg suggested standard values of 85, 60, and 3 mg per 150-ml (approximately 5 oz) cup. By way of comparison, caffeine content values for coffee reported by the FDA (1980b) and by Gilbert (1981) are also shown in Table 1.

2.2 Tea

Burg (1975) also obtained standard caffeine content values for tea. His results are shown in Table 1, and again the values reported by the FDA and by Gilbert are listed for comparison. Burg notes that his data lead to a standard caffeine value for instant tea of about 30 mg per 5-oz cup, but he did not propose a standard value for brewed tea. Caffeine content data for brewed tea include a range of 30–48 mg per cup as cited by Burg, 28–44 mg per cup as cited by the FDA (1980b), and 8–91 mg per cup as cited by Gilbert et al. (1976) and Gilbert (1981).

2.3 Cocoa and Chocolate Products

Caffeine content data on chocolate products are fairly limited but also show quite variable levels. Burg (1975) noted the differences in caffeine content of African cocoa and South American cocoa (6 mg vs 42 mg per 5-oz cup respectively). The FDA (1980b) cites a single value of 5 mg per cup, and Gilbert (1981) states that cocoa usually contains less than 40 mg per cup. Zoumas et al. (1980), using high-performance liquid chromatography (HPLC), obtained an average of 4 mg per 5-oz cup (range 2–7 mg) for five different brands of commercial cocoa. These authors question the accuracy of earlier analyses, pointing out the inability of classical methods to quantitate caffeine and theobromine separately. Zoumas et al. (1980) also report average caffeine contents of 6 mg per 1-oz serving for milk chocolate, 20 mg per 1-oz serving for sweet (dark, bittersweet, or semisweet) chocolate, and 5 mg per 8-oz glass of chocolate milk. Cocoa and chocolate product caffeine content values are summarized in Table 1.

2.4 Soft Drinks

As with other beverages, differing caffeine levels have been reported for soft drinks in the literature. The most recent of such data are those reported by the National Soft Drink Association (1982). Table 1 shows the ranges of caffeine content for different brands of soft drinks of each type based on the National Soft Drink Association (NSDA) data. In general, only the cola-type soft drinks contain caffeine, although some non-colas also do. Caffeine levels in the colas range primarily from about 15 to 29 mg per 6-oz serving, with a typical value of about 3 mg per fl oz. Recently, the major soft drink companies have introduced caffeine-free or decaffeinated (containing only a trace of caffeine) colas.

2.5 Drug Products

There are a wide variety of drug products that contain caffeine. According to the FDA, about 1000 prescription drug products and about 2000 OTC (nonprescription) drug products contain caffeine (FDA 1980b). Typical prescription drugs contain on the order of 30–100 mg caffeine per tablet or capsule. Caffeine levels in OTC drugs also vary widely (typically from 15 to 200 mg per tablet or capsule) and depend not only on the type of product, but also on the brand involved.

2.6 Standard Caffeine Content Values

Recognizing that there can be significant variability in caffeine content for a given source, it is nonetheless useful to have representative values for each of the major sources. Based on the data cited above, we have selected the following standard values:

Coffee
    Ground roasted   85 mg/5-oz cup
    Instant   60 mg/5-oz cup
    Decaffeinated   3 mg/5-oz cup
Tea
    Leaf or bag   40 mg/5-oz cup
    Instant   30 mg/5-oz cup
Cola (except caffeine-free)   18 mg/6-oz glass
Cocoa, hot chocolate   4 mg/5-oz cup
Chocolate milk   5 mg/8-oz glass

3 Consumption Data Sources

As is the case with most other dietary constituents, data on the human consumption of caffeine are quite limited and are based either on overall product usage data or on a small number of dietary consumption surveys. A gross estimate of consumption can be derived by considering per capita intake. As Graham (1978) has pointed out, essentially all U.S. dietary caffeine is imported in the form of coffee, tea, cocoa, kola nuts, and caffeine itself. In this context coffee is the most important caffeine source, accounting for approximately 75% of per capita caffeine intake; tea adds another 15%. According to Gilbert (1981), 60% of Canadian per capita intake of caffeine is from coffee and 30% is from tea. Thus, for both the U.S. and Canada, coffee and tea combined account overall for the vast majority of per capita caffeine intake.

In its evaluation report on caffeine, the Federation of American Societies for Experimental Biology (FASEB; 1978) utilized consumption estimates derived from data on frequency of consumption collected by the Market Research Corporation of America (MRCA) in a national household menu census covering a 14-day period in 1972–1973, together with estimated serving sizes derived from the United States Department of Agriculture (USDA) 1965 survey of food intake of individuals in the

United States (24-h recalls of food consumption). The FASEB also referred to summary data from the MRCA survey as reported by Arthur D. Little, Inc. (1977).

The MRCA data were obtained using a sample of 12,337 individuals who participated in MRCA's Fourth National Household Menu Census Study. Selection of households was controlled by region, city size, household size, age of housewife, and income. Each individual's food consumption during a 14-day period was recorded by a designated family member. Diary entries included foods consumed both at home and away from home.

Utilizing the USDA data on the amounts of various food items consumed per eating occasion, average serving sizes were computed for individuals classified into several age-groups.

Based on the number of eating occasions, the average serving sizes for each age-group, and the caffeine content of the foods consumed, the amounts of caffeine ingested by each individual over the 14-day period were then estimated. These caffeine intakes (in milligrams) were then converted to a body-weight basis (milligrams per kilogram body weight) utilizing the actual weights of each individual in the MRCA survey.

Caffeine consumption estimates for 5- to 18-year-old children as reported by Morgan et al. (1982) were derived from data compiled by Market Facts in September 1977. (The Market Facts Survey also obtained consumption data for adults, but to date, estimates have been reported only for children.) The Market Facts survey utilized 7-day food consumption diaries recorded by 1434 families throughout the U.S. These survey families were balanced by geographic area, population density, degree of urbanization, income, and age. Data for 1135 5- to 18-year-old children were obtained from the diaries, and included sex, age, and weight and amounts of each food and beverage item consumed during each meal or snack for 7 days. Based on the caffeine content of the coffee, tea, chocolate and chocolate products, and soft drinks consumed, caffeine intakes were calculated on a total and on a body-weight basis.

Another basic source of consumption data is the 1977–1978 Nationwide Food Consumption Survey (NFCS). Average intakes per day and per eating occasion from the NFCS are given in a USDA report by Pao et al. (1982). The NFCS is the most recent of the six nationwide household food consumption surveys conducted by the USDA and the second survey in which data were collected on the food intake of individual members of households. Both households and individuals are from a stratified area probability sample of the 48 conterminous states and thus can be considered representative of the continental U.S. population. Dietary information in the NFCS is based on a 24-h dietary recall followed by a 2-day dietary record, thus providing data for 3 consecutive days.

The NFCS includes data on dietary intakes from food consumption at home and away from home. Dietary information includes the kind and amount of food eaten, the time of day it was eaten, and the eating occasion.

Food items of interest relative to caffeine in the NFCS include coffee (ground roasted and instant), tea (leaf and bag, instant, tea mix, and iced tea), cocoa and hot chocolate, chocolate milk, chocolate cake and cupcakes, and cola soft drinks. Caffeine intake estimates from these sources were obtained by the authors using the caffeine content of each product and the amounts consumed.

One additional source of caffeine intake information is the annual winter coffee drinking study, conducted annually for 40 years. The most recent was conducted in 1982 (International Coffee Organization 1982), and involved telephone interviews with 7500 individuals aged 10 years and over representative of the population of the 48 continental states. Respondents in each case were asked about coffee and other beverages consumed "yesterday." Questions included the amounts consumed, where consumed, in what period of the day consumed, type of coffee used, and method of preparation.

Data on the consumption of caffeine from drugs is essentially nonexistent in the literature. This is not surprising, since for the most part, drugs are ingested intermittently rather than consistently as is the case with dietary constituents. Significant amounts of caffeine can be consumed by some individuals from drugs at particular times, and some individuals habitually consume OTC products containing caffeine. However, as Gilbert (1981) has noted, caffeine intake for the general population is primarily from coffee and tea and is relatively negligible from other sources such as drugs.

4 Consumption Estimates

Looking at caffeine from a global perspective, Gilbert (1981) estimated that the average daily consumption by the world's 4.4 billion inhabitants is about 50 mg per person per day, based on world production of coffee and tea. Judging that approximately 90% of caffeine consumed is contained in coffee and tea, Gilbert characterizes other sources as negligible by comparison. A similar estimate of nearly 90% derivation from coffee and tea has been calculated by Graham (1978).

Graham estimated U.S. daily caffeine consumption as 206 mg per person based on 1972 usage data for all sources of caffeine. Gilbert estimated it at 200 mg per adult based on 1979 consumption of coffee and tea.

4.1 Market Research Corporation of America Survey

For all subjects in the survey, the MRCA data show a mean daily caffeine intake from all sources of 2.6 mg/kg body weight for adults (18 years of age and above). Corresponding consumption estimates for children are 1.2 mg/kg, 0.85 mg/kg, and 0.74 mg/kg for 1–5, 6–11, and 12–17 year olds respectively. For infants (less than 1 year old) the caffeine consumption estimate is 0.18 mg/kg (Table 2).

The 90th percentile for adult caffeine consumers is 5.4 mg/kg. For 1–5, 6–11, and 12–17-year-olds the 90th percentiles are 3.2, 2.1, and 1.9 mg/kg respectively.

Mean estimated intake among the heaviest 10% of consumers has also been calculated from the MRCA data. For adults it is 7.0 mg/kg, in 1–5, 6–11, and 12–17-year-olds respectively it is 4.7, 3.2, and 2.9 mg/kg (Table 3). With reference to either mean consumption (Table 2) or heaviest consumption (Table 3), tea is the major source of caffeine for children. For adults, coffee is the predominant source.

65

Table 2. Mean daily consumption of caffeine (mg/kg body weight) by source for all MRCA survey subjects

Age (years)	Source				
	All sources	Coffee	Tea	Soft drinks	Chocolate
Under 1	0.18	0.009	0.13	0.02	0.02
1– 5	1.20	0.11	0.57	0.34	0.16
6–11	0.85	0.10	0.41	0.21	0.13
12–17	0.74	0.16	0.34	0.16	0.08
18 and over	2.60	2.1	0.41	0.10	0.03

Source: Arthur D. Little, Inc. (1977)

Table 3. Mean daily consumption of caffeine (mg/kg body weight) by MRCA subjects in the 90th to 100th percentiles of caffeine intake from all sources

Age (years)	Source				
	All sources	Coffee	Tea	Soft drinks	Chocolate
1– 5	4.7	0.49	3.2	0.79	0.22
6–11	3.2	0.43	2.1	0.52	0.19
12–17	2.9	0.96	1.5	0.33	0.092
18 and over	7.0	6.55	0.35	0.069	0.036

Source: Arthur D. Little, Inc. (1977)

Table 4. Mean daily caffeine consumption by Market Facts Subjects who consumed caffeine for days when consumed and for all 7 days of the survey

Age-group (years)	Number of subjects	Consumption (mg/kg)	
		Days of consumption	All 7 days
All ages	966	1.1	0.9
5– 6	141	1.3	1.1
7– 8	147	0.9	0.7
9–10	151	1.0	0.8
11–12	140	1.2	1.0
13–14	148	1.0	0.8
15–16	136	1.1	0.8
17–18	103	1.2	0.9

Source: Morgan et al. (1982)

4.2 Market Facts Survey

The mean consumption of caffeine over 7 days in the Market Facts survey was re-ported by Morgan et al. (1982). For the 1135 5- to 18-year-old children in the survey it is 37.4 mg per day (47.9 mg per day based on days of consumption only). Con-sumption appears to increase with increasing age.

Caffeine consumption on a body-weight basis from the Market Facts survey is shown in Table 4. The mean daily intake for consumers of caffeine is 0.9 mg/kg

Table 5. Mean daily caffeine consumption by source for all Market Facts survey subjects and for caffeine consumers on days of consumption

Source	Consumption (mg)		Proportion of total caffeine consumed: all subjects (%)
	Consumers on days of consumption	All subjects ($n = 1135$)	
Soft drinks	33.3 ($n = 825$)	9.8	26.4
Tea	59.5	12.8	34.2
Coffee	193.4 ($n = 134$)	8.3	22.1
Chocolate and chocolate-containing foods and beverages	11.7 ($n = 1053$)	6.4	17.3

Source: Morgan et al. (1982)

(1.1 mg/kg based on days of consumption only). It can be seen from Table 4 that caffeine intake on a body-weight basis is approximately 1 mg/kg for all ages from 5 to 18 years. As is the case with the MRCA data, the major source of caffeine for children in the Market Facts survey is tea, which accounts for 34.2% of the total consumed for all subjects. However, the average caffeine intake on days of consumption was higher for consumers of coffee than for consumers of other caffeine sources (Table 5).

4.3 Nationwide Food Consumption Survey

Average daily caffeine consumption estimates from coffee, tea, and cola are shown in Tables 6, 7, and 8 respectively. The estimates in each case are for those survey respondents who consumed the particular beverage at least once in 3 days. Estimates of caffeine intakes on a body-weight basis were calculated by the authors from the median weights by age and sex developed in the National Health Survey (National Center for Health Statistics 1977, 1979).

It should be noted that the NFCS data for coffee refer to liquid coffee made from ground roasted coffee, powdered instant coffee, liquid coffee concentrate, and coffee that was either acid-neutralized or decaffeinated. Based on the percentages of drinking occasions reported by USDA for each type of coffee, we estimated that 52% of the coffee was ground roasted, 38% was instant, and 10% was decaffeinated, with caffeine contents of 85, 60, and 3 mg per cup respectively. Combining these percentages and content values, a weighted average of 67.2 mg per 5-oz cup was calculated and used to estimate caffeine intake (Table 6).

NFCS tea consumption data refer to tea bags and loose leaf tea, powdered instant tea, frozen concentrate, and ready-to-drink cans. The percentage of drinking occasions was identified only for instant tea (20%) and leaf tea (34%). Based on the relative frequency of consumption for these two major types of tea, we assumed that 37% of drinking occasions involved instant tea and 63% leaf tea, with caffeine contents of 30 and 40 mg per cup respectively. A weighted average of 36.3 mg per 5-oz

Table 6. Average daily caffeine consumption from coffee for coffee drinkers (NFCS)

Age (years)	Sex	Total subjects	Coffee drinkers (%)	Caffeine[a]	
				mg	mg/kg
Under 1	M + F	498	0.0	0.0	0.0
1– 2	M + F	1045	1.0	46.9	4.2
3– 5	M + F	1719	1.2	38.9	2.4
6– 8	M + F	1841	2.0	48.2	2.1
9–14	M	2089	4.7	63.0	1.6
	F	2158	4.1	57.6	1.6
15–18	M	1394	16.4	108.5	1.7
	F	1473	17.1	119.3	2.2
19–34	M	3928	53.9	211.7	2.7
	F	5346	53.0	202.3	3.4
35–64	M	4929	84.2	282.7	3.6
	F	7069	82.4	253.3	4.0
65–74	M	1118	84.7	237.2	3.2
	F	1738	85.0	198.3	3.0
75 and over	M	536	85.1	215.7	2.9
	F	993	81.7	187.6	2.9
All coffee drinkers	M + F	37874	51.1	233.2	–

Source: Pao et al. (1982)
[a] Calculations made by authors: see text for explanation.

Table 7. Average daily caffeine consumption from tea for tea drinkers (NFCS)

Age (years)	Sex	Total subjects	Tea drinkers (%)	Caffeine[a]	
				mg	mg/kg
Under 1	M + F	498	4.9	28.3	5.2
1– 2	M + F	1045	19.9	32.7	2.9
3– 5	M + F	1719	22.4	42.1	2.6
6– 8	M + F	1841	24.5	45.7	2.0
9–14	M	2089	27.4	62.4	1.6
	F	2158	29.3	55.9	1.6
15–18	M	1394	30.1	80.6	1.2
	F	1473	33.5	66.1	1.2
19–34	M	3928	38.3	87.1	1.1
	F	5346	46.8	80.6	1.4
35–64	M	4929	41.0	87.1	1.1
	F	7069	48.4	81.3	1.3
65–74	M	1118	39.5	79.9	1.1
	F	1738	50.5	74.8	1.1
75 and over	M	536	32.6	69.0	0.9
	F	993	47.3	71.9	1.1
All tea drinkers	M + F	37874	38.5	76.2	–

Source: Pao et al. (1982)
[a] Calculations made by authors: see text for explanation.

Table 8. Average daily caffeine consumption from cola for cola drinkers (NFCS)

Age (years)	Sex	Total subjects	Cola drinkers (%)	Caffeine[a]	
				mg	mg/kg
Under 1	M + F	498	2.2	7.5	1.4
1– 2	M + F	1045	31.0	11.4	1.0
3– 5	M + F	1719	37.8	14.4	0.88
6– 8	M + F	1841	38.2	16.5	0.71
9–14	M	2089	44.9	21.9	0.55
	F	2158	44.4	21.3	0.59
15–18	M	1394	54.8	31.5	0.48
	F	1473	54.8	27.9	0.51
19–34	M	3928	57.3	33.9	0.44
	F	5346	46.1	27.9	0.47
35–64	M	4929	30.3	25.5	0.32
	F	7069	26.4	21.9	0.34
65–74	M	1118	12.8	20.4	0.27
	F	1738	10.4	17.1	0.26
75 and over	M	536	9.2	21.9	0.29
	F	993	8.2	15.3	0.23
All cola drinkers	M + F	37874	36.1	25.2	–

Source: Pao et al. (1982)
[a] Calculations made by authors: see text for explanation.

cup was then calculated and used to estimate the caffeine intake from tea as shown in Table 7.

Cola consumption data from the NFCS represent carbonated soft drinks specified as colas (about two-thirds of total carbonated soft drink drinking occasions). Caffeine consumption estimates for colas are based on a standard caffeine content value of 3 mg per fl oz (Table 8).

For cocoa and hot chocolate consumers in the NFCS, caffeine intakes ranged from 0.06 to 0.22 mg/kg for children and averaged about 0.05 mg/kg for adults. Chocolate milk contributed 0.02–0.06 mg/kg for adults and 0.05–0.19 mg/kg for children. Assuming a caffeine content of 0.15 mg/g for chocolate cake and cupcakes (Morgan et al. 1982), consumers had a caffeine intake from those sources of 0.06–0.10 mg/kg for adults and 0.10–0.30 mg/kg for children.

In the case of children, the NFCS generally showed similar intakes of caffeine by consumers of the two major sources, coffee and tea. Adult consumers of coffee had a higher caffeine intake from coffee than did tea drinkers from tea (Tables 6–8).

4.4 1982 Coffee Drinking Study

The 1982 coffee drinking study (International Coffee Organization 1982) gave 1.90 as the estimated average number of cups of coffee consumed per person per day. Of these, 1.33 cups were regular (from ground roasted coffee) and 0.56 cups were from instant coffee. Overall consumption of coffee continued its downward trend from

2.35 cups in 1972. Decaffeinated coffee accounted for 20% or 0.38 cups of the total of 1.90 cups.

Among the 56.3% of the population over 10 years of age who were coffee drinkers in 1982, the average number of cups consumed per day was 3.38. Decaffeinated coffee drinkers increased from one out of every 25 persons in 1962 to one out of every seven in 1982.

The 80% of the coffee which contains caffeine is composed of 63% ground roasted and 17% instant. Using caffeine content values of 85, 60, and 3 mg per cup for ground roasted, instant, and decaffeinated coffee respectively, we estimated a caffeine intake for all coffee drinkers of 217 mg daily.

4.5 Standard Consumption Estimates

Comparison of the various caffeine consumption estimates from the available sources shows a fair amount of agreement considering the different characteristics associated with those sources. Graham (1978) estimated daily consumption of 206 mg caffeine per person based on overall usage data. A similar estimate by Gilbert (1981) is 200 mg caffeine per adult. For adults weighing 60–70 kg these estimates correspond to a daily average for the total population of about 3 mg/kg. Consistent with that estimate, the mean daily caffeine intake for all adults was estimated to be 2.6 mg/kg based on the MRCA data.

The NFCS data, which refer only to consumers of caffeine-containing products (rather than all individuals), produce similar estimates for adults. Depending on age and sex, the mean daily caffeine intake from coffee for adult coffee drinkers ranged from 2.74 to 3.98 mg/kg. Adult consumers of tea had caffeine intakes of 0.9 to 1.4 mg/kg from tea, and the corresponding range for colas is 0.23 to 0.46 mg/kg. Comparable intakes from the various chocolate products were in each case 0.1 mg/kg or less. Such estimates would, of course, be expected to be somewhat higher than the average for all adults, including nonconsumers.

The 1982 coffee drinking study, with an estimated 1.52 cups of (caffeine-containing) coffee per person per day, yields an estimated 129 mg of caffeine per person per day. Among coffee drinkers only, average caffeine intake from coffee is estimated as approximately 217 mg/day which, for a 60-kg individual, is equivalent to 3.6 mg/kg.

For the heaviest adult consumers of caffeine, the MRCA data yield an intake estimate of 7 mg/kg from all sources. This estimate represents the mean daily intake by consumers in the 90th–100th percentiles. Estimates from the NFCS data show a range of 4.88–7.46 mg/kg, depending on age and sex, for the 90th percentile caffeine consumption in coffee by coffee drinkers.

Based on the preceding, it appears reasonable to establish 3 mg/kg body weight as the mean caffeine intake for adults in the total population. For adult consumers of caffeine (primarily in the form of coffee, tea, and cola drinks) the mean intake is on the order of 4 mg/kg. For the heaviest consumers of caffeine from all sources (90th–100th percentiles) the estimated mean intake is on the order of 7 mg/kg.

In the case of children (under 18 years of age) caffeine consumption estimates are much more variable than in adults. Based on MRCA data, the mean daily intakes for children of all age-groups are approximately 1 mg/kg. The Market Facts data show a mean daily caffeine consumption of 37.5 mg for 5- to 18-year-old children, an intake again approximating 1 mg/kg. In light of this consistency, the estimates for children from the NFCS data, shown in Tables 6, 7, and 8, are surprising. The NFCS mean estimates for coffee, for example, are so large that they correspond to the 90th–100th percentile intakes from all sources for the MRCA data.

The differences between the NFCS consumption data for children and similar data from other surveys is probably due to several factors. For instance, in some cases the number of children represented in the NFCS is too small to yield meaningful estimates. Additionally, the NFCS is based on only a 3-day period (2 days of dietary record and 1 day of recall) in contrast to the MRCA survey, which is based on a 14-day period (dietary record), and the Market Facts survey, which used a 7-day period (dietary record). The greater variability in consumption which could occur with children as opposed to adults would more likely be evened out in 7 or 14 days than in 3 days. Another difficulty is that the classes of consumption items (e. g., "coffee") in the NFCS are broader, making it difficult to assign an appropriate caffeine content value.

In light of the foregoing, the mean daily intake of caffeine for all children (consumers plus nonconsumers) is considered to be on the order of 1 mg/kg body weight. For the heaviest consumers of caffeine (90th–100th percentiles) the estimated daily intakes are considered to approximate to 3–5 mg/kg.

4.6 Consumption by Pregnant Women

Few data are available on the total intake of caffeine from all sources by pregnant women. The FDA (1980a) has cited daily intake of 2.9 mg/kg from coffee alone, this estimate being derived by the Interagency Epidemiological Working Group (IEWG) using data which have not been made public from the MRCA. These MRCA data are different from those utilized in the FASEB (1978) report. According to the IEWG, in a sample of 116 pregnant women, 46.5% did not consume coffee, while 53.5% consumed coffee ranging from one serving to 38 servings over a 14-day period. Average frequency of consumption among the consumers was 0.8 times per day. The mean daily consumption of caffeine for coffee consumers was 193 mg. Using the average weight of the pregnant women of 64.7 kg (range 44.4–100.6 kg), the IEWG calculated its daily average exposure of 2.9 mg/kg.

Data from the MRCA survey utilized by FASEB to estimate human exposure to caffeine (a different but similar survey to that used by the IEWG) permits examination of caffeine intake from coffee as well as from other sources. These data, covering 86 pregnant or nursing women, showed a mean daily caffeine intake for all individuals of 2.11 mg/kg. Of this total, coffee contributed 1.45 mg/kg (68.7%), tea 0.40 mg/kg (19.0%), soft drinks 0.20 mg/kg (9.5%), and chocolate 0.045 mg/kg (2.1%). For consumers of caffeine the mean daily total intake was 2.16 mg/kg, and the 90th and 95th percentiles were 5.03 and 6.35 mg/kg respectively.

It would seem, at least from the latter data, that daily average caffeine consumption may be less for pregnant women than for the general adult population (2.11 mg/kg vs 2.6 mg/kg). Such a conclusion, although based on limited data, is

Table 9. Daily patterns of beverage consumption for 5- to 18-year-old children (Market Facts)

Meal	Number consuming (n = 1135)			Average amount consumed by consumers (ml)		
	Tea	Coffee	Soft drinks	Tea	Coffee	Soft drinks
Breakfast	69	113	20	76.9	106.5	44.4
Morning snack	10	11	105	44.4	68.0	59.1
Lunch	218	11	434	73.9	53.2	68.0
Afternoon snack	76	5	423	68.0	65.1	68.0
Dinner	368	10	551	141.9	85.5	79.8
Evening snack	74	12	490	62.1	44.4	76.9

Source: Barone (1981)

consistent with the findings of Rosenberg et al. (1982), who noted in their study of 2030 births that pregnant women tend to be more moderate consumers of coffee and tea than those who are not pregnant.

5 Time Distribution of Caffeine Intake

In toxicological studies, animals are often exposed to large bolus doses of caffeine. In humans, caffeine ingestion generally occurs gradually and is spread throughout the day, multiple servings being consumed. Thus, human ingestion of caffeine is in many cases very different from that of test animals in terms of exposure. This fact must be considered in evaluating the significance of animal data and their relationship to human exposure.

The distribution of human caffeine intake over the course of a day is illustrated by the intake patterns for coffee, tea, and soft drinks derived from the Market Facts survey shown in Table 9. The number of 5- to 18-year-old children consuming these beverages at least once during the 7-day survey period at the noted meal/snack times are given along with the average amounts consumed. As can be seen from the table, the patterns of consumption vary with the beverage concerned, but in each case consumption occurs throughout the day. Distribution of caffeine intake from coffee, tea, and soft drinks throughout the day is also evidenced by data on beverage consumption patterns from the NFCS (Pao 1980).

6 Summary

For the major dietary caffeine sources, we suggest standard caffeine content values as follows: 85, 60, and 3 mg of caffeine per 5-oz cup for ground roasted, instant, and decaffeinated coffee respectively; 40 and 30 mg per 5-oz cup for leaf or bag tea and instant tea respectively; 18 mg per 6-oz glass for colas; 4 mg per 5-oz cup for cocoa or hot chocolate; and 5 mg per 8-oz glass for chocolate milk.

From product usage and consumption survey data, it would appear that the mean daily intake of caffeine is approximately 3 mg/kg for all adults in the general population and approximately 4 mg/kg for consumers of caffeine. Among the heaviest

10% of adult consumers, mean intake approximates 7 mg/kg daily. For children under 18 years of age the mean daily intake is approximately 1 mg/kg. The heaviest 10% of child consumers have a mean intake of about 3–5 mg/kg. Limited evidence from survey data indicates a daily caffeine intake by pregnant women lower than that of the general population (a mean of 2.1 vs 2.6 mg/kg). Human consumption of caffeine is distributed to some extent throughout the day, in contrast to the many animal studies which involve single bolus doses.

References

American Council on Science and Health (1983) The health effects of caffeine, 2nd edn. New York

Barone JJ (1981) Consumption and the Food and Drug Administration's proposal to remove caffeine in cola beverages from the list of substances generally recognized as safe (Docket No. 80 N-0418). Coca-Cola, Atlanta

Burg AW (1975) How much caffeine in the cup. Tea Coffee Trade J 147/1: 40–42, 88

Federation of American Societies for Experimental Biology (1978) Evaluation of the health aspects of caffeine as a food ingredient. A report to the Food and Drug Administration by the Select Committee on GRAS substances (FASEB/SCOGS), Bethesda, Md

Food and Drug Administration (1980a) Caffeine: Deletion of GRAS status, proposed declaration that no prior sanction exists, and use on an interim basis pending additional study. Fed Regist 45/205: 69817–69838

Food and Drug Administration (1980b) Caffeine content of various products. FDA, Washington (FDA Talk Paper, T 80-45)

Gilbert RM (1981) Caffeine: Overview and anthology. In: Miller SA (ed) Nutrition and behavior. Franklin Institute Press, Philadelphia, pp 145–166

Gilbert RM, Marshman JA, Schwieder M, Berg R (1976) Caffeine content of beverages as consumed. Can Med Assoc J 114: 205–208

Graham DM (1978) Caffeine – Its identity, dietary sources, intake, and biological effects. Nutr Rev 36/4: 97–102

International Coffee Organization (1982) United States of America, Coffee drinking study – winter 1982. London

Kaplan E, Holmes JH, Sapeika N (1974) Caffeine content of tea and coffee. S Afr J Nutr 10: 32–33

Little AD Inc (1977) Comments on the health aspects of caffeine, especially the contribution of soft drinks with particular reference to the report of the Select Committee on GRAS substances. Little, Cambridge/Mass

Morgan KJ, Stults VJ, Zabik ME (1982) Amount and dietary sources of caffeine and saccharin intake by individuals ages 5 to 18 years. Regul Toxicol Pharmacol 2: 296–307

National Center for Health Statistics (1977) NCHS growth curves for children, birth to 18 years, United States. (DHEW Publication (PHS) 78–1650) US Government Printing Office, Washington

National Center for Health Statistics (1979) Weight and height of adults, 18–74 years of age, United States, 1971–1974 (DHEW Publication (PHS) 79–1659) US Government Printing Office, Washington

National Soft Drink Association (1982) What's in soft drinks, 2nd edn. Washington

Pao EM (1980) Eating patterns and food frequencies of children in the United States. US Department of Agriculture, Hyattsville/MD. US Government Printing Office, Washington

Pao EM, Fleming KH, Guenther PM, Mickle SJ (1982) Foods commonly eaten by individuals: amount per day and per eating occasion (USDA Home Economics Research Report no 44). US Government Printing Office, Washington

Rall TW (1980) The xanthines. In: Gilman AG, Goodman LS, Gilman A (eds) The pharmacological basis of therapeutics, 6th edn. MacMillan, New York, pp 592–607

Roden C (1977) Coffee. Farber and Farber, London

Rosenberg L, Mitchell AA, Shapiro S, Slone D (1982) Selected birth defects in relation to caffeine-containing beverages. JAMA 47/10: 1429–1432

Ukers WH (1935) All about tea. Tea and Coffee Trade Journal Company, New York

Zoumas BL, Kreiser WR, Martin RA (1980) Theobromine and caffeine content of chocolate products. J Food Sci 45: 314–316

Section III
Physiological and Behavioral Effects

V The Cardiovascular Effects of Caffeine

D. Robertson and P. W. Curatolo*

1 Introduction

The effect of caffeine on the heart and blood vessels has attracted the attention of investigators for more than 100 years. The earliest studies are reviewed in some detail by Bock (1920) and Eichler (1938). In the second edition of his monograph on caffeine, Eichler (1976) reviewed the literature on the cardiovascular effects of caffeine up to the year 1974. Much of the available data comes from animal studies. In some cases the human pharmacology of caffeine has been inferred from studies with theophylline. The first part of this chapter will deal with in vitro and animal studies. In the last part of the chapter the effects of the drug in man will be treated.

Coffee has been shown to be made up of hundreds of chemical constituents, all with potential pharmacological effects (Vitzthum 1975). It would be remarkable if caffeine proved to be the only substance of significance. Unfortunately, the limited knowledge concerning the vast majority of these constituents prevents us from drawing firm conclusions about their contributions to the effect of coffee ingestion in man. Certainly the recent demonstration of a principle in coffee that acts as an opiate antagonist (Boublik et al. 1983), presumably at concentrations achievable with ordinary coffee consumption, provides a sobering reminder of just how much remains to be learned about the physiological effects of the beverage.

The mechanism of action of caffeine is treated in detail in Chaps. 9 and 10 of this book. Caffeine probably exerts most of its effects through antagonism of adenosine receptors (Fredholm and Persson 1982; Daly et al. 1981; Burnstock 1972), although phosphodiesterase inhibition (Beavo et al. 1971) and calcium mobilization (Guthrie and Naylor 1967) may be important at some concentrations of caffeine. The relative importance of these various mechanisms has been reviewed by Rall (1980).

* The author's work was supported in part by US Public Health Service grants HL 14192 and GM 15431 and by grants from the Hrafn Sveinbjarnrson Foundation and the International Life Sciences Institute. Dr. Robertson is the recipient of a Research Career Development Award from the National Institute of Health.

2 Myocardial Contractility

In studies in many species of animals there is usually an increase in myocardial contractility with caffeine. Thus in the superfused frog heart, tension development is enhanced by caffeine in a reversible manner (Chapman and Miller 1971). In the papillary muscle from the right ventricle of the cat, caffeine at concentrations of 0.02% elicited an increase in the amplitude of contraction (Krop 1944). Similar results have been seen in guinea pig atrium, where caffeine concentrations of 0.25–1.50 mM increased contractility, while higher concentrations had a lesser effect (De Gubareff and Sleator 1965). Pretreatment of the animals with 5 mg/kg reserpine, which reduced myocardial catecholamine content to 5% of normal, lessened but did not abolish the effect of caffeine on contractility. In general, theophylline has been shown to be more potent than caffeine in eliciting myocardial effects in virtually all species tested (Rall 1980).

3 Heart Rate

The effect of caffeine on heart rate is variable. It seems to depend not only on dose but also on route and manner of administration. Smaller doses tend to elicit a slight bradycardia in dogs, while larger doses increase heart rate. Since the bradycardia can be blocked by cutting the vagus nerve or by the administration of atropine, it is presumably mediated by parasympathetic activation (Bock and Buchholtz 1920). However this does not appear to be the sole explanation for the bradycardia, since it is also observed in isolated rabbit hearts, albeit to a lesser degree (Vittorio 1923).

An increase in heart rate following caffeine administration to dogs via the left coronary artery occurred with small doses which induced a primary hypotensive response (Raff 1971). With doses of 10 mg or greater there was no increase in heart rate. The administration of 50 mg/kg caffeine to rats also led to a transient tachycardia which was more prominent in older than younger animals (Ammon and Estler 1969).

In spite of the widespread conviction that caffeine provokes arrhythmias, there is limited animal data addressing this rather critical issue. There is a prolongation of the left atrial action potential in bullfrogs and guinea pigs with 3.0 mM caffeine (Kimoto et al. 1974). Dogs with myocardial infarctions induced by arterial ligature had lower fibrillation thresholds when given 25 mg/kg caffeine sodium benzoate intravenously (Bellet et al. 1972). Caffeine doses of 25–100 mg/kg intravenously in dogs caused the development of ventricular irregularities that could be partially attenuated by pretreatment with barbiturate, by pretreatment with reserpine, and by bilateral vagus section.

4 Blood Pressure

Caffeine doses above 10 mg/kg increase stroke volume in dogs (Pilcher et al. 1927). With the Starling heart-lung preparation, in which the complicating influence of autonomic reflexes can be removed, it is possible to observe an increase in stroke volume of up to 30% with reduced end-systolic volume and an increase in cardiac output of up to 50% (Flaum and Rössler 1933).

The blood pressure effect of caffeine in animals is somewhat variable. The intravenous administration of 2.5–10.0 mg/kg caffeine to dogs results in a transient (15-s) vasodepressor response followed by a mild pressor response (Raff 1971). The depressor response is lost with progressively higher doses of caffeine intravenously and also if the caffeine is administered orally. Qualitatively similar biphasic responses are observed in rats (Strubelt and Siegers 1968) and cats (Hahn 1941). Both increases and decreases in blood pressure have been described when electrical stimulation of the medulla oblongata is carried out before and after the administration of caffeine 10 mg/kg (Bondaryov 1967). It is known that central catecholamine turnover is increased following caffeine in rats, and that down-regulation of rat brain beta receptors occurs with chronic administration of caffeine (Goldberg et al. 1982).

In isolated arteries, caffeine tends to dilate (Chytkowski et al. 1970). In addition, the response to a number of other vasoactive substances is altered by caffeine. The effects of catecholamines on smooth muscle tend to be potentiated. It has been proposed that the latter is accomplished by inhibition of the enzyme catechol-O-methyltransferase (Kalsner 1971), which normally inactivates norepinephrine released from the nerve ending. However, the importance of this mechanism to the clinical effects of caffeine remains to be established.

Recently is has been shown that infusions of adenosine into rats at rates that increase plasma adenosine only very slightly result in considerable reductions in blood pressure; caffeine antagonizes this effect very potently (von Borstel and Wurtman 1983; this volume, Chap. X). This raises the possibility that most or all of the ability of caffeine to raise blood pressure relates to antagonism of adenosine.

The effect of caffeine on the coronary artery is dilatation in the isolated preparation (Anrep and Stacey 1927). The same is probably true in the intact animal, but whether this is a direct or indirect effect is uncertain. Adenosine, a potent coronary vasodilator, has been proposed as an endogenous mediator of metabolic vasodilatation (Berne and Rubio 1974). Caffeine as an antagonist at the adenosine receptor would be expected to counteract this effect directly. Since this is rarely observed, it is generally assumed that the highly significant increase in myocardial work induced by caffeine leads to an indirect metabolic coronary artery dilatation that the direct vascular effect of the drug cannot completely counteract.

5 Clinical Pharmacology

There have been relatively few studies of the cardiovascular effects of caffeine in man, which is remarkable when one considers how widely it is used in Western society. The clinical pharmacology of caffeine is the subject of a recent review (Curatolo and Robertson, to be published). Unfortunately, there are often contradictions in the clinical studies which have been carried out. For instance, in 1911, Sollman and Pilcher reported that caffeine ingestion lowered arterial blood pressure and raised heart rate. Some years later, Horst et al. (1936) found that caffeine raised blood pressure and lowered heart rate. The following year Starr et al. (1937) report-

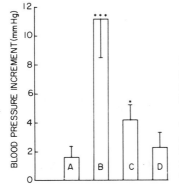

Fig. 1. Increase in systolic blood pressure during the 2 h following ingestion of *A* placebo beverage; *B* caffeine (250 mg) beverage in non-coffee drinkers; *C* caffeine (250 mg) beverage in coffee drinkers with initial caffeine levels < 1 µg/ml; *D* caffeine (250 mg) beverage in coffee drinkers with initial caffeine levels > 1 µg/ml. Each value represents the difference between pre-intake sphygmomanometric systolic blood pressure determinations and the mean of eight quarter-hourly blood pressure determinations for each subject. *, *P*<0.05; ***, *P*<0.01. *A, n*=17; *B, n*=17; *C, n*=8; *D, n*=8

ed that caffeine had no effect on either blood pressure or heart rate. A major reason for these discrepancies appears to be the failure in many of the early studies to distinguish between nonconsumers and habitual consumers of caffeinated beverages; tolerance to the cardiovascular effects of caffeine in man has now been clearly demonstrated (Robertson et al. 1978, 1981) and undoubtedly confounded early results.

Some of these issues are now clearer (Fig. 1). In nine healthy caffeine-naive subjects, either 250 mg oral caffeine in a methylxanthine-free beverage or methylxanthine-free beverage alone was administered in a double-blind protocol (Robertson et al. 1978). One hour following the ingestion of caffeine, systolic blood pressure had increased by 10 mm Hg. Heart rate decreased during the 1st h after caffeine administration, then increased above baseline during the subsequent 2 h. Plasma norepinephrine and epinephrine and plasma renin activity were significantly raised at 1 and 3 h after caffeine. However, the increase in catecholamines and plasma renin activity following caffeine is not present in all subjects. Furthermore, release of norepinephrine and epinephrine and plasma renin activity do not appear essential to the pressor effect of caffeine, since patients lacking a functioning autonomic nervous system have a normal or even exaggerated pressor response (Robertson, unpublished work). The ingestion of the methylxanthine-free beverage alone did not significantly affect these variables.

The effects of chronic caffeine were examined in a second study (Robertson et al. 1981). Caffeine (250 mg) or placebo was administered to 18 healthy habitual coffee drinkers who had abstained from all methylxanthine-containing beverages for 3 weeks. A randomized, double-blind protocol was used. The acute effects of caffeine were similar to those observed in the first study (increased blood pressure, plasma epinephrine and norepinephrine, renin activity). Again, some subjects seemed resistant to these effects of caffeine. In the initially sensitive subjects also, essentially complete tolerance developed to all these effects after 1–4 days regular caffeine (250 mg thrice daily) consumption (Fig. 2). Similar results have been observed in hypertensive subjects (Robertson et al. 1983).

Caffeine increases cardiac output significantly (Starr et al. 1937; Grollmann 1930). In five normal subjects, 158 mg caffeine increased stroke index as much as 33% (Gould et al. 1973). Unfortunately, it was not possible to perform these studies

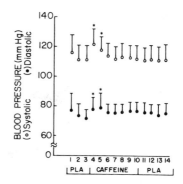

Fig. 2. Blood pressure response to caffeine. Numbers on the horizontal axis indicate days of study. On days 1–3, subjects were given placebo beverage with each meal. On days 4–10, they received 250 mg caffeine with each meal. On days 11–14, they again received placebo. Each point represents the mean of six upright and six supine sphygmomanometric systolic (○) and diastolic (●) blood pressure determinations. *, $P < 0.05$

in a blind fashion, and thus the exact magnitude of the caffeine response is difficult to assess.

Despite the lack of evidence for a hemodynamic effect of chronic caffeine ingestion, coffee consumption has been purported to have a number of toxic effects on the cardiovascular system. Specifically, caffeine consumption has been considered a risk factor for myocardial infarction and arrhythmias.

A positive association between coffee consumption and ischemic heart disease was first reported in 1963 by Paul et al. In a prospective study of 1951 men employed at Western Electric in Chicago, they found a significant correlation between coffee consumption and the later development of ischemic heart disease. However, the same group subsequently demonstrated that this association could be entirely accounted for by tobacco use (Paul et al. 1968).

Two recent studies by the Boston Collaborative Drug Surveillance Program have again suggested that coffee consumption is associated with an increased risk of myocardial infarction (Boston Program 1972; Jick et al. 1973). The Boston investigations were based on a survey conducted at 24 metropolitan hospitals during 1972 which attempted to relate the use of many different drugs, including caffeine, to various disease states. The initial Boston study of 276 cases and 1104 matched controls reported that drinking more than six cups of coffee daily was associated with a risk of myocardial infarction more than twice as great as normal. This association could not be accounted for by smoking, but this study failed to control for many other significant variables, such as sugar use and previous ischemic heart disease. Therefore, a second, more comprehensive study of 12759 hospitalized patients (including 440 with myocardial infarction) was undertaken, controlling for age, sex, past ischemic heart disease, hypertension, congestive heart failure, obesity, diabetes, smoking, and other risk factors. This investigation also demonstrated a more than doubled risk of myocardial infarction among patients who consumed more than six cups of coffee a day.

The reports of the Boston group generated much lively debate in the medical community. Numerous retrospective (Walker and Gregoratos 1967; Klatsky et al. 1973; Hennekens et al. 1976; Rosenberg et al. 1980) and prospective (Dawber et al. 1974; Tibblin et al. 1975; Wilhelmsen et al. 1977; Yano et al. 1977; Heyden et al. 1978; Murray et al. 1981) investigations have been conducted, mostly since that time to examine the reported correlation between coffee consumption and myocardial infarction. These studies consistently failed to uphold the findings of the Boston study. In the Framingham study, Dawber et al. (1974) found no association between coffee consumption and ischemic heart disease, other cardiovascular disease, or death from all causes. Tibblin et al. (1975) found that coffee consumption did not relate to nonfatal myocardial infarction, fatal myocardial infarction, or death from all causes in a prospective study of 855 men in an industrial city in Sweden. In a prospective study of Japanese men living in Hawaii, Yano et al. (1977) found no association between coffee intake and risk of ischemic heart disease. Finally, Heyden et al. (1978) demonstrated that coffee consumption had no influence on total mortality, ischemic heart disease mortality, or cerebrovascular mortality in a prospective study in Evans county, Georgia.

The discrepancy between the findings of the Boston program and subsequent investigations probably results from several factors. Rosenberg et al. (1980) demonstrated that among hospitalized women, those admitted for chronic conditions reported that they drank significantly less coffee than those admitted for acute conditions; it was therefore suggested that the results of the Boston program may have been distorted by the inclusion of hospitalized patients with chronic conditions among the controls. Wilhelmsen et al. (1977) found that retrospective estimations of coffee consumption by patients suffering a myocardial infarction were significantly higher than prospective estimations of coffee consumption by subjects who later suffered a myocardial infarction. Kannel and Dawber (1973) stated that "... the subjects investigated [in the Boston study] constituted only those with myocardial infarction, who survived long enough to be hospitalized. This group of patients experienced a mortality rate of only 4 percent. Such a sample is hardly representative of this highly lethal disease." Further, Kannel and Dawber point out that "... Jick used discharged hospitalized patients [for the control group]. Such a population may contain an excessive number of subjects with gastrointestinal or other diseases in which coffee drinking has been either abandoned or medically proscribed. Thus, the coffee consumption of a hospitalized population cannot be accepted unequivocally as representative of the habits of the general population."

Hennekens et al. (1976) proposed that the Boston program did not control for enough variables. In their own case-controlled study of coffee and myocardial infarction, they demonstrated a nearly twofold increase in risk of death from ischemic heart disease in heavy coffee drinkers when controlling only for those variables used in the Boston study, but when they controlled for additional variables such as physical activity and coffee additives, no increase in risk was found. Other unrecognizable and unavoidable sources of bias undoubtedly influenced the Boston studies. All in all, the consistent failure of numerous investigations to demonstrate any correlation between coffee consumption and myocardial infarction appears to justify the conclusion that coffee intake is not a risk factor in this disease.

One of the most universally applied dicta in medical practice is the proscription of caffeine for individuals with cardiac arrhythmias. The published evidence relating to this question is surprisingly shallow, however. Polonowski et al. (1952) observed increased extrasystoles in individuals given 200 mg of caffeine as coffee. We did not observe such a response in five healthy normal subjects who wore a Holter monitor for 24 h before caffeine and then for 24 h in which they received three 250-mg doses of caffeine. We have not tested this question in patients, in elderly persons, or in subjects with a history of arrhythmias. However, in approximately 50 blind studies, we have encountered one case of paroxysmal atrial tachycardia which developed in a 26-year-old woman within 1 h of the administration of 250 mg caffeine. The electrophysiological effect of caffeine in man is primarily to lengthen the effective refractory period of the left atrium while shortening that of many other cardiac tissues (Dobmeyer et al. 1983). The ingestion of caffeine increased the tendency of susceptible individuals to develop arrhythmias following electric shock, although these results were interpreted cautiously (Dobmeyer et al. 1983; Graboys and Lown 1983).

In spite of the dearth of information concerning arrhythmias induced by caffeine, it is impossible not to be swayed by epidemiological (Prineas et al. 1980) and other evidence that excessive caffeine may be deleterious in individuals prone to arrhythmias. The widespread belief that coffee intake is associated with arrhythmias may have deterred investigators from pursuing this question with greater vigor; it may also have prevented case reports of such an association. These considerations must not, however, continue to cause us to neglect the study of this potentially important issue. Until more studies of the effect of caffeine on the electrical activity of the heart are carried out, the real risk, if any, of caffeine in these circumstances cannot be assessed.

References

Ammon HPT, Estler CJ (1969) The influence of caffeine on carbohydrate and lipid metabolism in alloxan-diabetic mice. Med Exp 19: 161–169

Anrep GV, Stacey RF (1927) Comparative effect of various drugs upon the coronary circulation. J Physiol 64: 187–192

Beavo JA, Rogers NL, Crofford OB, Baird CE, Hardman JG, Sutherland EW, Newman EV (1971) Effects of phosphodiesterase inhibitors on cyclic AMP levels and on lipolysis. Ann NY Acad Sci 185: 129–136

Bellet S, Horstman E, Roman LR, de Guzman NT, Kostis JB (1972) Effect of caffeine on the ventricular fibrillation threshold in normal dogs with acute myocardial infarction. Am Heart J 84: 215–227

Berne RM, Rubio R (1974) Regulation of coronary blood flow. Adv Cardiol 12: 303–317

Bock J (1920) Die Purinderivate. In: Heffter A, Heubner W (eds) Handbuch der experimentellen Pharmakologie, vol 2/1. Springer, Berlin, pp 508–598

Bock J, Buchholtz J (1920) Henriques-Methode über das Minutenvolumen des Herzens beim Hunde und über den Einfluß des Coffeins auf die Größe des Minutenvolumens. Arch Exp Pharmacol 88: 192–215

Bondaryov MG (1967) The influence of analeptic drugs on the pontine vasomotor center. Prog Brain Res 20: 171–186

Boston Collaborative Drug Surveillance Program (1972) Coffee drinking and acute myocardial infarction. Lancet 2: 1278–1281

Boublik JH, Quinn MJ, Clements JA, Herington AC, Wynn KN, Funder JW (1983) Coffee contains potent opiate receptor binding activity. Nature 301: 246–248

Burnstock G (1972) Purinergic nerves. Pharmacol Rev 24: 509–581

Chapman RA, Miller DJ (1971) The action of caffeine on frog myocardial contractility. J Physiol (Lond) 217: 64P–66P

Chytkowski A, Panczenko B, Krupinska J, Bieron K, Zmuda A (1970) Circulatory action of 7(beta-methyl,thio-ethyl)-theophylline. Diss Pharm Pharmacol 22: 199–207

Curatolo PW, Robertson D (1983) The health consequences of caffeine. Ann Intern Med 98: 641–653

Daly JW, Bruns RF, Snyder SH (1981) Adenosine receptors in the central nervous system: relationship to the central actions of methylxanthines. Life Sci 28: 2083–2097

Dawber TR, Kannel WB, Gordon T (1974) Coffee and cardiovascular disease: observations from the Framingham study. N Engl J Med 291: 871–874

De Gubareff T, Sleator W Jr (1965) Effects of caffeine on mammalian atrial muscle and its interaction with adenosine and calcium. J Pharmacol Exp Ther 148: 202–214

Dobmeyer DJ, Stine RA, Leier CV, Greenberg R, Schall SF (1983) The arrhythmogenic effects of caffeine in human beings. N Engl J Med 308: 814–816

Eichler O (ed) (1938) Kaffee und Coffein. Springer, Berlin

Eichler O (ed) (1976) Kaffee und Coffein, 2nd edn. Springer, Berlin Heidelberg New York

Flaum E, Rössler R (1933) Über die Herzwirkung der Purinkörper. Klin Wochenschr 11: 1489

Fredholm BB, Persson CGA (1982) Xanthine derivatives as adenosine receptor antagonists. Eur J Pharmacol 81: 673–676

Goldberg MR, Curatolo PW, Tung C-S, Robertson D (1982) Caffeine reduces beta-adrenoceptor density in rat cerebral cortex. Neurosci Lett 31: 47–53

Gould L, Venkataraman K, Goswami M, Gomprecht RF (1973) The cardiac effects of coffee. Angiology 24: 455–463

Graboys TB, Lown B (1983) Coffee, arrhythmias, and common sense. N Engl J Med 308: 835–837

Grollmann A (1930) The action of alcohol, caffeine, and tobacco on the cardiac output (and its related functions) of normal man. J Pharmacol Exp Ther 39: 313–327

Guthrie JR, Naylor WG (1967) Interaction between caffeine and adenosine on calcium exchangeability in mammalian atria. Arch Int Pharmacodyn 170: 249–255

Hahn F (1941) Vergleichende Untersuchungen über die Krampf- und Blutdruckwirkung verschiedener Analeptica. Arch Exp Pathol Pharmacol 198: 491–508

Hennekens CH, Drolette ME, Jesse MF, Davies JE, Hutchinson GB (1976) Coffee drinking and death due to coronary heart disease. N Engl J Med 294: 633–636

Heyden S, Tyroler HA, Heiss G, Hames CG, Bartel A (1978) Coffee consumption and mortality: total mortality, stroke mortality, and coronary heart disease mortality. Arch Intern Med 138: 1472–1475

Horst K, Wilson RJ, Smith RG (1936) The effect of coffee and decaffeinated coffee on oxygen consumption, pulse rate and blood pressure. J Pharmacol Exp Ther 58: 294–304

Jick H, Miettinen OS, Neff RK, Shapiro S, Heinonen OP, Slone D (1973) Coffee and myocardial infarction. N Engl J Med 289: 63–67

Kalsner S (1971) Mechanism of potentiation of contractor responses to catecholamines by methylxanthines in aortic strips. Br J Pharmacol 43: 379–388

Kannel WB, Dawber TR (1973) Coffee and coronary disease (Editorial). N Engl J Med 289: 100–101

Kimoto Y, Saito M, Goto M (1972) Effects of caffeine on the membrane potentials, membrane currents and contractility of the bullfrog atrium. Jap J Physiol 22: 225–238

Klatsky AL, Friedman GD, Siegelaub AB (1973) Coffee drinking prior to acute myocardial infarction: results from the Kaiser-Permanente epidemiological study of myocardial infarction. JAMA 226: 540–543

Krop ST (1944) The influence of heart stimulants on the contraction of isolated mammalian cardiac muscle. J Pharmacol 82: 48–62

Murray SS, Bjelke E, Gibson RW, Schuman LM (1981) Coffee consumption and mortality from ischemic heart disease and other causes: results from the Lutheran Brotherhood Study, 1966–1978. Am J Epidemiol 113: 661–667

Paul O, Leper MH, Phelan WH, Dupertuis GW, MacMillan A, McKean H, Park H (1963) A longitudinal study of coronary heart disease. Circulation 28: 20–31

Paul O, MacMillan A, McKean H, Park H (1968) Sucrose intake and coronary heart disease. Lancet 2: 1049–1051

Pilcher C, Wilson CP, Harrison TR (1927) The action of drugs on cardiac output. Am Heart J 2: 618–630

Polonowski M, Donzelot E, Briskas S, Doliopoulos T (1952) The comparative effects of coffee and soluble extracts of coffee on normal persons and on cardiacs. Cardiologia 21: 809–816

Prineas RJ, Jacobs DR, Crow RS, Blackburn H (1980) Coffee, tea and VPB. J Chronic Dis 33: 67–72

84

Raff WK (1971) Wirkung des Coffeins auf Herz und Kreislauf. Arzneimittelforsch 21: 1177–1179

Rall TW (1980) The xanthines. In: Gilman AG, Goodman LS, Gilman A (eds) The pharmacological basis of therapeutics, 6th edn. Macmillan, New York, pp 592–607

Robertson D, Frolich JC, Carr RK, Watson JT, Hollifield JW, Shand DG, Oates JA (1978) Effects of caffeine on plasma renin activity, catecholamines and blood pressure. N Engl J Med 298: 181–186

Robertson D, Wade D, Workman R, Woosley RL, Oates JA (1981) Tolerance to the humoral and hemodynamic effects of caffeine in man. J Clin Invest 67: 1111–1117

Robertson D, Wade D, Smith WB (to be published) Caffeine and hypertension

Rosenberg I, Stone D, Shapiro K, Kaufman DW, Stolley PD, Miettinen OS (1980) Coffee drinking and myocardial infarction in young women. Am J Epidemiol 111: 675–681

Sollman T, Pilcher JD (1911) The actions of caffeine on the mammalian circulation. J Pharmacol Exp Ther 3: 19–92

Starr I, Gamble CJ, Margolies A (1937) A clinical study of the action of 10 commonly used drugs on cardiac output, work, and size: on respiration, on metabolic rate, and on the electrocardiogram. J Clin Invest 16: 799–823

Strubelt O, Siegers C-P (1968) Die Beteiligung endogener Catecholamine an den Wirkungen des Kaffees auf Energieumsatz und Herzfrequenz. Arzneimittelforsch 18: 1278–1281

Tibblin G, Wilhelmsen L, Werko L (1975) Risk factors for myocardial infarction and death due to ischemic heart disease and other causes. Am J Cardiol 35: 514–522

Vittorio S (1923) Action of caffeine on the frequency of the cardiac pulse (in Italian) Arch Int Pharmacodyn 27: 265–282

Vitzthum OG (1975) Chemie und Bearbeitung des Kaffees. In: Eichler O (ed) Kaffee und Coffein. Springer, Berlin Heidelberg New York

von Borstel R, Wurtman RJ, Conlay LA (1983) Chronic caffeine consumption potentiates the hypotensive action of circulating adenosine. Life Sci 32: 1151–1158

Walker WJ, Gregoratos MG (1967) Myocardial infarction in young men. Am J Cardiol 19: 339–343

Wilhelmsen L, Tibblin G, Elmfeldt D, Wedel H, Werko L (1977) Coffee consumption and coronary heart disease in middle-aged Swedish men. Acta Med Scand 201: 547–552

Yano K, Rhoads GG, Kagan A (1977) Coffee, alcohol, and risk of coronary heart disease among Japanese men living in Hawaii. N Engl J Med 297: 405–409

VI Behavioral Effects of Caffeine*

P. B. Dews

1 Introduction

Caffeine was a favored agent for study by pharmacologists in the early years of pharmacology as a scientific discipline, and there are many papers on caffeine in the literature from the last decades of last century and the first decades of this century. The twentieth century brought a spate of new chemical entities to be studied as to their pharmacology, and toxicology and caffeine became relatively neglected, although clinical pharmacological studies on methylxanthines, for the most part theophylline, continued and increased in number. There has been a renewed interest in caffeine in the past 10 years, partly as a result of the general intensified public interest in the effects on health of all components of the diet, along with other environmental influences such as air and water quality and radiation, and partly because hypotheses of the mechanism of action of caffeine have been generated which intrigue the modern pharmacologist.

The pharmacology of caffeine was reviewed exhaustively as recently as 1976 (Eichler). This chapter will emphasize the possible effects of sane dietary intakes of caffeine, rather than the putative therapeutic and possible toxicological effects of the agent.

One of the difficulties in the way of public appreciation of the effects of dietary caffeine arises from the terms that professional pharmacologists have used to describe those effects. If a reference source is consulted, the reader will be told that caffeine is a stimulant or even "a powerful stimulant of the central nervous system" (Rall 1980). The term "stimulant" is undefined and is, indeed, hard or even impossible to define. Under the heading "stimulant" are drugs as diverse as strychnine (which interferes with the transmission of inhibitory influences to motoneurons in the spinal cord and causes few behavioral effects short of tonic convulsions), picrotoxin (which also may interfere with inhibitory influences and also has little behavioral effect in doses less than those causing epileptiform convulsions), and cocaine (which inhibits the uptake of biogenic amines into certain neurons and can produce a behavioral syndrome resembling mania). We therefore agree with Salter (1952) who says in his textbook: "The word 'stimulant' has been used in so many senses that, like the word 'morals' in the lay press, it has become a source of confusion." It

---

* Preparation of this paper was supported in part by grants from the U.S. Public Health Service (MH 02094, MH 07658, DA 00499, and DA 02658).

may be noted in passing that the term "depressant" as applied to central nervous system agents is almost equally meaningless. Take, for example, the studies of Waldeck (1974) on locomotor activity in mice. A dose of 25 mg/kg caffeine increased activity, but so did 1–2 g/kg ethyl alcohol, and the two together caused a still larger increase. The author comments: "A popular belief is that the stimulant drug, caffeine, antagonizes the depressant action of ethanol." The popular belief is clearly misleading. While it is always possible to contrive an ad hoc "explanation" of why a "stimulant" or "depressant" does not do what it is supposed to do in a particular situation, it is ineluctably true that whenever the terms "stimulant" and "depressant" are used it will continue to be the popular expectation that "stimulants" will stimulate and "depressants" will depress any activity under study and that they will antagonize one another's effects. Such expectations will usually be unfulfilled, so the descriptors are at best untrustworthy and at worst misleading.

2 Man

A great many primarily psychological studies have included administration of caffeine as an additional independent variable giving rise to extensive literature. Caffeine is chosen for many reasons, among them that it is readily available, generally recognized as safe, has a rapid onset and an appropriate duration of action (half-life about 4 h), and is active by mouth. A disadvantage is that caffeine in the amounts that are given has effects so slight and subtle that the investigator is usually glad to be able to detect them (at $P < 0.05$ from an analysis of variance!) and their nature can rarely be specified except in arbitrary terms. The effects of caffeine on performance have been studied in many tests designed to assess different putative factors in human psychological performance. Despite the large number of papers, it is proving hard to arrive at a coherent account of the behavioral effects of caffeine, even at a descriptive level. In the following paragraphs a few selected findings will be presented to provide the reader with an appreciation of the nature of the information available. A more exhaustive review would not add materially to coherence.

2.1 Performance in Laboratory Tests

It has been reported that an absolute visual luminance threshold was lowered by about 0.08 log millilamberts after 90 mg caffeine and about 0.14 log millilamberts after 180 mg caffeine, without regard to the area of the stimulus (Diamond and Cole 1970). The effects are surprisingly large, representing about 20% and 38% falls in threshold. Placebo and caffeine were given to three subjects, always in the same order in the session, and there were no controls for sequential effects. As the subjects had to report whether or not they could see the stimulus, performance variables were involved as well as sensitivity of the afferent visual system. The condition of the subjects, fresh or fatigued, is not reported, though it is presumed to be the former. How long the testing required is not stated. In a study by Baker and Theologus (1972) subjects were required to watch two red lights for 4 h and to report each time they started to move apart, which they did with an angular velocity of about 5°/min at random intervals of 1.5–3.5 min. While most latencies were in the range 3–5 s, occasional latencies were more than twice the average minimum, and the mean frequency of long latencies increased slightly from just under three in the 1st h to just over four in the 4th h under control conditions. When 200 or 400 mg caffeine was given at the end of the 1st or 2nd h, the subsequent mean frequency of long latencies decreased to just under two. There was little difference in the effects of the two doses, so perhaps the maximum effect on this function was already attained at 200 mg. There are anomalies in the data; the number of long latencies fell in the 2nd h in both groups that were going to receive caffeine at the end of that hour, while it increased in the placebo group.

In one of the few studies on effects of caffeine on hearing, "Caffeine in doses from 75 to 300 mg increased auditory vigilance compared to lactose dummy. Auditory reaction times were shortened, tapping rates increased and subjects 'felt more alert.' No changes occurred in 'short term memory,' arithmetic or digit symbol substitution." (Clubley et al. 1979; internal quotes added to indicate interpretive rather than descriptive terms). The changes were no more than a few percent and did not even show a trend of dose dependency, i.e., there were no greater effects with larger doses.

A single dose of caffeine citrate, even as high as 500 mg, given alone in a capsule had equivocal effects on performance in a variety of tests (reading, counting, arithmetic, naming) carried out with delayed auditory feedback, a disruptive influence (Forney and Hughes 1965). In these tests the subjects had to respond by speaking into a microphone, and their speech was fed into their earphones after a delay. The length of the delay is not given, but in previous work the authors used 280 ms, which is longer than the optimum for disruption but presumably still quite disruptive. Alcohol in a dose of 45 ml/150 lb body weight (which should give a blood and brain alcohol level of about 1 mg/ml: many jurisdictions forbid automobile driving at this level) caused a substantial deterioration of performance, consistent in all the tests. When both alcohol and caffeine were given, in some tests the caffeine partially ameliorated the deleterious effects of the alcohol (reverse reading and counting, subtraction, color discrimination); in others, the caffeine increased the deleterious effects of the alcohol (verbal output, addition and subtraction of 7 s); and in yet others, the combination was less deleterious than either alcohol or caffeine alone (progressive counting, addition). Again, such antagonism as exists between alcohol and caffeine is neither specific nor general nor very effective.

Increase in skin conductance when a tone was played into earphones was reinforced by caffeine in people diagnosed as "extroverts" by the Eysenck Personality Inventory, but not in "introverts" (Smith et al. 1983). As the two groups differed in their placebo response, the difference in the effect of the caffeine may be related to differences in the skin response rather than to differences in "version." Caffeine reduced the tendency of subjects to press a key that they had been told would subtract money from or administer blasts of white noise to another subject who was not present, and in fact was nonexistent, while increasing their frequency of pressing another key that gave a real subject a monetary return (Cherek et al. 1983). The effect was dose related over the 1, 2, and 4 mg/kg range studied and is described as a "suppressive effect of caffeine on aggressive responding."

88

In a study involving a 2-h cycle endurance test, Ivy et al. (1979) found that 250 mg caffeine 1 h before the test and another 250 mg total in divided doses every 15 min during the test led to consistently higher work output throughout the test. The average increase in total work output in the nine subjects was about 7%. At the other end of the scale from endurance, the effects of caffeine on hand steadiness have been studied in students by having them hold a 1-mm stylus in a 2.5-mm hole, avoiding, as much as possible, contacts between stylus and edges of hole (Smith et al. 1977). The mean number of contacts in 20 s increased after 200 mg caffeine from 41 to 53, so performance went from terrible to slightly worse. In other tests, a conditional reaction time and a hand movement time decreased by 10% and 22% after caffeine. Intake of 0.3 mg or 1.3 mg nicotine from a cigarette had similar but lesser effects, except on hand steadiness where the effects were greater. Pulse rate was increased by all treatments, but not statistically significantly so.

Effects of 200 mg caffeine on performance in Graduate Record type tests have been studied and related to inventory of personality (Revelle et al. 1980). Only transformed results are given, and they are presented so inextricably enmeshed in theoretical constructs that it is difficult to discern the actual effects of caffeine; it appears that the effects were inconsistent, varying with time of day as well as with putative personality variables. Experiments were conducted on 2 days. The authors comment: "In the morning of the first day, low impulsives were hindered and high impulsives helped by caffeine. This pattern reversed in the evening of the first day, and it reversed again in the evening of Day 2." One has the impression that if the results were considered as a whole there would be no difference attributable to caffeine.

The foregoing results were obtained in deliberate experiments on subjects in more or less controlled laboratory circumstances. How does caffeine as ordinarily consumed affect behavior in everyday life? Academic grades in a psychology course have been reported to be significantly negatively correlated with increasing daily intake of caffeine in a sample of 159 students (Gilliland and Andress 1981). But of course, as the authors point out, such findings give no information on causality, as the caffeine consumption was self-selected. Caffeine consumption is correlated with a host of other variables characterizing the "style of life," any of which or any combination may be causally related to the observed correlation. For example, caffeine consumption may be negatively correlated with good study routines without causal relationship, in that reduction in caffeine consumption would not, in itself, improve study routines. A correlation that is notoriously misleading is the positive association between caffeine intake and cigarette smoking. In the case of behavioral effects of caffeine, as distinction from physiological effects, the problem of associations is especially formidable, as caffeine consumption is itself a behavioral activity, so that differences in caffeine intakes in itself indicates differences in behavioral propensities before the pharmacological effects of caffeine are considered. The slightness of the effects of dietary caffeine increases the likelihood that the observed changes will be due to other unidentified factors. As a consequence, without extensive ancillary studies the demonstration of a relationship between self-determined intake of caffeine and any change does not indicate an effect of caffeine itself. In general, definitive determination of effects of dietary caffeine on activities of everyday life will come only from a combination of objective assessments and interventions, in the form of deliberate changes in the caffeine consumptions of individuals in the study. Such studies are extremely expensive to conduct and to monitor for compliance. We must anticipate few such studies; in the absence of clear indications of a significant impact of caffeine consumption on the health of the public, people will prefer to use resources on illumination of demonstrated problems.

2.2 Individual Variation

One of the most ubiquitous beliefs about caffeine is that its effects vary greatly from individual to individual in the normal population. If the matter comes up for discussion among a group of people, almost always some individuals will testify to great sensitivity, being disturbed by even a single cup of coffee, while in contrast, others will testify that several cups of coffee in the late evening have no effect on going to sleep. Carefully controlled experiments, however, do not predict such great variability in the direct effects of caffeine. For example, in 20 subjects the coefficient of variation of time taken to go to sleep was the same whether they had taken lactose or 300 mg caffeine before retiring, although the mean time in all 20 was longer after caffeine (Goldstein et al. 1965; Dews 1982). How is the widespread impression of great variability to be explained?

First there is the obvious but often overlooked dosage factor. Other factors being equivalent, the same intake of caffeine will produce about twice the brain levels in a 50 kg individual as it would in a 100 kg individual. Second, although caffeine is well absorbed and readily distributed, differences in rate of stomach emptying and intestinal absorption will contribute to individual differences. The first and second factors jointly lead to substantial differences in the plasma levels generated by an intake of caffeine. In nine normal young subjects fasted from midnight and then given 250 mg caffeine dissolved in 300 ml fluid, the resulting peak plasma caffeine levels varied from 4.2 to 26 mg/l, a sixfold variation (Robertson et al. 1978). In everyday life, caffeine is ingested sometimes with cream, sometimes in ice-cold carbonated solution, sometimes with food, sometimes with fatty food, and so on, all factors that will add to the already large variation seen by Robertson et al. (1978).

Third, tolerance develops to the effects of caffeine. Interestingly, there is a dearth of quantitative information on the development of tolerance to its behavioral effects. Goldstein et al. (1969) showed clear differences between the behavioral effects of 150 or 300 mg caffeine in people who were regular consumers of caffeine and people who were not, but of course consumers and nonconsumers were self-selected, so to what extent the differences was due to factors that had led to consumption pattern and how much was due to tolerance cannot be distinguished. It is hard to believe, however, that acquired tolerance was not involved in the differences. The development of tolerance to the cardiovascular effects of caffeine has been demonstrated unequivocally (Robertson et al. 1981). Characteristically, people who report great sensitivity to caffeine tend to be nonconsumers or low consumers. They will, therefore, be more sensitive than most of the population by reason of lack of tolerance.

90

Fourth, in a lot of studies many environmental circumstances are controlled, whereas in everyday life many factors besides caffeine affect the same behavioral activities. The effects of dietary levels of caffeine are subtle, and other factors have effects as large. "Influences such as slight discomfort, nonoptimal temperature, or noise can postpone sleep and may greatly amplify the effects of caffeine" (Dews 1982, p.329). When a nonconsumer takes caffeine it is almost invariably under unusual circumstances, for example, before an examination or at a late-night party, and other features of the unusual circumstances themselves may contribute substantially to the disturbances attributed to the ingested caffeine. For all these reasons, then, the apparent great variations in individual sensitivity to effects of caffeine may be reconcilable with only a very modest variation in inherent sensitivity to the direct effects of caffeine. The question of variability is of some practical importance. If some individuals are inherently exquisitely sensitive to caffeine, they might be expected to be similarly sensitive to the potentially dangerous effects of caffeine, such as arrhythmogenesis in a damaged heart, and it would be important to identify and warn them. If, however, as argued above, inherent sensitivity varies little from individual to individual, then no special handling of a minority is required and people should continue to be allowed to self-determine their intake, except that chronic low consumers may need to avoid sprees of caffeine consumption. The routine proscription of caffeine by some physicians for a variety of conditions, usually intractable, may be a reflection of the desire of the physician to make some sort of recommendations for treating the conditions while honoring the rule of *primum non nocere*. Cessation of caffeine intake can hardly be harmful.

2.3 Effects in Children

Special concern has been expressed about the effects of dietary caffeine in children. Unusually thorough assessment of behavior of prepubertal boys revealed no significant changes after 3 mg/kg, although there were effects after 10 mg/kg (Elkins et al. 1981). Salivary levels of caffeine [which have been shown to reflect plasma levels sufficiently accurately for practical purposes (Cook et al. 1976)] were measured in some of the children 1 h after ingestion. They averaged 3.1 mg/l after the 3 mg/kg dose and 10.4 mg/l after the 10 mg/kg dose. Ratings of mood, side effects, and total motor activity (objectively with an inertial device), and visual evoked potentials were made. In further experiments, a direct comparison of the effects of caffeine in prepubertal boys and college students was made in the same laboratory. Again doses of 3 mg/kg and 10 mg/kg were given, and again a variety of objective measurements as well as behavior ratings were made (Rapoport et al. 1981). After the lower dose the effects were minimal in adults as well as in children, the latter result confirming the previous finding. At the higher dose, the authors conclude that the children showed more objective effects of the caffeine than did the adults, although most of the effects might be considered beneficial, for example, increased speech rate, decreased reaction time, and decreased errors of omission in a continuous performance test. Recall in a verbal memory test was decreased. Comparison between the two groups is complicated by large differences between the groups under placebo conditions in some of the measurements; for example, activity was some three times higher in the children than the adults, while verbal memory recall was two times higher in the adults than the children. Against these group differences the effects of even the higher dose of caffeine, which were in the range of 0%–25% in both groups, appear modest. Side effects were less in children. The results reinforce the conclusion that the differences in sensitivity of children and adults to measured effects of caffeine are not of a magnitude to prompt special concern for the effects in the former.

In six hyperactive children, 6 mg/kg caffeine slightly increased reaction time, while in six normal children the reaction time was slightly decreased (Reichard and Elder 1977). The changes were not statistically significant. Hyperactive children averaged some 20% slower than normals under control conditions. The authors comment: "This, although clinically significant, did not reach statistical significance." What is meant presumably is that a difference of 20% would be clinically significant if it in fact existed; the lack of statistical significance means that the difference observed could well have been due to chance rather than any real difference between the groups. Garfinkel et al. (1975) also showed an inappreciable difference in behavior rating scores in eight hyperactive children when they were given 75 mg/day caffeine and when they were given placebo. The main interest of these studies of hyperactive children is to confirm the lack of greater sensitivity of children, including hyperactive children, to the effects of caffeine.

2.4 Adverse Effects in Man

Ill effects of caffeine have been described in psychiatric patients in hospital. For example, Greden et al. (1978) reported an association between intake of caffeine and State-Trait Anxiety Index scores in 83 sequentially admitted psychiatric patients, but the difference between consumers of less than 250 mg and more than 750 mg was slight, about 10%. Differences in Beck Depression Scale scores were substantial, going from 40% to 83% for "moderate depression" and from 17% to 50% for "serious depression." The problem is, of course, that consumption of caffeine was self-determined, and so again the studies do not show a causal relationship. Improvement in scores on the Nurses Observation Scale for Inpatient Evaluation and the Brief Psychiatric Rating Scale was claimed by De Freitas and Schwartz (1979) when 14 psychiatric patients had their regular coffee replaced by decaffeinated coffee for 3 weeks, but the authors did not present the numerical scores on which the claim was based. There are scattered case reports of deleteriously large intakes of caffeine in people sequestered in hospitals or prisons. Taken together, the reports are convincing. It is to be expected that excessive intakes of caffeine, say, several grams per day, will have adverse effects and will produce symptoms; excessive intake of any food component will have adverse effects (how else can excessive be defined?). Sequestered patients and occasional free-living individuals can ritualize their lives to include very large intakes of caffeine. Such excessive consumption is usually evident, and the effects rapidly reversible when intake is reduced.

2.5 Comments on Studies of Behavioral Effects in Human Subjects

From the foregoing description of the behavioral effects of caffeine, no particular psychological attributes among those measured emerge as the selective target of caffeine. Even a complete review of the literature provides no clearer picture (Weiss and Laties 1962; Eichler 1976).

Three effects of sufficient doses of caffeine are clear. One is a tendency to postpone sleep (Dews 1982). The second is reduction of deterioration of performance due to fatigue, boredom, and the like. The third is a decrease in hand steadiness. It seems likely that the last would be one manifestation of a generalized effect on fine motor control, but this has not been established, and no impairment of the relatively fine motor control required for skilled automobile driving has been reported. Before attempting to characterize further the behavioral effects of caffeine, some studies in experimental animals will be described.

3 Experimental Animals

3.1 Mice

When mice are allowed to move around, they generally do so. Such activity has been variously called spontaneous motor activity (SMA), emphasizing that the factors that determine and control it are unknown; locomotor activity; and exploratory activity, giving an anthropomorphic interpretation. SMA has been measured objectively in a variety of ways, e. g., counting interruptions of a beam of light to a photocell by a mouse passing by or remaining in the beam (Dews 1953); changes of ultrasound shadows due to mouse movement (Winter and Flataker 1951); accelerational devices (Schulte et al. 1939); running wheels; and a number of others (Finger 1972). Typically, SMA in a constant environment decreases with time over the short run, reaching an asymptote at a relatively low fraction of the original rate in very roughly an hour (see, for example, Takagi et al. 1971) although the time varies a great deal from method to method. Doses of caffeine as low as 2–3 mg/kg can increase SMA significantly, and doses causing peak effects (which vary from report to report from 10 to 200 mg/kg) can cause a severalfold increase in SMA, making SMA, with sleep postponement in humans, among the most sensitive and quantitatively largest of the behavioral effects of caffeine. The maximum effect at 200 mg/kg was found under special circumstances, in mice that had been subjected to 4 h in an oscillating shaker moving 12.3 cm 129 times per minute (Takagi et al. 1972).

Despite the many years over which the effect of caffeine on SMA has been studied, even questions on simple descriptive aspects remain unanswered, such as whether the effect is entirely or primarily a prevention of the rapid decrement of SMA with time that occurs under control conditions. In addition, the lack of information on the factors that determine the initial level of SMA and then the rapid decline makes interpretation of the effects of caffeine in a wider context difficult.

In mice given 150 mg/kg per day of caffeine for 6 weeks in their drinking water, the SMA was similar to that in controls (Estler et al. 1978). Surprisingly, the subcu-

93

taneous injection of 50 mg/kg of caffeine into the mice pretreated for 6 weeks caused a large increase in SMA. In the 2nd h of assessment, the SMA of control animals or animals after 6 weeks of caffeine was about 100; when 50 mg/kg caffeine was given immediately before the session the SMA in the 2nd h was about 300. In a separate experiment, 50 mg/kg is shown as increasing SMA in the 2nd h to about 150, from 30 in controls. The reason for the difference in the control values in the two experiments is not clear, but the effects of 50 mg/kg seems to have been to increase the 2nd-h SMA three- to fivefold, unaffected by 6 weeks of 150 mg/kg caffeine per day. There was, therefore, no evidence of development of tolerance under the chronic regime. A problem in interpreting the study is that no information is available on the actual plasma levels of caffeine that were produced by 150 mg/kg per day in the drinking water. The low licking rate of an unpalatable liquid can result in only low plasma levels and there is evidence in mice that the clearance rate for caffeine at low plasma levels is much greater than is implied by a half-life of 3 h. The concentrations of caffeine in the plasmas of ten mice at the end of 8 weeks of 125 mg/kg caffeine daily in the drinking water were measured at 4-h intervals for 24 h (Aeschbacher et al. 1978). No level as high as 7 mg/l was detected at any time in any mouse, and the great majority of values were less than 0.5 mg/l. These values imply a half-life of only a few minutes. Hence, even though the low rate of licking may be maintained over much of the time, the plasma level may never build up to the sort of level that might be necessary to produce tolerance to the effects of 50 mg/kg subcutaneously. The pretreated mice performed better (i. e., remained longer) on a rotating rod, but were less able to maintain their body temperature when exposed to an ambient temperature of 0 °C or immersed in water at 25 °C, and were unable to swim as long in the water. All these effects may be related to the lower mean weight of the mice treated with caffeine: 26 g as compared to 28.7 g for controls. Of course, 150 mg/kg daily is a level never approached in humans.

In view of the low plasma levels from ingestion of caffeine in the drinking water, it is perhaps not surprising that Dews and Wenger (1979) found no changes in the subsequent behavior of the offspring of mice treated through pregnancy and lactation with doses of up to 100 mg/kg per day in the drinking water. Acute effects of caffeine on schedule-controlled responding have been studied. An increase in the proportion of inter-response times shorter than 18 s in mice under a DRL 18-s schedule was produced by caffeine in doses from 3 to 24 mg/kg (Webb and Levine 1978). Increased rate of responding of mice under FI 600 s but insignificant increases under FR 30 were found by McKim (1980). The peak increase in rate, at 56 mg/kg, was to about 150% of control. Such an increase is much closer to the magnitude of effects that have been described on interesting behavioral functions in humans under optimum conditions than are the manyfold increases seen in SMA. Indeed, while SMA has proved to be a useful method of generating dose-effect curves for a variety of agents, and of determining relative potencies, the absolute quantitative findings on SMA are hard to interpret. SMA, as its name implies, is weakly determined behavior; its rapid decline with time is one indication of that. Because it is unregulated, it is easily subject to wide variations in measured magnitude. The magnitude of such variations provides little information on the magnitude of effects to be expected on regulated human behavioral activities. The effects on schedule-controlled behavior generally yield much more useful information on both the quantitative and the qualitative effects to be expected in interesting human behavior.

Castellano (1976) has reported that caffeine facilitated learning and consolidation processes in mice provided they were initially naive and were trained under a so-called D procedure, but not when they were trained under an L procedure. Both the L and D procedures comprised mice swimming in a Y water maze, one arm of which was lighted, toward an escape platform in the lighted arm (L procedure) or in the dark arm (D procedure). The mice exhibited an initial bias toward the lighted arm. If the mice had been previously trained, caffeine caused only decrements in subsequent sessions. Doses of 0.5 mg/kg, 1.0 mg/kg, and 2.0 mg/kg caffeine were studied. When the doses were given before the session, the results were attributed to effects on learning, whereas when the caffeine was given after the session, the results of subsequent sessions were attributed to effects on consolidation. Interpretation in terms of other of the many possible behavioral variables that might have been affected by caffeine was not considered. The large differences in effects with the relatively minor procedural difference (minor in terms of the putative main factors of learning and consolidation) between the L and D procedures suggest that the real determinants of the different effects of caffeine were among those other behavioral variables, rather than in the basic biological mechanisms of "learning" and "consolidation."

The number of holes a mouse puts its head into when placed on a board with many holes is greatly reduced by keeping the mouse in a cage alone for 29 days (Valzelli and Bernasconi 1973). Caffeine at 20 mg/kg had little effect on this activity in either normal or previously isolated mice. When three previously isolated mice are put together in a cage, they fight, a phenomenon glorified in the literature as "aggressiveness." This aggressiveness is reduced by caffeine in doses of 5, 10, and 20 mg/kg, though in a manner poorly related to dose (Valzelli and Bernasconi 1973). Comparative effects in nonisolated mice were not studied. The many behavioral differences between isolated and nonisolated mice, documented here by differences in head insertions, make claims that caffeine has a selective effect on aggression unwarranted.

3.2 Rats

Caffeine has been reported by Merkel et al. (1981) to increase the intake of food and water in a 3-h period following 21 h deprivation. Over a range of 3.12–50 mg/kg, they found an increase in food consumption of about 20% and an even bigger proportional increase in water consumption at the lower doses. Consumption of food was decreased at 100 mg/kg and of water at 50 and 100 mg/kg. The effects were greatest in previously untreated subjects, and were much reduced when the larger doses of caffeine had been given on previous occasions.

Caffeine has similar effects on SMA in rats to those described above in mice. For example, 5 mg/kg caffeine caused a more than doubling of SMA in rats in the 2nd h following administration by gavage (Collins et al. 1977).

A series of studies of effects of caffeine on activity, "social investigation," and other behaviors of neonatal, juvenile, and adult rats have been performed by Holloway and Thor (Holloway 1982; Holloway and Thor 1982, 1983 a, b). In general, acute doses of caffeine could increase both activity and social investigation in rats of all ages, and the differences at different ages were not conspicuous. In adult rats, chronic administration of about 15 or 57 mg/kg caffeine per day in the drinking water led to a surprisingly large increase in social investigation, although the acute effect of an injected dose of 20 mg/kg in increasing activity was not changed by 12 days of caffeine in the drinking water. This paper is unique in reporting a large sustained behavioral effect on rodents of caffeine taken in the drinking water.

As long ago as 1937, Skinner and Heron reported that caffeine increased the rate of responding of rats under an FI 240-s schedule or during extinction. A dose of 10 mg caffeine sodium benzoate per rat, caused about a 50% increase in responding. Similar effects on responding under a self-initiated FI 30-s schedule have been reported by Mechner and Latranyi (1963), who also found modest increases in responding under other schedules which they called "fixed number" and "fixed minimum interval" schedules. Both schedules required a response first on one lever and subsequently on a second lever: under the former schedule, 45 additional first-lever responses were necessary, and under the latter schedule, 12 s without a response had to elapse before a response on the second lever would trigger food delivery. Only decreases in rates of responding are reported by Barone et al. (1979) for rats under FT 60 s; with this schedule, food was delivered every 60 s without regard to lever pressing. The same laboratory reported a very small increase in rate under FI 60 s (Wayner et al. 1976). Doses of 30 mg/kg and greater were studied by Harris et al. (1978) on FR 30 and FI 120 s and only decreases in responding were seen. For rats responding under DRL schedules, Ando (1975) found inappreciable effects at 8 and 16 mg/kg caffeine and a decrease at 32 mg/kg. The four rats studied with caffeine showed appreciable reductions in responding following vehicle alone, not shown in other rats given other drugs in the study, so the apparent lack of effect of 8 and 16 mg/kg is hard to assess. It is clear, however, that the effects of caffeine were slight compared to the large increases caused by amphetamine. An increase of 50% of responding under DRL 20 s was found by Sanger (1980) at 40 mg/kg, with a smaller increase at 20 mg/kg and a decrease at 60 mg/kg. In addition, an enhancement by chlordiazepoxide of the effects of caffeine in increasing rates of responding was shown.

A modest increase in the rate of responding of rats under VI 120 s following 30 mg/kg caffeine was reported by Morrison (1969). In these experiments each delivery of water, the reinforcer, was accompanied by an 0.5-s electric shock of 0.2–0.4 ma. In rats responding at about 0.8 responses/s under an uncomplicated VI 30 s for food, caffeine given 45 min before the session in the range 1–3 mg/kg caused a modest increase in responding, no more than 20%–25%, while 32 mg/kg reduced responding to roughly 25% of the control rate (Carney 1982). When the 32 mg/kg was repeated daily, the suppressant effect declined, until after 7 days suppression was no longer apparent and the whole dose-effect curve for caffeine was shifted 0.5–1.0 log units to the right, i.e., from three to ten times as much caffeine was required for a given effect as in rats not exposed to repeated daily doses of caffeine. The findings constitute a clear quantitative determination of tolerance to behavioral effects of caffeine. It is interesting that tolerance, known to occur in humans, was seen in this schedule-controlled behavior, in contrast to the lack of tolerance reported above in SMA (if that finding can be accepted at face value). The tolerance was obtained with only a single daily dose of caffeine. The half-life of caffeine in rats is about 3 h, so the concentration would have fallen to only about $1/20$ of its original level after 12 h. The tolerance therefore developed despite the rats being essentially caffeine-free for much of each 24 h.

Rats that had had caffeine solution of 0.17, 0.34, or 0.5 mg/ml flavored by mocha as sole source of drinking water for 14 days subsequently drank about the same amounts of water, mocha-flavored water, and the concentration of caffeine they had been on when given equal access to all three concentrations, except that the 0.5 mg/ml caffeine group drank significantly less mocha-flavored water and insignificantly more caffeine solution (Vitiello and Woods 1975). Taken as a whole, the findings are taken to indicate that withdrawal from forced drinking of caffeine solution does not provoke an abstinence syndrome that can be discriminably attenuated by a flavor associated with caffeine or by caffeine itself, but the data do not warrant confident generalization.

The offspring of rats treated throughout pregnancy with caffeine in the drinking water showed no convincing behavioral abnormalities (Sobotka et al. 1979). Although the doses ranged up to 90 mg/kg daily, lack of information on the plasma levels produced leads to uncertainties in the interpretation of the negative results, as in the case of the mouse experiments above. A report by Peters (1967) that rats given large doses of caffeine sometimes self-mutilate by biting and even destroying parts of the body, notably feet, has been confirmed by Mueller et al. (1982) who found that six of 15 rats injected with 140 mg/kg caffeine daily bit their feet in a few days. Drugs such as amphetamine (more effective than caffeine) and pemoline also produce the phenomenon. Despite its superficial similarity to the Lesch-Nyhan syndrome seen in children with certain metabolic abnormalities, the mechanism of the phenomenon in rats has not been elucidated and its significance as a test system remains undemonstrated.

Fundaro et al. (1983) trained rats to press the left-hand lever of two levers under FR 10 for food, then gave them pure drinking water or water with 6 mg/l or 18 mg/l caffeine daily (other drugs were studied too). After 8 days, the FR 10 was shifted from the left lever to the right lever, and subsequently back to the left, to the right again, and then finally to the left. Caffeine made no difference to the total number of responses made after the first reversal, but the number of responses made after the subsequent reversals was decreased in the rats taking 18 mg/kg daily but not in those taking 6 mg/kg daily. It is difficult to think of a direct pharmacological effect that would not occur on the first reversal but would emerge on subsequent reversals. The number of responses made by the controls more than doubled from the first to the fourth reversal, whereas the number remained fairly constant for the 18 mg/kg daily group, suggesting large variations which might have been inappropriately attributed to drug effects. Also in a two-lever situation, rats were trained to press one lever when they had been injected with saline and the other when they had been given 32 mg/kg caffeine (Modrow et al. 1981). In subsequent sessions, when the rats were given saline essentially 100% of the responses were made on the saline lever, and when they were given 32 mg/kg caffeine essentially 100% of the responses were made on the caffeine lever. In sessions following smaller doses of caffeine the proportion of responses on the caffeine lever decreased, to about 75% after 20 mg/kg,

50% after 10 mg/kg, and 30% after 3.2 mg/kg. Injection of any of a range of doses of amphetamine, methylphenidate, and nicotine did not produce as much as 30% responses on the caffeine lever. A dose of 75 mg/kg theophylline produced 74% responses on the caffeine lever. The selective pharmacological effects of the caffeine and theophylline clearly powerfully controlled which lever the animal would press. The decreasing proportion of responses on the caffeine lever as the dose of caffeine was reduced could have been due to the lessened "discriminability" from saline of the lower doses. They could be due at least partly, however, to the quantitative differences in the pharmacological "cues" with lower doses from those to which the animals had been trained. Certainly, stimulus generalization gradients may be obtained in psychophysical experiments around the stimulus magnitude of training, for example in visual experiments, even though all the magnitudes studied are greatly above the discriminability threshold.

Atkinson and Enslen (1976) were unable to maintain responses in rats by self-administration of intravenous injections of caffeine at levels above injections of saline.

3.3 Other Species

Griffiths et al. (1979) found that 3.2 mg/kg caffeine citrate injections "maintained steady or erratic patterns of self-administration in all 3 baboons tested." The mean response rates with caffeine, however, were still within the saline control range. The marginal ability of caffeine to maintain self-administration responses has been confirmed by Spealman (personal communication) in squirrel monkeys: seemingly, responses under a second-order schedule of FR 10 units were maintained under FI 3000 s but not under FI 300 s. In rhesus monkeys, Hoffmeister and Wüttke (1973) found not only that caffeine did not maintain self-administration, but also that when added to codeine it reduced the otherwise high rate of self-administration of the codeine. The ineffectiveness of caffeine in maintaining self-administration is surprising in that caffeine clearly possesses two of the major attributes of those agents that very effectively maintain self-administration: ability to cross the blood-brain barrier rapidly and discriminability, the latter as shown by Modrow et al. (1981). In this matter, caffeine very clearly differs from the so-called drugs of abuse.

The influence of caffeine on discriminative responses among golden hamsters was studied by Rahmann (1963). Very low doses of caffeine were given – 0.25 mg/kg to a high of 3.0 mg/kg – and no effects on performance were detected during 7 consecutive days of injections. Testing was then continued for several weeks in the absence of caffeine. The author claims that animals that had previously received 0.5 mg/kg showed speeded "learning" and improved "retention," while animals that had previously received 1.0 mg/kg and 3.0 mg/kg had dose-dependent effects in the opposite direction. The effects were slight even in the 1 and 3 mg/kg groups and unconvincing at the lower doses. Furthermore, the complex design of the experiment makes interpretation difficult. No effects were detected while the caffeine was actually being given, but the subsequent effects are claimed to persist for weeks. An effect on a discrimination subsequent to training under an agent rather than while the agent is being given is reminiscent of effects attributed to "dissociation" rather than a direct pharmacological effect (Overton 1971). Subjects trained under one set of circumstances (such as while being injected with caffeine) may show a change in performance when the injections are discontinued simply because the circumstances are changed rather than because of persistent pharmacological consequences. The use of words such as "learning" and "retention" to describe results of studies such as this is justified only if the terms are regarded as loosely descriptive. Performance variables and indicators of putative underlying changes in learning and retention are inextricably confounded in these experiments. Different groups of animals were studied at the different dose levels, and considerable variability is seen in the graphs showing the repeated testing over the several weeks of the experiments. No standard deviation or other measure of variability is presented. In view of these considerations the biological reality of the effects following 0.5 mg/kg, opposite in direction to the effects following 1.0 or 3.0 mg/kg, cannot be considered as established. Even the effects following 1 and 3 mg/kg are dubious and uninterpretable in these experiments.

There have been relatively few studies of caffeine on subhuman primates. In squirrel monkeys, caffeine in doses of 3–10 mg/kg caused a modest (about 10%) increase in FI 180 s responses, most of the increase occurring in the first half of the FI, and in responses to postpone an electric shock (Davis et al. 1973). Essentially no effect was seen on FR responses or on a work activity requiring climbing up and down a pole. Steadiness, as measured by how infrequently the monkey caused a stylus protruding through a hole to touch the edges of the hole, was slightly decreased. Only a decrease in responses was found by Stinnette and Isaac (1975) in the squirrel monkey under FI 80 s with doses of 2–8 mg/kg caffeine citrate (equivalent to about half the dosage of base), but dose-effect relationships were either unapparent, when the animals were working in the dark, or reversed (highest dose being closest to the control), when they were working in the light. Amphetamine also caused only decreases in responses. The reason for the unusual results is not apparent. In both young and old rhesus monkeys doses of 2–16 mg/kg caffeine had "rather unimpressive and often inconstant" effects on a delayed response procedure (Bartus 1979). No dose-effect relationship was apparent. Performance was, if anything, impaired, but not convincingly so; the same was true for pemoline and a pentylenetetrazole – niacin mixture. Methylphenidate convincingly impaired performance to a progressively greater degree as the dose was increased from 2 to 8 mg/kg.

4 Conclusions

The dose range that can produce measurable selective changes in behavior is quite similar across all the species studied, from mice to humans, being in the range of 1–10 mg/kg, perhaps going as high as 30 mg/kg. Still higher doses produce a relatively nonspecific decrease in effective behavioral activities while maintaining wakefulness. No qualitative differences between the behavioral effects of caffeine in man and in experimental animals have been demonstrated or even indicated. Yet even when all available information from humans and experimental animals is combined, a coherent account of the salient selective effects of caffeine on behavior cannot be given to the extent that an account can be given of the behavioral effects of chlordiazepoxide, chlorpromazine and even amphetamine. Part of the problem is that the behavioral effects of caffeine at levels causing selective changes are modest and even subtle. Small effects are harder to analyze than big effects. Another problem is that much of our information on caffeine has come from studies whose main purpose was not the study of the pharmacology of caffeine. As we have seen, effects on learning, consolidation, aggression, and the like have been reported; none of these attributions bears scrutiny. It is clear that caffeine is not a simple stimulant, whatever that means. Indeed, it may not be a stimulant at all in any meaningful way. The evidence at present is compatible with the view that the selective effects of caffeine is not determined by the nature of the behavior on which it is imposed, but by the condition of freshness or fatigue of the subject. In recent years we have become familiar with drug effects that are apparent only when function is disordered or suboptimal. Examples are histamine α-receptor blockers, whose effect in this regard in an intact subject is manifest only when there has been abnormal release of histamine, and acetylsalicylic acid, whose action in inhibiting prostaglandin synthetase is manifest only when the synthetase activity has been increased by a pathological process. It may be speculated that caffeine may antagonize the effects of some agent that is present in pharmacologically active amounts only under conditions of fatigue or deteriorated performance of other origin. Whether the concept is valid for caffeine, and if so, whether the substance in question is adenosine, can hardly be addressed, far less assessed, on the evidence presently available. There have been few systematic, qualitative studies on the effects of caffeine in fatigued or bored subjects in comparison to fresh, alert subjects in either man or experimental animals. Only by systematic studies can even the first question be answered definitively: Are the selective behavioral effects of caffeine confined, largely or totally, to restorative effects on decremented performance?

Acknowledgment. I thank Mrs. R. Share for help in preparation of the manuscript.

References

Aeschbacher HU, Milon H, Wurzner HP (1978) Caffeine concentrations in mice plasma and testicular tissue and the effect of caffeine on the dominant lethal test. Mutat Res 57: 193–200

Ando K (1975) Profile of drug effects on temporally spaced responding in rats. Pharmacol Biochem Behav 3: 833–841

Atkinson J, Enslen M (1976) Self-administration of caffeine by the rat. Arzneimittelforsch 26: 2059–2061

Baker WJ, Theologus GC (1972) Effects of caffeine on visual monitoring. J Appl Psychol 56: 422–427

Barone FC, Wayner MJ, Kleinrock S (1979) Effects of caffeine on FT-1 min schedule-induced drinking at different body weights. Pharmacol Biochem Behav 11: 347–350

Bartus RT (1979) Four stimulants of the central nervous system: effects on short-term memory in young versus aged monkeys. J Am Geriatr Soc 7: 289–297

Carney JM (1982) Effects of caffeine, theophylline and theobromine on schedule controlled responding in rats. Br J Pharmacol 75: 451–454

Castellano C (1976) Effects of caffeine on discrimination learning, consolidation, and learned behavior in mice. Psychopharmacology 48: 255–260

Cherek DR, Steinberg JL, Brauchi JT (1983) Effects of caffeine on human aggressive behavior. Psychiatry Res 8: 137–145

Clubley M, Bye CE, Henson TA, Peck AW, Riddington CJ (1979) Effects of caffeine and cyclizine alone and in combination on human performance, subjective effects and EEG activity. Br J Clin Pharmacol 7: 157–163

Collins C, Richards PT, Starmer GA (1977) Caffeine-phenacetin interaction in the rat: effects on absorption, metabolism and locomotor activity. J Pharm Pharmacol 29: 217–221

Cook CE, Rallent CR, Amerson EW, Myers MW, Kepler JA, Taylor GF, Christensen HD (1976) Caffeine in plasma and saliva by a radioimmunoassay procedure. J Pharmacol Exp Ther 199: 679–686

Davis TRA, Kensler CJ, Dews PB (1973) Comparison of behavioral effects of nicotine, d-amphetamine, caffeine and dimethylheptyl tetrahydrocannabinol in squirrel monkeys. Psychopharmacologia 32: 51–65

De Freitas B, Schwartz G (1979) Effects of caffeine in chronic psychiatric patients. Am J Psychiatry 136: 1337–1338

Dews PB (1953) The measurement of the influence of drugs on voluntary activity in mice. Br J Pharmacol 8: 46–48

Dews PB (1982) Caffeine. Ann Rev Nutr 2: 323–341

Dews PB, Wenger GR (1979) Testing for behavioral effects of agents. Neurobehav Toxicol [Suppl 1] 1: 119–127

Diamond AL, Cole RE (1970) Visual threshold as a function of test area and caffeine administration. Psychon Sci 20: 109–111

Eichler O (ed) (1976) Kaffee und Coffein, 2nd edn. Springer, Berlin Heidelberg New York

Elkins RN, Rapoport JL, Zahn TP, Buchsbaum MS, Weingartner H, Kopin IJ, Langer D, Johnson C (1981) Acute effects of caffeine in normal prepubertal boys. Am J Psychiatry 138: 178–183

Estler CJ, Ammon HPT, Herzog C (1978) Swimming capacity of mice after prolonged treatment with psychostimulants. I. Effect of caffeine on swimming performance and cold stress. Psychopharmacology 58: 161–166

Finger FW (1972) Measuring behavioral activity. In: Myers RD (ed) Methods in psychobiology, vol 2. Academic, London New York, pp 1–19

Forney RB, Hughes FW (1965) Effect of caffeine and alcohol on performance under stress of audiofeedback. Q J Stud Alcohol 26: 206–212

Fundaro A, Ricci GS, Molinengo L (1983) Action of caffeine, d-amphetamine, diazepam and imipramine in a dynamic behavioral situation. Pharmacol Res Commun 15: 71–84

Garfinkel BD, Webster CD, Sloman L (1975) Methylphenidate and caffeine in the treatment of children with minimal brain dysfunction. Am J Psychiatry 132: 723–728

Gilliland K, Andress D (1981) Ad lib caffeine consumption, symptoms of caffeinism, and academic performance. Am J Psychiatry 138: 512–514

Goldstein A, Warren R, Kaizer S (1965) Psychotropic effects of caffeine in man. I. Individual differences in sensitivity to caffeine-induced wakefulness. J Pharmacol Exp Ther 149: 156–159

Goldstein A, Kaizer S, Whitby O (1969) Psychotropic effects of caffeine in man. IV. Quantitative and qualitative differences associated with habituation to coffee. Clin Pharmacol Ther 10: 489–497

Greden JF, Fontaine P, Lubetsky M, Chamberlin K (1978) Anxiety and depression associated with caffeinism among psychiatric inpatients. Am J Psychiatry 135: 963–966

Griffiths RR, Brady JV, Bradford LD (1979) Predicting the abuse liability of drugs with animal drug self-administration procedures: psychomotor stimulants and hallucinogens. In: Thompson T, Dews PB (eds) Advances in behavioral pharmacology, vol 2. Academic, London New York, pp 163–208

Harris RA, Snell D, Loh HH (1978) Effects of stimulants, anoretics, and related drugs on schedule-controlled behavior. Psychopharmacology 56: 49–55

Hoffmeister F, Wüttke W (1973) Self-administration of acetylsalicylic acid and combinations with codeine and caffeine in rhesus monkeys. J Pharmacol Exp Ther 186: 266–275

Holloway WR (1982) Caffeine: effects of acute and chronic exposure on the behavior of neonatal rats. Neurobehav Toxicol Teratol 4: 21–32

Holloway WR, Thor DH (1982) Caffeine sensitivity in the neonatal rat. Neurobehav Toxicol Teratol 4: 331–333

Holloway WR, Thor DH (1983a) Caffeine: effects on the behaviors of juvenile rats. Neurobehav Toxicol Teratol 5: 127–134

Holloway WR, Thor DH (1983b) Caffeine and social investigation in the adult male rat. Neurobehav Toxicol Teratol 5: 119–125

Ivy JL, Costill DL, Fink WJ, Lower RW (1979) Influence of caffeine and carbohydrate feedings on endurance performance. Med Sci Sports 11: 6–11

McKim WA (1980) The effect of caffeine, theophylline and amphetamine on operant responding of the mouse. Psychopharmacology 68: 135–138

Mechner F, Latranyi M (1963) Behavioral effects of caffeine, methamphetamine, and methylphenidate in the rat. J Exp Anal Behav 6: 331–342

Merkel AD, Wayner FB, Jolicoeur FB, Mintz R (1981) Effects of caffeine administration on food and water consumption under various experimental conditions. Pharmacol Biochem Behav 14: 234–240

Modrow HE, Holloway FA, Christensen HD, Carney JM (1981) Relationship between caffeine discrimination and caffeine plasma levels. Pharmacol Biochem Behav 15: 323–325

Morrison CF (1969) The effects of nicotine on punished behaviour. Psychopharmacologia 14: 221–232

Mueller K, Saboda S, Palmour R, Nyhan WL (1982) Self-injurious behavior produced in rats by daily caffeine and continuous amphetamine. Pharmacol Biochem Behav 17: 613–617

Overton DA (1971) Discriminative control of behavior by drug states. In: Thompson T, Pickens R (eds) Stimulus properties of drugs. Appleton-Century-Crofts, New York, pp 87–110

Peters JM (1967) Caffeine-induced hemorrhagic automutilation. Arch Int Pharmacodyn 169: 139–146

Rahmann H (1963) Einfluß von Coffein auf das Gedächtnis und das Verhalten von Goldhamstern. Pflügers Arch 276: 384–397

Rall TW (1980) Central nervous system stimulants. The xanthines. In: Gilman AG, Goodman LS, Gilman A (eds) The pharmacological basis of therapeutics, 6th edn. Macmillan, New York, pp 592–607

Rapoport JL, Jensvold M, Elkins R, Buchsbaum MS, Weingartner H, Ludlow C, Zahn T, Berg CJ, Neims AH (1981) Behavioral and cognitive effects of caffeine in boys and adults. J Nerv Ment Dis 169: 726–732

Reichard CC, Elder ST (1977) The effects of caffeine on reaction time in hyperkinetic and normal children. Am J Psychiatry 134: 144–148

Revelle W, Humphreys MS, Simon L, Gilliland K (1980) The interactive effect of personality, time of day, and caffeine: a test of the arousal model. J Exp Psychol [Gen] 109: 1–31

Robertson D, Frolich JC, Carr RK, Watson JT, Hollifield JW, Shand DG, Oates JA (1978) Effects of caffeine on plasma renin activity, catecholamines and blood pressure. N Engl J Med 298: 181–186

Robertson D, Wade D, Workman R, Woosley RI (1981) Tolerance to the humoral and hemodynamic effects of caffeine in man. J Clin Invest 67: 1111–1117

Salter WT (1952) A textbook of pharmacology. Saunders, Philadelphia

Sanger D (1980) The effects of caffeine on timing behavior of rodents: comparison with chlordiazepoxide. Psychopharmacology 68: 305–330

Schulte JW, Tainter ML, Dille JM (1939) Comparison of different types of central stimulation from analeptics. Proc Soc Exp Biol Med 42: 242–248

Skinner BF, Heron WT (1937) Effects of caffeine and benzedrine upon conditioning and extinction. Psychol Rec 1: 340–346

Smith DL, Tong JE, Leigh G (1977) Combined effects of tobacco and caffeine on the components of choice reaction-time, heart rate, and hand steadiness. Percept Mot Skills 15: 635–639

Smith BD, Wilson RJ, Jones BE (1983) Extraversion and multiple levels of caffeine-induced arousal: effects on overhabituation and dishabituation. Psychophysiology 20: 29–34

Sobotka TJ, Spaid SL, Brodie RE (1979) Neurobehavioral teratology of caffeine exposure in rats. Neurotoxicology 1: 403–416

Stinnette MJ, Isaac W (1975) Behavioral effects of d-amphetamine and caffeine in the squirrel monkey. Eur J Pharmacol 30: 268–271

Takagi K, Watanabe M, Saito H (1971) Studies of the spontaneous movement of animals by the hole cross test; effect of 2-dimethylaminoethanol and its acyl esters on the central nervous system. Jpn J Pharmacol 21: 797–810

Takagi K, Saito H, Lee CH, Hayashi T (1972) Pharmacological studies on fatigue I. Jpn J Pharmacol 22: 17–26

Valzelli L, Bernasconi S (1973) Behavioral and neurochemical effects of caffeine in normal and aggressive mice. Pharmacol Biochem Behav 1: 251–254

Vitiello MV, Woods SC (1975) Caffeine: preferential consumption by rats. Pharmacol Biochem Behav 3: 147–149

Waldeck B (1974) Ethanol and caffeine: a complex interaction with respect to locomotor activity and central catecholamines. Psychopharmacologia 36: 209–220

Wayner MJ, Jolicoeur FB, Rondeau DB, Barone FC (1976) The effects of acute and chronic administration of caffeine on schedule dependent and schedule induced behavior. Pharmacol Biochem Behav 5: 343–348

Webb D, Levine TE (1978) Effects of caffeine on DRL performance in the mouse. Pharmacol Biochem Behav 9: 7–10

Weiss B, Laties VG (1962) Enhancement of human performance by caffeine and the amphetamines. Pharmacol Rev 14: 1–36

Winter CA, Flataker L (1951) The effect of cortisone, desoxycorticosterone and adrenocorticotrophic hormone upon the responses of animals to analgesic drugs. J Pharmacol Exp Ther 103: 93–105

Section IV

Mechanisms of Effects

VII Effects of Caffeine on Monoamine Neurotransmitters in the Central and Peripheral Nervous System*

J. D. Fernstrom and M. H. Fernstrom

1 Introduction

Over the past 10–15 years, interest in the behavioral and autonomic effects of caffeine has led neuropharmacologists, psychopharmacologists, and autonomic physiologists to explore for effects of this and related methylxanthines on the formation and release of neurotransmitters. Probably because of the availability of techniques and observed autonomic effects, most early studies focused on the catecholamines, and to a lesser extent on serotonin. In fact, the bulk of the neuropharmacologic literature on caffeine (which is small) considers effects related to these transmitters. Fewer and more recent studies have explored the possibility that caffeine effects may be mediated by other mechanisms, such as via an interaction with putative adenosine receptors. And only a handful of articles deal with effects of caffeine on such other transmitters as gamma-aminobutyric acid (GABA) and acetylcholine. For this reason, this review focuses primarily on the effects of caffeine on the monoamine neurotransmitters. Some information, however, is also presented on caffeine's proposed effects on adenosine receptors, inasmuch as this is one possible route by which the methylxanthine exerts its actions on catecholamine neurons (as well as other cells). Reference to work on other transmitters is also made, but only in passing, to give the reader access to some of the available literature.

2 Effects on Brain Monoamines

2.1 Serotonin

The acute administration of caffeine has been reported by several laboratories to elevate brain levels of serotonin (5-HT) and 5-hydroxyindoleacetic acid (5-HIAA) (Berkowitz and Spector 1971a; Corrodi et al. 1972; Valzelli and Bernasconi 1973; Geyer et al. 1975; Curzon and Fernando 1976; Schlosberg et al. 1981). The effects are observed both in whole brain and in such brain regions as the brainstem and cerebral cortex (Berkowitz and Spector 1973). In at least one case, they have been shown to persist when the compound is administered chronically (Berkowitz and

* The studies described from the authors' laboratory were supported in part by grants from the National Institute of Mental Health (MH 38 178) and the International Life Sciences Institute

Spector 1973). Theophylline and aminophylline have also been shown to increase brain 5-hydroxyindole concentrations, suggesting that the methylxanthines as a class may have these effects on serotoninergic neurons in brain (Karasawa et al. 1976; Paalzow and Paalzow 1974; Sakata et al. 1975; Curzon and Fernando 1976).

The mechanism by which caffeine injection elevates brain levels of 5-HT and 5-HIAA is, to say the least, unclear. The potential mechanisms include:

1. increase of 5-HT synthesis rate,
2. reduction of 5-HT catabolic and/or release rate,
3. reduction in 5-HIAA clearance from the central nervous system, and
4. some combination of the above.

If 5-HT synthesis rate were increased, how might this effect be elaborated? At least two possibilities seem clear. First, caffeine might somehow induce tryptophan hydroxylase; second, it might elevate brain levels of tryptophan, which would then lead indirectly to a stimulation of 5-HT synthesis. We have obtained data suggesting that caffeine does not directly influence tryptophan hydroxylase activity (Fernstrom et al., to be published). When the methylxanthine was added to brain homogenates, in concentrations up to 50 mg/g (a concentration about that found following injection of 100 mg/kg caffeine), no effect on either the K_m or the V_{max} of the enzyme was apparent.

Other data suggest that caffeine might act via the second postulated mechanism. Specifically, a repeatedly observed effect following caffeine administration is a rise in brain tryptophan levels (Curzon and Fernando 1976; Schlosberg et al. 1981). [The rise in brain tryptophan level may follow from the ability of high doses of caffeine to induce insulin secretion, thereby so altering the plasma amino acid pattern as indirectly to favor tryptophan transport into brain (see Schlosberg et al. 1980). However, other mechanisms have also been postulated, such as a reduction in the binding of tryptophan to albumin in blood (Curzon and Fernando 1976). It seems likely that a multiplicity of known and unknown factors may contribute to the caffeine-induced rise in brain tryptophan, because of the relatively high doses required to obtain this effect.] Curzon and Fernando (1976) in fact speculated that caffeine or aminophylline increases 5-HT synthesis, since the injection of each increases brain tryptophan levels. Normally, a rise in tryptophan levels enhances 5-HT synthesis rate by increasing the degree of substrate saturation of tryptophan hydroxylase, the enzyme that catalyzes the rate-limiting step in 5-HT formation (e.g., see Carlsson and Lindqvist 1978). However, we have recently measured the in vivo rate of 5 HT synthesis, using a variety of techniques, and find *no* increase (Fernstrom et al., to be published). This result is somewhat surprising, since the elevation in brain tryptophan level probably should increase 5-HT production. If so, then the absence of such increases suggests that in vivo, some indirect effect of caffeine (caffeine does not appear directly to inhibit tryptophan hydroxylase) causes an inhibition of hydroxylation sufficient to offset any increase due to the rise in brain tryptophan. Another, simpler possibility is that the rise in brain tryptophan occurs in brain regions that contain no 5-HT cell bodies or terminals. Both possibilities warrant testing.

If caffeine administration does not enhance the 5-HT synthesis rate, then the 5-HT catabolic rate must be reduced in order for the 5-HT level to be increased. While the in vivo catabolic rate has not been directly measured, caffeine has been studies for its effects in vitro on monoamine oxidase (MAO) activity. The methylxanthine does exert a modest inhibitory influence on MAO (Galzigna et al. 1971; Bellin and Sorrentino 1974), and at a concentration that is found in brain soon after the injection of a 100 mg/kg dose (Fernstrom et al., to be published). Consistent with this finding are the results of Corrodi et al. (1972) and Berkowitz et al. (1973), showing that the acute fall-off in brain 5-HT level following inhibition of tryptophan hydroxylase (with alpha-propyldopacetamide or parachlorophenylalanine) is below normal in rats treated with caffeine. [Berkowitz' and Spector's (1973) results with pargyline and caffeine might even be interpreted to support this view, if the dose of pargyline used failed fully to inhibit brain MAO.] Taken together, these results therefore support the notion that the 5-HT level in brain is elevated following caffeine injection because the catabolic rate is reduced [though it should be noted that Berkowitz and Spector (1973) did not draw this conclusion from their data].

However, if the rate of 5-HT oxidation is reduced following caffeine administration, how could the level of 5-HIAA be increased, as is known to be the case? The most straightforward explanation would be that caffeine somehow reduces the rate of 5-HIAA efflux from the central nervous system. If it did, then this might explain why Valzelli and Bernasconi (1973) and we (Fernstrom et al., to be published) found the 5-HT turnover rate to be below normal in rats treated with caffeine. The method employed to estimate 5-HT turnover involves estimating the rate of 5-HIAA fall-off following inhibition of MAO. This rate is slower than normal in caffeine-treated rats. If caffeine inhibited 5-HIAA efflux, then one would expect to see 5-HIAA fall-off following pargyline to be less than normal. However, in this case the result would indicate nothing about turnover rate. An implicit assumption in using this method is that the 5-HIAA efflux rate is unaffected by the treatment under study. No data are available that bear on this issue, so the analysis is speculative. However, it is difficult to imagine how the 5-HIAA level could be elevated in the presence of reduced 5-HT catabolism if the rate of 5-HIAA removal were not also reduced. It is hoped that future studies will resolve this issue.

Overall, caffeine's effects on 5-HT synthesis and turnover appear more complex than initially perceived. It is disconcerting to have to postulate multiple sites of action in producing such effects. This concern is not new, as earlier investigators have sought for a single explanation for all of the effects discussed here. One notion apparent to Berkowitz and Spector (1973) and Bernasconi and Valzelli (1973), as well as to us, that might yield a common mechanism for all of the 5-HT effects is that caffeine slows the rate of 5-HT release from the neuron by reducing firing rate. It would therefore be interesting to know, for example, if caffeine administration slows raphe unit firing.

One indirect approach to this issue that has been attempted is to study whether caffeine administration alters any physiologic functions or behaviors thought to be controlled in part by 5-HT neurons in brain. For example, Spindel et al. (1980) studied the effect of caffeine on growth hormone (GH) secretion. The release of GH by the pituitary is thought to be controlled in part by 5-HT neurons (See Martin 1976). Serotoninergic neurons are thought to impinge on cells in the hypothalamus that release either of two factors into the hypothalamic-pituitary blood supply. These factors interact with GH-secreting cells, either to stimulate (GH-releasing factor) or to suppress (somatostatin) GH secretion. Spindel et al. (1980) observed that the intraperitoneal administration of caffeine suppressed the pulsatile secretion of GH in rats for several hours. This effect on GH could be antagonized if the rats were also given an injection of antisomatostatin serum. This result fits with the notion that caffeine turns off 5-HT neurons, inasmuch as other data suggest that when 5-HT is released by neurons, somatostatin secretion is suppressed (see Arnold and Fernstrom 1980).

2.2 Catecholamines

Caffeine has frequently been studied for its effects on catecholamine neurons in brain. Early reports by Berkowitz et al. (1970) indicated that caffeine injection enhances norepinephrine (NE) synthesis and turnover. The increase in turnover suggested to these investigators that caffeine enhanced NE release from nerve terminals. Using similar paradigms, other groups obtained findings with caffeine and other methylxanthines that were compatible with this view [Waldeck 1971; Corrodi et al. 1972; Goldberg et al. 1982; though Waldeck reported in a later paper (1974) either a rise or no change in catecholamine synthesis rate, depending on the method employed, no clear explanation for the differences being offered]. Grant and Redmond (1982) studied the effect of another methylxanthine, isobutylmethylxanthine (IBMX), on the spontaneous firing rate of neurons in the locus ceruleus, a major site of NE cell bodies in the brain. [IBMX and caffeine may have the common feature of blocking adenosine receptors (see below; Daly et al. 1981; Snyder et al. 1981).] Grant and Redmond observed that IBMX increased firing rate, an effect that could be blocked with clonidine. In related studies, Galloway and Roth (1982, 1983) demonstrated that IBMX also elevated the in vivo rate of tyrosine hydroxylation, and methoxyhydroxyphenylethyleneglycol (MHPG) levels in several brain regions containing terminal projections of locus ceruleus cells. These biochemical results suggest to neuropharmacologists that methylxanthines may increase the firing rate of NE-containing neurons in brain, thereby leading to increases in both NE synthesis and turnover. They are thus consistent with this same notion put forth by Berkowitz et al. (1970) over 10 years ago.

The mechanism by which caffeine stimulates NE neurons in brain is unknown. One hypothesis currently popular is that the methylxanthine acts by blocking an adenosine receptor, perhaps located on NE neurons. [Adenosine may be a neurotransmitter or neuromodulator in the central nervous system (Daly et al. 1981).] Presumably, stimulation of the adenosine receptor inhibits the activity of NE neurons. Inasmuch as caffeine and related methylxanthines act as antagonists at these receptors (e.g., Daly et al. 1981; Snyder et al. 1981), their administration should block such inhibitory receptors and thereby increase neuronal activity. Like some other receptors (e.g., the beta-adrenergic receptor; see Cooper et al. 1982), stimulation or blockade of an adenosine receptor appears to be translated within the cell into changes in cyclic 3',5'-adenosine monophosphate (cAMP) production. The change in cAMP formation is believed to mediate the observed cellular responses (see Daly et al. 1981). A second, equally plausible hypothesis is that these compounds exert their effects via another cAMP-linked phenomenon, inhibition of phosphodiesterase. That is, caffeine and related compounds may stimulate NE neurons in brain by

110

inhibiting the phosphodiesterase within them, such that the catabolism of cAMP might be reduced and cAMP levels therefore increased (see Cooper et al. 1982). This might lead to enhanced responsiveness of these neurons. According to Daly et al. (1981), however, behavioral effects of caffeine and theophylline occur at doses too small to inhibit phosphodiesterase. Hence, these authors favor the view that these actions are probably related to occupancy of an adenosine receptor, not inhibition of phosphodiesterase. Of course, both mechanisms are at present still speculative, and others are possible. However, a mechanism involving some connection with cAMP production seems likely, inasmuch as a good deal of other data exist that the cAMP production to the state of activation of tyrosine hydroxylase and the rate of catecholamine synthesis in brain (e. e., Harris et al. 1974).

Unfortunately, few data are available concerning the consequences to brain function of a caffeine-induced increase in NE release. Immediately postsynaptically, caffeine has been noted to cause beta- (but not alpha-) receptor density to decrease somewhat (Goldberg et al. 1982). This result is compatible with the view that downregulation of the receptor population has occurred in the face of increased transmitter release (Goldberg et al. 1982). A similar effect has been noted with another methylxanthine, pentoxyfylline (Lowenstein et al. 1982). But by and large, the most convincing postsynaptic effects of caffeine have been studied in relation to the sympathetic nervous system function; they are discussed below.

Dopamine (DA) synthesis in brain is also influenced by the administration of caffeine and other methylxanthines. Injection of caffeine is reputed to cause an acute (30-min) increase in the rate of DA formation in vivo (Waldeck 1971); theophylline has a similar effect in vitro (Gysling and Bustos 1977). However, the increase is thought to be followed rapidly by a decrease in the rate of DA formation (measured over a 4-h period following caffeine injection; Corrodi et al. 1972). The reduction in DA synthesis is thought by some to occur in conjunction with a reduction in DA turnover (Paalzow and Paalzow 1974) and release (Corrodi et al. 1972). Some psychopharmacologic data support the view that DA release has been reduced. For example, caffeine was found to antagonize the amphetamine-induced increase in turning behavior exhibited by rats with unilateral lesions of the nigrostriatal tract (Corrodi et al. 1972). Since amphetamine is believed (among other things) to stimulate DA neurons to release their transmitter, antagonism of turning behavior by caffeine could be interpreted as indirect evidence that the xanthine somehow decreased DA neuron activity (Corrodi et al. 1972). Consistent with this interpretation was the finding by the same investigators that caffeine administration did not block the effect of a direct-acting (and presumably postsynaptic) DA receptor agonist on turning behavior.

However, total agreement is lacking as to caffeine's effect on the DA neuron in brain. Caffeine injection usually increases locomotor activity (LMA) at reasonable doses (Waldeck 1973; White et al. 1978; Estler 1979), an effect that is said to be blocked by pimozide, a DA receptor antagonist (Waldeck 1973; Estler 1979). This finding would tend to suggest that caffeine increases, not decreases, DA release. Also, caffeine has no effect on serum prolactin levels, even at quite high doses (Spindel et al. 1980). Since some DA neurons in brain are in part responsible for controlling prolactin secretion, this latter result suggests that the methylxanthine has no influence on the release of DA from some neurons in brain.

Another approach to studying the effect of caffeine on DA neurotransmission bypasses these disparate effects on the DA neuron itself and looks instead for post-synaptic effects of the compound on DA receptor "sensitivity." Such studies have generally been psychopharmacologic in nature. For example, Waldeck (1973) reported that in animals given combined treatment with reserpine and alpha-methyl-paratyrosine (AMPT) to deplete neurons of their catecholamines and to block further synthesis, caffeine enhanced the increase in LMA produced by an injection of clonidine and ET-495 (direct-acting NE and DA agonists respectively). Since these compounds are agonists (the clonidine dose was high, and thus probably acted both pre- and postsynaptically), any effect of caffeine was presumably mediated postsynaptically. In this case, the investigator concluded that caffeine enhanced receptor sensitivity and suggested phosphodiesterase inhibition (and increased cAMP levels) as a possible mechanism. Of course, this study, by its very design, could not distinguish NE from DA effects; the drugs employed acted on both DA and NE neurons. Besides, one should be suspicious of studies in which more than one or two drugs were administered to the same animal (in this case, *five* were ultimately given to each animal!). Fuxe and Ungerstedt (1974) conducted experiments similar in design, but using animals with unilateral lesions of the nigrostriatal tract. Such animals constitute a well-characterized behavioral model for the study of DA receptors in situ (see Cooper et al. 1982). Fuxe and Ungerstedt observed that caffeine administration would increase the turning behavior elicited by a minimally effective dose of *L*-dopa or by combined treatment with apomorphine and ET-495 (both compounds are direct-acting DA receptor agonists). Like Waldeck, these investigators concluded that caffeine acted postsynaptically, perhaps via cAMP changes, to enhance DA receptor sensitivity. They also suggested that the biochemical effects obtained by Corrodi et al. (1972) could be interpreted in this context, since one consequence of increased DA receptor sensitivity should be increased feedback inhibition of DA synthesis. Other investigators, using similar behavioral paradigms, have also obtained data consistent with a change in DA receptor responsiveness following caffeine administration (e.g., Anden and Jackson 1975; Stricker et al. 1977; Wanatabe et al. 1981; Joyce and Koob 1981).

While this review focuses principally on the monoamines, it should be noted that caffeine and other methylxanthines may influence the activities of brain neurons utilizing other transmitters. For example, a limited number of studies show methylxanthine effects in GABA (e.g. Sytinskii and Priyatkina 1966; Scholfield 1982), on the ability of drugs to influence acetylcholine release (Jhamandas et al. 1978), and on the central nervous system actions of benzodiazepines (e.g., Marangos et al. 1979; Polc et al. 1981). Perhaps future studies will show these foci of methylxanthine action to be important in mediating some or all of the central nervous system effects of caffeine.

3 Effects on Catecholamines in the Peripheral Nervous System

Caffeine and other methylxanthines influences catecholamine neurons in the peripheral as well as the central nervous system. In particular, caffeine (and/or coffee) administration has been noted to increase blood (Robertson et al. 1978) and urinary

(Levi 1967; Bellet et al. 1969) levels of epinephrine and norepinephrine in man. Theophylline and aminophylline are reputed to have qualitatively similar effects to caffeine (Atuk et al. 1967; Higbee et al. 1982; Vestal et al. 1983). Such results suggest that caffeine stimulates the release of catecholamines from both the adrenal gland and sympathetic nerves. Studies in animals provide support for this notion, showing that epinephrine is released directly from the adrenal gland following treatment with caffeine or closely-related methylxanthines (e. g., DeSchaepdryver 1959; Berkowitz and Spector 1971 b; Peach 1972; Poisner 1973 a,b) and that caffeine can influence a variety of variables consistent with an increase in sympathetic function [e. g., it can enhance transmission through sympathetic ganglion in vitro (Skok et al. 1978), and theophylline, a closely related methylxanthine, can enhance (a) the stimulation-induced release of NE and dopamine beta-hydroxylase from the hypogastric nerve in vitro (Wooten et al. 1973), and (b) the release of NE from an in vitro kidney preparation (Hedqvist et al. 1978)]. Of course, part of the mechanism by which caffeine stimulates epinephrine release by the adrenal may involve stimulation of the sympathetic nerves to the adrenal medulla, with a resultant increase in tyrosine hydroxylase activity and catecholamine synthesis (Snider and Waldeck 1974). However, more data are needed to determine the extent to which each site of caffeine action contributes to the overall rise in adrenal catecholamine release.

Two questions (at least) arise from the finding that caffeine increases the release of sympathetic catecholamines. First, are there predictable consequences of caffeine administration to body functions normally influenced by the release of catecholamines in the periphery? And second, what is the mechanism by which caffeine has these effects?

Predictable consequences of an increase in sympathetic activation and catecholamine release should include increased gluconeogenesis, lipolysis, and metabolic rate, increased cardiac function, and enhanced secretory rates for such compounds as renin. In fact, such changes have been documented following caffeine administration. For example, caffeine has been shown to increase metabolic rate in man (Acheson et al. 1980) and rats (Strubelt and Siegers 1969). A portion of the effect in rats has been tied to the release of catecholamines (Strubelt and Siegers 1969; Lin et al. 1980). Caffeine also elevates serum levels of glucose (Strubelt 1969) and nonesterified fatty acids (Bellet et al. 1968). The glucose effect also appears to be related to the increased release of catecholamines induced by caffeine (Strubelt 1969). Acute caffeine administration is also known to have positive inotropic and chronotropic effects on the heart (e. g., DeGubareff and Sleator 1965; Robertson et al. 1978), to elevate blood pressure (Robertson et al. 1978), and to stimulate the release of renin (Robertson et al. 1978). Similar effects are reported following administration of other methylxanthines (e. g., Vestal et al. 1983).

Caffeine may cause these peripheral effects *directly,* by some action on the end organ itself, *indirectly,* via the release of catecholamine and its interaction with end organs (e. g., such as for the glucose and metabolic rate effects noted above), or by some *combination* of these two mechanisms. Regardless, the methylxanthine must somehow elicit a cellular response, be it on a sympathetic neuron or on some end organ cell. It may have this effect by acting

1. on or within cells via adenosine receptors (whether neurons releasing catecholamines or acetylcholine, or effector cells directly);
2. within cells via phosphodiesterase inhibition;
3. by some combination of the above; or
4. by other, as yet unknown mechanisms.

At best, only incomplete information is available for some of the actions of methylxanthines. For example, methylxanthines may increase sympathetic nerve activity by blocking adenosine receptors. Nerve activity presumably increases, because the effects of an inhibitory compound (adenosine) are thereby blocked (e. g., see Hedqvist and Fredholm 1976; Hedqvist et al. 1978). In at least one study (Hedqvist et al. 1978), such effects of methylxanthines were shown *not* to be related to inhibition of phosphodiesterase activity, thereby reducing the likely importance of this mechanisms, and increasing the likelihood that an adenosine receptor is involved. As another example, a significant literature exists concerning direct effects of methylxanthines on adipocyte lipolysis. One currently popular view is that methylxanthines stimulate lipolysis by reversing the inhibition of adenyl cyclase caused by endogenous adenosine (interacting with a so-called P adenosine receptor, presumed to be intracellular: see Londos et al. 1978; Daly et al. 1981). The increased production of cAMP resulting from this effect would promote lipolysis. However, this view is not compatible with all available data, and alternative possibilities have been expressed (see Fain et al. 1979).

Beyond these and a few other examples, the *mechanisms* by which caffeine interacts with particular postsynaptic cells are either not studied or incompletely understood. However, it is at least clear from limited data that caffeine effects on certain cells *are present,* and in certain cases they may be mediated by adenosine receptors. The existing data suggest the possible fruitfulness of further investigation. For example, though the blood pressure and cardiac effects of caffeine may in part follow from the sympathetic effects, available data suggest that they may also in part be the consequence of direct actions of caffeine on blood vessels (e. g., see Hedqvist et al. 1978; Scholtholt et al. 1972) and the heart (e. g., to increase sinoatrial node depolarization rate; Chiba et al. 1972). It would be interesting to know whether these effects of caffeine are mediated via an adenosine receptor on the relevant cell types, or by some other mechanism. In addition other data are available which indicate that the gut is differentially responsive to the direct application of adenosine and methylxanthines. The results generally support direct postsynaptic actions of the methylxanthines on this tissue, and suggest them to be mediated by adenosine receptors (e. g., Ally and Nakatsu 1976). Again, however, additional data are required to establish rigorously whether or not the methylxanthines act on this end organ via an adenosine receptor.

Regardless of the ultimate mechanisms shown to account for their end organ effects in the periphery, it appears that methylxanthines such as caffeine exert such effects via *combined* actions on the sympathetic nervous system and the release of catecholamines and on the end organs themselves.

Finally, while not the focus of this review, it should be noted that caffeine can also influence cholinergic neurotransmission in the peripheral nervous system. It may affect both acetylcholine release onto muscle (e. g., Hofmann 1969; Elmquist and

Feldman 1965) and the properties of contraction within the muscle itself (Varagic and Zugic 1971; Cohen et al. 1970). Acetylcholine release by methylxanthines may also be mediated via an action on an adenosine receptor, as discussed above for other transmitters (Sawynok and Jhamandas 1976), though other possibilities cannot at present be excluded.

References

Acheson KJ, Zahorska-Markiewicz B, Pittet P, Anantharaman K, Jequire E (1980) Caffeine and coffee: their influence on metabolic rate and substrate utilization in normal weight and obese individuals. Am J Clin Nutr 33: 989–997

Ally AI, Nakatsu K (1976) Adenosine inhibition of isolated rabbit ileum and antagonism by theophylline. J Pharmacol Exp Ther 199: 208–215

Anden NE, Jackson DM (1975) Locomotor activity stimulation in rats produced by dopamine in the nucleus accumbens: potentiation by caffeine. J Pharm Pharmacol 27: 666–670

Arnold MA, Fernstrom JD (1980) Administration of antisomatostatin serum to rats reverses the inhibition of pulsatile growth hormone secretion produced by an injection of metergoline, but not yohimbine. Neuroendocrinology 31: 194–199

Atuk, NO, Blaydes MC, Westervelt FB, Wood JE (1967) Effect of aminophylline on urinary excretion of epinephrine and norepinephrine in man. Circulation 35: 745–753

Bellet S, Kershbaum A, Finck EM (1968) Response of free fatty acids to coffee and caffeine. Metabolism 17: 702–707

Bellet S, Roman L, DeCastro O, Kim KE, Kershbaum A (1969) Effect of coffee ingestion on catecholamine release. Metabolism 18: 288–291

Bellin JS, Sorrentino GM (1974) Activation of brain monoamine oxidase by some CNS depressants. Res Commun Chem Pathol Pharmacol 9: 673–680

Berkowitz BA, Spector S (1971a) The effect of caffeine and theophylline on the disposition of brain serotonin in the rat. Eur J Pharmacol 16: 322–325

Berkowitz BA, Spector S (1971b) Effect of caffeine and theophylline on peripheral catecholamines. Eur J Pharmacol 13: 193–196

Berkowitz BA, Spector S (1973) The role of brain serotonin in the pharmacologic effects of the methyl xanthines. In: Barchas JD, Usdin E (eds) Serotonin and behavior. Academic, New York, pp 137–147

Berkowitz BA, Tarver JH, Spector S (1970) Release of norepinephrine in the central nervous system by theophylline and caffeine. Eur J Pharmacol 10: 64–71

Carlsson A, Lindqvist M (1978) Dependence of 5-HT and catecholamine synthesis on concentrations of precursor amino acids in rat brain. Naunyn Schmiedebergs Arch Pharmacol 303: 157–164

Chiba S, Hashimoto K, Hashimoto K (1972) Pharmacological analysis of chromatographic responses of the S-A node to caffeine. Eur J Pharmacol 18: 116–120

Cohen Y, Lesne M, Valette G, Wepierre J (1970) Etude de l'interaction entre les xanthines et la noradrenaline ³H, au niveau du coeur isolé de rat. Biochem Pharmacol 19: 2117–2124

Cooper JR, Bloom FE, Roth RH (1982) The biochemical basis of neuropharmacology, 4th edn. Oxford, New York

Corrodi H, Fuxe K, Jonsson G (1972) Effects of caffeine on central monoamine neurons. J Pharm Pharmacol 24: 155–158

Curzon G, Fernando JCR (1976) Effect of aminophylline on tryptophan and other aromatic amino acids in plasma, brain, and other tissues, and on brain 5-hydroxytryptamine metabolism. Br J Pharmacol 58: 533–545

Daly JW, Bruns RF, Snyder SH (1981) Adenosine receptors in the central nervous system: relationship to the central action of methylxanthines. Life Sci 28: 2083–2097

DeGubareff T, Sleator W (1965) Effects of caffeine on mammalian atrial muscle and its interaction with adenosine and calcium. J Pharmacol Exp Ther 148: 202–214

DeSchaepdryver AF (1959) Physio-pharmacological effects on suprarenal secretion of adrenaline and noradrenaline in dogs. Arch Int Pharmacodyn 119: 517–518

Elmquist D, Feldman DS (1965) Calcium dependence of spontaneous acetylcholine release at mammalian motor nerve terminals. J Physiol (Lond) 181: 487–497

Estler CJ (1979) Influence of pimozide on the locomotor hyperactivity produced by caffeine. J Pharm Pharmacol 31: 126–127

Fain JN, Li SY, Moreno FJ (1979) Regulation of cyclic AMP metabolism and lipolysis in isolated rat fat cells by insulin. N^6-(phenylisopropyl)adenosine and 2′,5′-dideoxyadenosine. J Cyclic Nucleotide Res 5: 189–196

Fernstrom MH, Bazil CW, Fernstrom JD (to be published) Lack of effect of caffeine injection on serotonin synthesis rate in rat brain.

Fuxe K, Ungerstedt U (1974) Action of caffeine and theophylline on supersensitive dopamine receptors: considerable enhancement of receptor response to treatment with dopa and dopamine receptor agonists. Med Biol 52: 48–54

Galloway MP, Roth RH (1982) Clonidine prevents methylxanthine stimulation of norepinephrine metabolism. Trans Am Soc Neurochem 13: 392

Galloway MP, Roth RH (1983) Clonidine prevents methylxanthine stimulation of norepinephrine metabolism in rat brain. J Neurochem 40: 246–251

Geyer MA, Dawsey WJ, Mandell AJ (1975) Differential effects of caffeine, d-amphetamine, and methylphenidate on individual raphe cell fluorescence: a microspectrofluorimetric demonstration. Brain Res 85: 135–139

Galzigna L, Maina G, Rumney G (1971) Role of L-ascorbic acid in the reversal of the monoamine oxidase inhibition by caffeine. J Pharm Pharmacol 23: 303–305

Goldberg MR, Curatolo PW, Tung CS, Robertson D (1982) Caffeine down-regulates beta adrenoreceptors in rat forebrain. Neurosci Lett 31: 47–52

Grant SJ, Redmond DE (1982) Methylxanthine activation of noradrenergic unit activity and reversal by clonidine. Eur J Pharmacol 85: 105–109

Gysling K, Bustos G (1977) Effect of ethanol on dibutyryl cyclic adenosine monophosphate- and theophylline-induced stimulation of dopamine biosynthesis by rat striatal slices. Biochem Pharmacol 26: 559–562

Harris JE, Morgenroth VH, Roth RH, Baldessarini RJ (1974) Regulation of catecholamine biosynthesis in the rat brain in vitro by cyclic AMP. Nature 252: 156–158

Hedqvist P, Fredholm BB (1976) Effects of adenosine on adrenal neurotransmission: prejunctional inhibition and post-junctional enhancement. Naunyn Schmiedebergs Arch Pharmacol 293: 217–223

Hedqvist P, Fredholm BB, Olundh S (1978) Antagonistic effect of theophylline and adenosine on adrenergic neuroeffector transmission in the rabbit kidney. Circ Res 43: 592–598

Higbee MD, Kumar M, Galant SP (1982) Stimulation of endogenous catecholamine release by theophylline: a proposed additional mechanism of action for theophylline effects. J Allergy Clin Immunol 70: 377–382

Hofmann WW (1969) Caffeine effects on transmitter depletion and mobilization at motor nerve terminals. Am J Physiol 216: 621–629

Jhamandas K, Sawynok J, Sutak M (1978) Antagonism of morphine action on brain acetylcholine release by methylxanthines and calcium. Eur J Pharmacol 49: 309–312

Joyce EM, Koob GF (1981) Amphetamine-, scopolamine-, and caffeine-induced locomotor activity following 6-hydroxydopamine lesions of the mesolimbic dopamine system. Psychopharmacology (Berlin) 73: 311–313

Karasawa T, Furakawa K, Yoshida K, Shimizu M (1976) Effect of theophylline on monoamine metabolism in the rat brain. Eur J Pharmacol 37: 97–104

Levi L (1967) The effect of coffee on the function of the sympathoadrenomedullary system in man. Acta Med Scand 181: 431–438

Lin MT, Chandra A, Liu GG (1980) The effects of theophylline and caffeine on thermoregulatory functions of rats at different ambient temperatures. J Pharm Pharmacol 32: 204–208

Londos C, Cooper DMF, Schlegel W, Rodbell M (1978) Adenosine analogs inhibit adipocyte adenylate cyclase by a GTP-dependent process: basis for actions of adenosine and methylxanthines on cyclic AMP production and lipolysis. Proc Natl Acad Sci USA 75: 5362–5366

Lowenstein PR, Vacas MI, Cardinali DP (1982) Effect of pentoxifylline on alpha- and beta-adrenoceptor sites in cerebral cortex, medial basal hypothalamus, and pineal gland of the rat. Neuropharmacology 21: 243–248

116

Marangos PJ, Paul SM, Parma AM, Goodwin FK, Syapin P, Skolnick P (1979) Purinergic inhibition of diazepam binding to rat brain (in vitro). Life Sci 24: 851–858

Martin JB (1976) Brain regulation of growth hormone secretion. In: Martini L, Ganong WF (eds) Frontiers in neuroendocrineology, vol 4. Raven, New York, pp 129–168

Paalzow G, Paalzow L (1974) Theophylline increased sensitivity to nociceptive stimulation and regional turnover of rat brain 5-HT, noradrenaline and dopamine. Acta Pharmacol Toxicol (Copenh) 34: 157–173

Peach MJ (1972) Stimulation of release of adrenal catecholamine by adenosine 3':5'-cyclic monophosphate and theophylline in the absence of extracellular Ca^{2+}. Proc Natl Acad Sci USA 69: 834–836

Poisner AM (1973a) Caffeine-induced catecholamine secretion: similarity to caffeine-induced muscle contraction. Proc Soc Exp Biol Med 142: 103–105

Poisner AM (1973b) Direct stimulant effect of aminophylline on catecholamine release from the adrenal medulla. Biochem Pharmacol 22: 469–476

Polc P, Bonetti EP, Pieri L, Cumin R, Angioi RM, Mohler H, Haefely WE (1981) Caffeine antagonizes several central effects of diazepam. Life Sci 28: 2265–2275

Robertson D, Frolich JC, Carr K, Watson JT, Hollifield JW, Shand DG, Oates JA (1978) Effects of caffeine on plasma renin activity, catecholamines and blood pressure. N Engl J Med 298: 181–186

Sakata T, Fuchimoto H, Kodama J, Fukushima M (1975) Changes of brain serotonin and muricide behavior following chronic administration of theophylline in rats. Physiol Behav 15: 449–453

Sawynok J, Jhamandas KH (1976) Inhibition of acetylcholine release from cholinergic nerves by adenosine, adenine nucleotides, and morphine: antagonism by theophylline. J Pharmacol Exp Ther 197: 379–390

Schlosberg AJ, Fernstrom JD, Kopczynski MC, Cusack BM, Gillis MA (1981) Acute effects of caffeine injection on neutral amino acids and brain monoamine levels in rats. Life Sci 29: 173–183

Scholfield CN (1982) Antagonism of gamma-aminobutyric acid and muscimol by picrotoxin bicuculline, strychnine, bemegride, leptazol, D-tubocurarine and theophylline in the isolated olfactory cortex. Naunyn Schmiedebergs Arch Pharmacol 318: 274–280

Scholtholt J, Nitz RE, Schraven E (1972) On the mechanism of the antagonistic action of xanthine derivatives against adenosine and coronary vasodilators. Arzneimittelforsch 22: 1255–1259

Skok VI, Storch NN, Nishi S (1978) The effect of caffeine on the neurons of a mammalian sympathetic ganglion. Neuroscience 3: 697–708

Snider SR, Waldeck B (1974) Increased synthesis of adrenomedullary catecholamines induced by caffeine and theophylline. Naunyn Schmiedebergs Arch Pharmacol 281: 257–260

Snyder SH, Katims JJ, Annau Z, Bruns RF, Daly JW (1981) Adenosine receptors and behavioral actions of methylxanthines. Proc Natl Acad Sci USA 78: 3260–3264

Spindel E, Arnold M, Cusack B, Wurtman RJ (1980) Effects of caffeine on anterior pituitary and thyroid function in the rat. J Pharmacol Exp Ther 214: 58–62

Stricker EM, Zimmerman MB, Friedman MI, Zigmond MJ (1977) Caffeine restores feeding response to 2-deoxy-D-glucose in 6-hydroxydopamine-treated rats. Nature 267: 174–175

Strubelt O (1969) The influence of reserpine, propranolol, and adrenal medullectomy on the hyperglycemic actions of theophylline and caffeine. Arch Int Pharmacodyn 179: 215–224

Strubelt O, Siegers CP (1969) Zum Mechanismus der kalorigenen Wirkung von Theophyllin und Coffein. Biochem Pharmacol 18: 1207–1220

Sytinskii IA, Priyatkina TN (1966) Effect of certain drugs on the gamma-amino-butyric acid system of the central nervous system. Biochem Pharmacol 15: 49–54

Valzelli L, Bernasconi S (1973) Behavioral and neurochemical effects of caffeine in normal and aggressive mice. Pharmacol Biochem Behav 1: 251–254

Varagic VM, Zugic M (1971) Interactions of xanthine derivatives, catecholamines and glucose-6-phosphate on the isolated phrenic nerve diaphragm preparation of the rat. Pharmacology 5: 275–286

Vestal RE, Eiriksson CE, Musser B, Ozaki LK, Halter JB (1983) Effect of intravenous aminophylline on plasma levels of catecholamines and related cardiovascular and metabolic responses in man. Circulation 67: 162–171

Waldeck B (1971) Some effects of caffeine aminophylline on the turnover of catecholamines in the brain. J Pharm Pharmacol 23: 824–830

Waldeck B (1973) Sensitization by caffeine of central catecholamine receptors. J Neural Transm 34: 61–72

Waldeck B (1974) Ethanol and caffeine: a complex interaction with respect to locomotor activity and central catecholamines. Psychopharmacologia (Berlin) 36: 209–220

Wanatabe H, Ikeda M, Wanatabe K (1981) Properties of rotational behavior produced by methyl-xanthine derivatives in mice with unilateral striatal 6-hydroxydopamine-induced lesions. J Pharmacobiodyn 4: 301–307

White BC, Simpson CC, Adams JE, Harkins D (1978) Monoamine synthesis and caffeine-induced locomotor activity. Neuropharmacology 17: 511–513

Wooten GF, Thoa, NB, Kopin IJ, Axelrod J (1973) Enhanced release of dopamine beta-hydroxylase and norepinephrine from sympathetic nerves by dibutyryl cyclic adenosine 3′,5′-monophosphate and theophylline. Mol Pharmacol 9: 178–183

VIII Neuroendocrine Effects of Caffeine in Rat and Man*

E. R. Spindel and R. J. Wurtman

odify the biochemical composition of the brain or otherwise af-
sion can, as a consequence, alter one or more of the brain's three
behavior; hormone secretion from neuroendocrine organs; and
ed by autonomic nerves (e. g., cardiac rhythm). Caffeine adminis-
levels and turnover rates of catecholamines (Berkowitz and Spec-
rg et al. 1981) and serotonin (Fernstrom and Fernstrom, this vol-
NS and may also interrupt adenosine-mediated neurotransmis-
feine's brain effects are known to lead to the cardiovascular and
that are summarized in this volume by Robertson and Curatolo
p. 86) respectively. This chapter considers the evidence that caf-
ı can affect the brain's third output channel, neuroendocrine secretion, in experimental animals and in human subjects.

As described below, when rats are given very high caffeine doses (i. e., greater than 20 mg/kg, which is equivalent, for humans, to the amount that would be contained in 15 or more cups of coffee ingested at a time), profound neuroendocrine changes occur, causing the pattern of blood hormone levels to resemble that seen in stress [i. e., decreased thyrotropin (TSH), decreased growth hormone (GH), increased corticosterone and β-endorphin]. However, lower doses fail to affect the hormones. Studies on human subjects yield observations that correlate well with the findings in rats: low caffeine doses (equivalent to the amounts present in two to three cups of coffee) have no discernable effects on pituitary or "target organ" hormones, while higher doses can cause a stress-like stimulation of the pituitary-adrenal axis (Spindel et al., to be published).

2 Studies on Experimental Animals

Caffeine injected intraperitoneally into rats decreases serum levels of TSH and increases those of corticosterone, with 30–50 mg/kg doses needed to produce half maximal effects (Fig. 1). This ED_{50} is associated with peak serum caffeine levels

* Some of these studies were supported in part by grants from the International Life Sciences Institute

greater than 20 µg/ml; doses that do not elevate serum caffeine above 15 µg/ml fail to affect serum levels of either hormone (Spindel et al. 1980). Costa et al. (1977) and Sullivan et al. (1978) have similarly reported that caffeine increases corticosterone secretion in rodents. DePasquale et al. (1979) have suggested that this effect may be mediated by prostaglandins, since it could be blocked by indomethacin.

The effect of caffeine on TSH secretion is independent of the corticosterone response, inasmuch as it persists in adrenalectomized rats (Fig. 1; Spindel et al. 1983). This is in accord with the hypothesis that high caffeine doses produce a stress-like pattern of endocrine responses, since adrenalectomy also fails to block the decreases in serum TSH caused by other experimental stresses (Kraicer et al. 1963). Caffeine administration (and other stressors) also releases β-endorphin from the anterior pituitary into the serum (Arnold et al. 1982). This release of β-endorphin suggests that caffeine's effect on serum corticosterone is indirect and mediated through the secretion of pituitary adrenocorticotropin (ACTH), since β-endorphin and ACTH share a common peptide precursor and tend to be secreted together.

High doses of caffeine also inhibit the pulsatile secretion of GH from the rat's pituitary (Fig. 2). This effect lasts for several hours (similar to the time courses of caffeine's effects on TSH and corticosterone), a duration consistent with caffeins's serum half-life of 3–5 h (Aldridge et al. 1977). Caffeine's ED_{50} for inhibition of GH secretion is 30–50 mg/kg, the same as for suppression of TSH and stimulation of corticosterone secretion. The complete suppression of the pulsatile increases in serum GH levels that can be obtained with sufficient caffeine doses suggests that caffeine works by inhibiting the hormone's secretion, and not, for example, by accelerating its catabolism.

Rate characteristically suppress pulsatile GH release in response to stress (Rice and Critchlow 1976), and this suppression is thought to be mediated by the release of hypothalamic somatostatin (Terry et al. 1976). The mechanism by which caffeine inhibits GH secretion probably also involves stimulation of somatostatin release, inasmuch as passive immunization of rats with an antisomatostatin antiserum blocks caffeine's ability to inhibit hormone secretion (Spindel et al. 1980).

The effects of caffeine on the pattern of hormones present in rat serum deviate from the typical pattern engendered by stress only in that unlike stress (Mueller et al. 1976), high caffeine doses apparently do not elevate serum prolactin levels in male or female rats (Fig. 3; Spindel et al. 1980; Arnold et al. 1982). Interestingly, am-

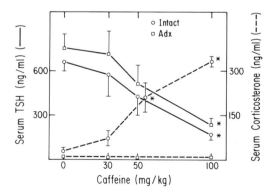

Fig. 1. Effect of caffeine on serum TSH and corticosterone levels in intact and adrenalectomized rats. Rats were killed 2 h after i.p. injection of caffeine at the dose shown. Each group contained six or seven animals. Data here and in other figures are expressed as mean ± SEM
* $P < 0.05$ compared to saline-treated group of the same adrenal status (Newman-Keuls test)

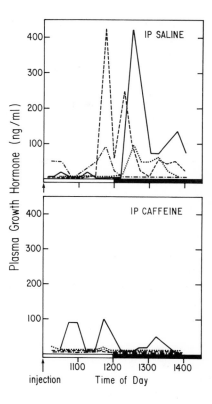

Fig. 2. Plasma GH profiles of four rats given saline or caffeine (80 mg/kg i. p., 2 days apart)

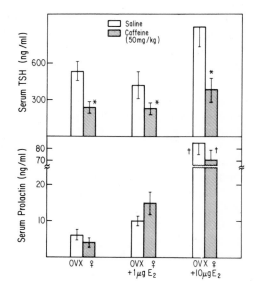

Fig. 3. Effect of caffeine on serum prolactin and TSH levels in ovariectomized female rats with (♀) or without *(DVX)* estrogen pretreatment. Rats were killed 2 h after i. p. injection of caffeine (50 mg/kg) or saline. Animals were also injected s. c. with sesame oil or estradiol benzoate *(E₂)* at the dose shown for 10 days. Each group contained seven or eight animals. * $P < 0.01$ for caffeine effect (two-way analysis of variance); † $P < 0.05$ compared to non-estradiol-treated rats (Newman-Keuls test)

121

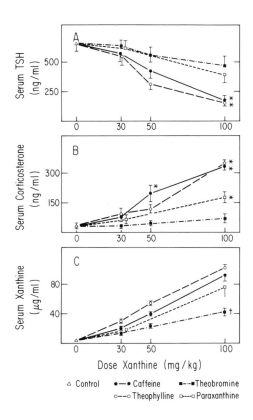

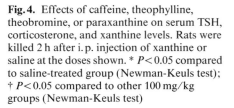

Fig. 4. Effects of caffeine, theophylline, theobromine, or paraxanthine on serum TSH, corticosterone, and xanthine levels. Rats were killed 2 h after i. p. injection of xanthine or saline at the doses shown. * $P < 0.05$ compared to saline-treated group (Newman-Keuls test); † $P < 0.05$ compared to other 100 mg/kg groups (Newman-Keuls test)

phetamine shares caffeine's effect on serum levels of TSH (Spindel et al. 1978, GH, and corticosterone (Cohen et al. 1981; Knych and Eisenberg 1979), and also fails to stimulate prolactin secretion (Ravitz and Moore 1977; Clemens and Fuller 1979). Perhaps these agents activate only part of the final common pathway that mediates endocrine stress responses.

The methylxanthines theophylline, theobromine, and paraxanthine have endocrine effects similar to those of caffeine, decreasing serum TSH and increasing serum corticosterone levels (Fig. 4; Spindel et al. 1983). Theophylline is equipotent with caffeine in producing these neuroendocrine changes, while theobromine and paraxanthine are less potent, perhaps because their peak serum levels after a given parenteral dose tend to be lower than peak levels after equivalent doses of caffeine or theophylline (Fig. 4). The relatively poor neuroendocrine potency of theobromine compared with caffeine also correlates with its 40-fold poorer solubility in water. Rats metabolize caffeine to theobromine, paraxanthine, 1,3,7-trimethyluric acid, and 4-amino-5[N-methylformylamino]-1,3-dimethyluracil (ADMU; Arnaud 1976a, b; Latini 1981). In contrast, man produces little theobromine or ADMU from caffeine, making instead relatively more paraxanthine, 1-methylxanthine, and 1-methyluric acid (Cornish and Christman 1957; Latini 1981; Tang-Liu et al. 1983). The low potencies of theobromine and paraxanthine make it unlikely that either of these metabolites mediated caffeine's endocrine effects.

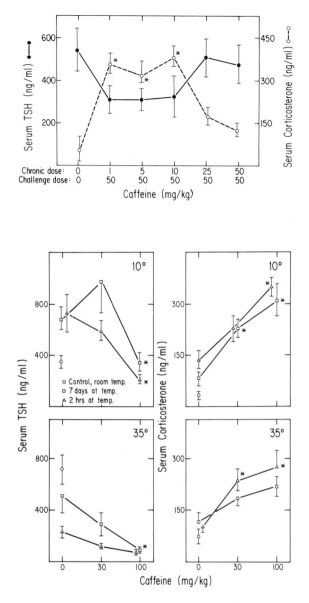

Fig. 5. Determination of the lowest dose of caffeine needed to produce neuroendocrine tolerance. Serum TSH and corticosterone levels were determined 2 h after i. p. injection of 50 mg/kg caffeine or saline. Rats had previously received 13 daily i. p. injections of caffeine at the doses shown. Each group contained seven or eight animals. * *P*<0.05 compared to saline-only controls (Newman-Keuls test)

Fig. 6. Effect of ambient temperature on caffeine-induced changes in serum TSH and corticosterone levels. Rats were killed 2 h after i. p. injection of caffeine or saline at the doses shown. The animals were acclimated for days 7 (□) or 2 h (△) at the temperature indicated before caffeine injection. * *P*<0.05 compared to corresponding saline-treated group (Newman-Keuls test)

Rats develop tolerance to the endocrine effects of caffeine within 2 weeks. The lowest dose of caffeine to induce tolerance is 25 mg/kg (Fig. 5). This tolerance is similar to the tolerance described for caffeine's cardiovascular effects (Robertson et al. 1981), its diuretic effects (Eddy and Downs 1928), and its effects on sleep (Colton et al. 1968; Goldstein et al. 1969). Caffeine is metabolized by the 3-methylcholan-threne-inducible cytochrome P-450 enzyme system (Aldridge et al. 1977). Tolerant rats, however, do not clear serum caffeine more rapidly.

Caffeine's neuroendocrine effects can be distinguished from those on body temperature. Caffeine, like amphetamine (Yehuda and Wurtman 1972; Moskowitz et al. 1977), produces hypothermia at low ambient temperatures; in warm environments, however, caffeine's effects differ from those of amphetamine, since it fails to elevate body temperature. Caffeine's effects on TSH are independent of body temperature and are simply additive to whatever changes in TSH secretion might be caused by the ambient temperature itself (Fig. 6). The interactions of caffeine and ambient temperature in modifying pituitary TSH secretion probably represent the summation of excitatory (e. g., cold) and inhibitory (e. g., warmth or caffeine) influences on brain neurons that ultimately control the release of thyrotropin-releasing hormone (TRH) and somatostatin into the pituitary portal vascular system.

The exact CNS neurons that mediate caffeine's neuroendocrine effects remain obscure. Clearly the locus of action does not appear to be directly on the anterior pituitary gland, since caffeine incubated directly with rat pituitaries in vitro has no direct effect on TSH release at concentrations known to influence TSH in vivo (Spindel et al. 1980). (At very high in vitro concentrations, caffeine actually *increases* TSH release from the pituitary.)

Caffeine and theophylline have been shown to antagonize adenosine receptors in rat brain, and also to interact with peripheral adenosine receptors (van Calker et al. 1979; Londos and Wolff 1977). The behavioral potencies of methylxanthines appear to correlate well with their affinities for adenosine receptors. Moreover both adenosine (Maitre et al. 1975) and adenosine agonists like *L*-phenylisopropyl adenosine (PIA) induce sedation that can be reversed by methylxanthines (Snyder et al. 1981). In preliminary studies, however, we found that neither PIA nor adenosine increased serum TSH or blocked the caffeine-induced decrease in TSH, despite causing profound sedation (Spindel et al. 1983). Similarly, another adenosine analog, 8-phenyl-theophylline, had no reproducible endocrine effects. These studies suggest that if caffeine's endocrine effects are indeed mediated by adenosine receptors, the mediation is complex: simply increasing the occupancy of adenosine receptors will not elevate serum TSH, nor will it block the effects of caffeine. In support of these findings, Dunwiddie and Worth (1982) could not reverse all aspects of theophylline toxicity with PIA.

In summary, high doses of caffeine provoke changes in circulating hormone levels resembling an endocrine stress response in rats, while lower doses lack clear endocrine effects. The neurons and the neurotransmitter mechanisms mediating these endocrine responses remain obscure, but must involve hypothalamic releasing factors like somatostatin.

3 Studies in Man

The magnitude of the caffeine dose that is needed to provoke endocrine response in rats suggests that commonly-consumed caffeine doses will have few, if any, endocrine effects in man. Moreover, serum TSH is much less labile in man than it is in rats: temperature variations and experimental stresses have rarely been found to change serum TSH levels in man, but have frequently been shown to do so in rats (Mueller et al. 1976; Martin et al. 1978). Furthermore, stress *increases* serum GH levels in man rather than suppressing release of the hormone as in rats (Martin et al. 1978). These data all suggest that caffeine will have little effect on TSH or GH levels in man.

There are, however, some similarities between the responses to caffeine of rats and man, and the human responses also bear some resemblance to the endocrine stress syndrome. As in rats, human subjects receiving caffeine (220–250 mg p.o.) display increased serum and urinary catecholamine levels (Levi 1967; Bellet et al. 1969a; Robertson et al. 1978; though Jung et al. 1981, saw no such increase). Like rats, people also develop tolerance to this effect; after 7 days of caffeine consumption with each meal, subjects no longer exhibited an increase in serum catecholamines after a 250-mg oral caffeine challenge (Robertson et al. 1981).

Just as stressed rats display activation of the pituitary-adrenal axis, humans also readily respond to stress by increasing the secretion of ACTH, β-endorphin, and cortisol (not corticosterone). Consistent with a stress effect, Bellet et al. (1969b) and Avogaro et al. (1973) reported that caffeine (200–250 mg p.o.) mildly elevated serum cortisol and urinary 11-hydroxycorticosteroid levels. Spindel et al. (to be published), Oberman et al. (1975), and Daubresse et al. (1973) found no such effect; however, Spindel et al. (to be published) did observe small increases in serum cortisol when larger caffeine doses (500 mg p.o.) were used (Fig. 7), suggesting that the 250-mg dose is of borderline effectiveness and will or will not stimulate cortisol secretion depending on such variables as the subject's normal daily caffeine intake.

A 250-mg caffeine dose had no effect on serum β-endorphin levels, while a 500-mg dose did slightly elevate the opiate peptide, with a time course slightly in advance of the increase in serum cortisol seen in Fig. 7 (Spindel et al., to be published). Similarly, Geffner et al. (1982) reported that theophylline infusions sufficient to produce serum theophylline levels of 10–18 µg/ml do elevate serum ACTH. Thus higher doses of caffeine in man clearly do activate the pituitary-adrenal axis, increasing serum levels of cortisol, β-endorphin, and ACTH.

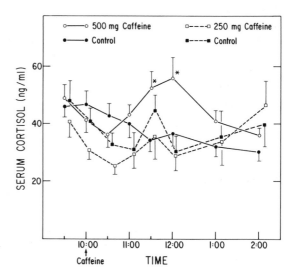

Fig. 7. Serum cortisol levels in man after caffeine or placebo. Eight to ten subjects per time point. * $P < 0.05$ compared to control time point (paired t-test)

Consistent with the above discussion, Spindel et al. (to be published) found no effect of either 250-mg or 500-mg caffeine doses on serum TSH or GH levels. Ensinck et al. (1970) did however observe that an intravenous infusion of 500 mg aminophylline did decrease serum GH – a somewhat surprising finding considering that stresses usually *increase* serum GH levels in humans.

4 Conclusions

High doses of caffeine in rats produce an endocrine stress syndrome characterized by decreased serum TSH levels, suppressed pulsatile secretion of GH, and elevated serum levels of corticosterone and β-endorphin. In man, 500-mg doses of caffeine given orally produce qualitatively similar responses in serum, cortisol, and β-endorphin. [A lower dose (250 mg) reportedly increases serum catecholamines.] Ingestion of 500 mg caffeine at a time constitutes a sizeable dose; in normal patterns of coffee consumption, 500 mg caffeine (five cups of coffee) is not usually consumed at one sitting. Thus it is not likely that normal patterns of coffee consumption would produce any of the endocrine effects described here. Indeed, people who habitually drink large amounts of coffee, who would also be most likely to consume large quantities of caffeine in a short time, would probably be *least* sensitive to caffeine's neuroendocrine effects because of the tolerance that develops to this methylxanthine. However, a non-coffee drinker who suddenly chose to drink large amounts of this beverage or of cola drinks, or who took caffeine-containing tablets for alertness, might well be expected to experience transient endocrine changes.

How caffeine produces its stress-like neuroendocrine effects remains to be determined. Does it act via adenosine receptors, or another neurotransmitter system, or does it nonspecifically affect many neurons? These are questions for future research.

References

Aldridge A, Parsons WD, Neims AH (1977) Stimulation of caffeine metabolism in the rat by 3-methylcholanthrene. Life Sci 21: 967–974

Arnaud MJ (1976a) Identification, kinetic and quantitative study of [12-^{14}C] and [1-Me-^{14}C]caffeine metabolites in rat's urine by chromatographic separations. Biochem Med 16: 67–76

Arnaud MJ (1976b) Metabolism of 1,3,7-trimethyldihydrouric acid in the rat: new metabolic pathways of caffeine. Experientia 32: 1238–1240

Arnold MA, Carr DB, Togasaki DM, Pian MC, Martin JB (1982) Caffeine stimulates β-endorphin release in blood but not in cerebrospinal fluid. Life Sci 32: 1017–1024

Avogaro P, Capri C, Pais M, Cazzolato G (1973) Plasma and urine cortisol behavior and fat mobilization in man after coffee ingestion. Isr J Med Sci 9: 114–119

Bellet S, Roman L, DeCastro O, Evin Kim K, Kershbaum A (1969a) Effect of coffee ingestion on catecholamine release. Metabolism 18: 288–291

Bellet S, Kostis J. Roman L, DeCastro O (1969b) Effect of coffee ingestion on adrenocortical secretion in young men and dogs. Metabolism 18: 1007–1012

Berkowitz BA, Spector S (1971) Effect of caffeine and theophylline on peripheral catecholamines. Eur J Pharmacol 13: 193–196

Clemens JA, Fuller RW (1979) Differences in the effects of amphetamine and methylphenidate on brain dopamine turnover and serum prolactin concentration in reserpine-treated rats. Life Sci 24: 2077–2082

Cohen MR, Nurnberger JI, Pickar D, Gershon E, Bunney WE (1981) Dextroamphetamine infusions in normals result in correlated increases of plasma β-endorphin and cortisol immunoreactivity. Life Sci 29: 1243–1247

Colton T, Gosselin RE, Smith RP (1968) The tolerance of coffee drinkers to caffeine. Clin Pharmacol Ther 9: 31–39

Cornish HH, Christman AA (1957) A study of the metabolism of theobromine, theophylline and caffeine in man. J Biol Chem 228: 315–323

Costa C, Trovato A, DePasquale A (1977) Effects of caffeine on corticosterone production in rats. Communication at Joint Meeting of German and Italian Pharmacologists, Venice

Daubresse JC, Luyckx A, Demey-Ponsart E, Fracnhimont P, Lefebvre P (1973) Effects of coffee and caffeine on carbohydrate metabolism, free fatty acid, insulin, growth hormone and cortisol plasma levels in man. Acta Diabetol Lat 10: 1069–1084

DePasquale A, Costa G, Trovato A, Ceserani R (1979) Effect of prostaglandins on the increased corticosterone output induced by caffeine in the rat. Prostaglandins Med 3: 97–103

Dunwiddie TV, Worth T (1982) Sedative and anti-convulsant effects of adenosine in mouse and rat. J Pharmacol Exp Ther 220: 70–76

Eddy NB, Downs AW (1928) Tolerance and cross-tolerance in the human subject to the diuretic effect of caffeine, theophylline and theobromine. J Pharmacol Exp Ther 33: 167–174

Ensinck JW, Stoll RW, Gale CC, Santen RJ, Touber JL, Williams RH (1970) Effect of aminophylline on the secretion of insulin, glucagon, luteinizing hormone and growth hormone in humans. J Clin Endocrinol Metab 31: 153–161

Geffner ME, Lippe BM, Kaplan SA, Itami RM (1982) The use of theophylline as an in vivo probe of adrenocortical function. J Clin Endocrinol Metab 55: 56–60

Goldstein A, Kaizer S, Whitby O (1969) Psychotropic effects of caffeine in man. IV. Quantitative and qualitative difference associated with habituation to coffee. Clin Pharmacol Ther 10: 489–497

Jung RT, Shetty PS, James WPT, Barrand MA, Callingham BA (1981) Caffeine: its effects on catecholamines and metabolism in lean and obese humans. Clin Sci 60: 527–535

Knych ET, Eisenberg RM (1979) Effects of amphetamine on plasma corticosterone in the conscious rat. Neuroendocrinology 29: 110–118

Kraicer J, Ducommun P, Jobin M, Rervp C, van Rees GP, Fortier C (1963) Pituitary and plasma TSH response to stress in the intact and adrenalectomized rat. Fed Proc 22: 507

Latini R (1981) Urinary excretion of an uracilic metabolite from caffeine by rat, monkey and man. Toxicol Lett 7: 267–272

Levi L (1967) The effect of coffee on the function of the sympathoadrenomedullary system in man. Acta Med Scand 181: 431–438

Londos C, Wolff J (1977) Two distinct adenosine-sensitive sites on adenylate cyclase. Proc Natl Acad Sci USA 74: 5482–5486

Maitre M, Ciesielski L, Lehmann A, Kempf E, Mandel P (1975) Protective effect of adenosine and nicotinamide against audiogenic seizure. Biochem Pharmacol 23: 2807–2816

Martin JB, Reichlin S, Brown GM (1977) Clinical neuroendocrinology. Davis, Philadelphia, pp 201–228

Moskowitz MA, Rubin D, Liebschutz J, Munro HN, Mowak TS, Wurtman RJ (1977) The permissive role of hypothermia in the disaggregation of brain polysomes by L-dopa or D-amphetamine. J Neurochem 28: 779–782

Mueller GP, Twohy CP, Chen JT, Advis JP, Meites J (1976) Effects of L-tryptophan and restraint stress on hypothalamic and brain serotonin turnover, and pituitary TSH and prolactin release in rats. Life Sci 18: 715–724

Oberman Z, Hershberg M, Jaskolka A, Havell A, Hoerer E, Laurian L (1975) Changes in plasma cortisol, glucose, free fatty acids after caffeine ingestion in obese women. Isr J Med Sci 11: 33–36

Ravitz AJ, Moore KE (1977) Effects of amphetamine, methylphenidate and cocaine on serum prolactin concentrations in the male rat. Life Sci 21: 267–272

Rice, RW, Critchlow V (1976) Extrahypothalamic control of stress-induced inhibition of GH secretion in the rat. Endocrinology 99: 970–976

Robertson D, Frolich JC, Carr RK, Watson JT, Hollifield JW, Shand DG, Oates JA (1978) Effects of caffeine on plasma renin activity, catecholamines and blood pressure. N Engl J Med 298: 181–186

127

Robertson D, Wade D, Workman R, Woosley RL, Oates JA (1981) Tolerance to the humoral and hemodynamic effects of caffeine in man. J Clin Invest 67: 1111–1117

Schlosberg AJ, Fernstrom JD, Kopczynski MC, Cusack BM, Gillis MA (1981) Acute effects of caffeine injections on neutral amino acids and brain monoamine levels in rats. Life Sci 29: 173–183

Snyder SH, Katims JJ, Annau Z, Bruns RF, Daly JW (1981) Adenosine receptors and behavioral actions of methylxanthines. Proc Natl Acad Sci USA 78: 3260–3264

Spindel ER, Mueller GP, Wurtman RJ (1978) D-Amphetamine: effects of TRH immunoreactivity in regions of rat brain and on plasma TSH (Abstr 398). Program of the 60th Annual Meeting of the Endocrine Society

Spindel ER, Arnold MA, Cusack B, Wurtman RJ (1980) Effects of caffeine on anterior pituitary and thyroid function in the rat. J Pharmacol Exp Ther 214: 58–62

Spindel ER, Griffith L, Wurtman RJ (1983) Neuroendocrine effects of caffeine. II. Effects on thyrotropin and corticosterone secretion. J Pharmacol Exp Ther 225: 346–350

Spindel ER, McCall A, Carr D, Arnold MA, Griffith L, Wurtman RJ (to be published) Neuroendocrine effects of caffeine. III. Anterior pituitary effects limited to stimulation of adrenal axis

Sullivan FM, McElhatton PR, Elmazar MM (1978) Studies on the teratogenicity of caffeine. Proceedings of First Annual Caffeine Committee Workshop, International Life Sciences Institute, Honolulu

Tang-Liu DD, Williams RL, Reigelman S (1983) Disposition of caffeine and its metabolites in man. J Pharmacol Exp Ther 224: 180–185

Terry LC, Willoughby JO, Brazeau P, Martin JB, Patel Y (1976) Antiserum to somatostatin prevents stress-induced inhibition of growth hormone secretion in the rat. Science 192: 565–567

van Calker D, Muller M, Hamprecht B (1979) Adenosine regulates, via two different types of receptors, the accumulation of cAMP in cultures brain cells. J Neurochem 33: 999–1005

Yehuda S, Wurtman RJ (1972) The effects of D-amphetamine and related drugs on colonic temperatures of rats kept at various ambient temperatures. Life Sci 11: 851–859

IX Adenosine as a Mediator of the Behavioral Effects of Xanthines*

S. H. Snyder

Though caffeine has been one of the most widely used psychoactive substances throughout history, it has been difficult to work out molecular mechanisms that account for its behavioral actions. One of the first widely considered mechanisms relates to cyclic AMP. Soon after the identification of phosphodiesterase as an enzyme degrading cyclic AMP, Sutherland and associates (Sutherland and Rall 1958; Butcher and Sutherland 1962) showed that xanthines, including caffeine and theophylline, inhibit phosphodiesterase. By inhibiting this enzyme xanthines might elevate levels of cyclic AMP. However, substantial inhibition of phosphodiesterase requires millimolar concentrations of caffeine, roughly 100 times the caffeine levels in the brain after ingestion of typical doses in man. Further, some inhibitors of phosphodiesterase that are 100–1000 times more potent than caffeine lack behavioral effects.

1 Physiologic Effects of Adenosine

Recently, a variety of evidence has accumulated suggesting strongly that adenosine may mediate the behavioral influences of xanthines. Adenosine (Fig. 1) is an intermediary in a wide range of metabolic pathways and is a constituent of ATP and nucleic acids. In addition, evidence has accumulated that adenosine can influence organs including the brain via receptors on the outside surface of cells (Burnstock and Brown 1981). Many effects of adenosine are opposite to those of xanthines, suggesting some type of antagonism. Moreover, most of the humoral effects of adenosine are blocked by xanthines.

Adenosine dilates blood vessels, especially in the coronary and cerebral circulation, and pharmaceutical companies over the years have attempted to develop coronary vasodilators by potentiating the actions of adenosine. The widely used coronary vasodilator dipyridamole is a potent inhibitor of adenosine accumulation into cells, though it is not established definitely that this accounts for its therapeutic effects.

Adenosine inhibits platelet aggregation, suggesting that adenosine-mimicking drugs might be useful in the prophylaxis of myocardial infarction. Adenosine

* These studies were supported by USPHS grants DA-00266, MH-18501, and NS-16375, RSA grant DA-00074, and grants from the McKnight Foundation and the International Life Sciences Institute, and conducted in collaboration with R. F. Bruns, J. W. Daly, R. R. Goodman, M. Gavish, J. J. Katims, and Z. Annau

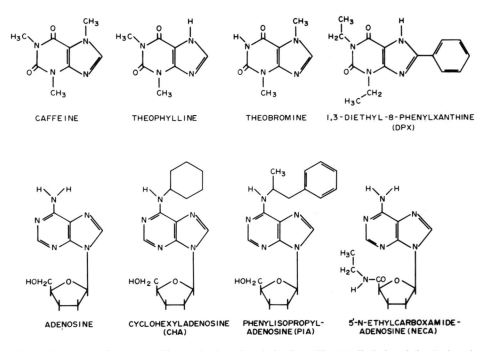

Fig. 1. Structures of some xanthine and adenosine derivatives. The 1,3-diethyl and the 8-phenyl substituents in DPX result in 1000-fold enhanced potency at adenosine receptors, so that [³H]DPX can be used to label adenosine A_1 receptors (Bruns et al. 1980; Murphy and Snyder 1982). The cyclohexyl and phenylisopropyl substituents in CHA and PIA respectively both protect adenosine from degradation by adenosine deaminase and increase affinity for adenosine A_1 receptors. PIA and CHA have much greater affinity for A_1 than A_2 receptors, and when labeled with tritium are useful tools for binding to adenosine A_1 receptors. NECA, on the other hand, has greater potency at A_2 than A_1 receptors

strongly inhibits hormone-induced lipolysis, and adenosine derivatives have been evaluated as agents to lower blood lipid levels.

Adenosine has a variety of actions on central neurons. In most instances it inhibits spontaneous neuronal firing (Phillis and Wu 1981; Stone 1981). The inhibitory actions of adenosine seem in large part to be presynaptic, i. e., due to the inhibition of release of excitatory neurotransmitters, though there are also postsynaptic effects (Okada and Ozawa 1980; Dunwiddie and Hoffer 1980). In biochemical investigations monitoring transmitter release directly, adenosine inhibits the release of almost all neurotransmitters evaluated, whether they are inhibitory or excitatory (Hollins and Stone 1980; Harms et al. 1979; Jhamandas and Sawynok 1976).

Though adenosine has clear-cut effects on neuronal functioning, it is not established whether extracellular adenosine has a physiologic role in the brain, in particular whether it is a neurotransmitter. Understanding the function of adenosine in the brain would be greatly facilitated by establishing whether it is contained in specific neuronal populations. The successful study of peptides as putative neurotransmitters has been based in large part on immunohistochemical mapping of peptide-containing neurons localized to specific regions of the brain. So far no such

130

Table 1. Regional adenosine (A_1) receptor densities

High	Moderate	Low	Very low
Cerebellum Molecular layer	Superior colliculus Superficial layer	Cerebral cortex Layers II, III, V	Hypothalamus
Hippocampus/dentate gyrus Molecular layers	Piriform cortex	Trigeminal nerve	Anterior commissure
Polymorphic layers	Olfactory tubercle	Spinal tract nucleus	Cerebellum White matter
Medical geniculate body	Cerebral cortex Layers I, IV, VI	Pontine nuclei Inferior colliculus	Superior cerebellar peduncle
Thalamic nuclei Medial Gelatinosus Lateral	Cerebellum Granule cell layer	Periaqueductal gray matter	Pyramidal tract
	Nucleus accumbens	Corpus callosum	Trigeminal nerve Spinal tract
Lateral septum		Reticular formation Pontine	
	Caudate nucleus/putamen	Medullary	Spinal tract
Spinal cord Substantia gelatinosa	Amygdala Central nucleus		
	Thalamic nuclei Ventral		

Adapted from Goodman and Snyder (1982)

techniques are available for localizing adenosine. If a neurotransmitter pool of adenosine involves only a small percentage of endogenous brain adenosine, one might have difficulty visualizing putative adenosinergic neurons.

2 Adenosine Receptor Localization

One alternative approach has been to visualize the localization of adenosine receptors. As will be discussed below, adenosine receptors can be labeled with a variety of ligands, [³H]cyclohexyladenosine ([³H]CHA) being particularly effective and widely used (Bruns et al. 1980). Applying the technique of in vitro autoradiography (Young and Kuhar 1979), we have been able to map in detail the localization of adenosine receptors in the central nervous system (Goodman and Snyder 1981, 1982). There are marked differences in the concentration of adenosine receptors in different brain areas. The highest densities occur in specific areas such as the molecular layer of the cerebellum, the molecular and polymorphic layers of the hippocampus and dentate gyrus, the medial geniculate body, certain thalamic nuclei, and the lateral septum (Table 1). In a preliminary study others detected similar localizations (Lewis et al. 1981).

Table 2. Lesion and mutant studies localizing adenosine receptors to excitatory axon terminals

Condition	Abnormality	[³H]CHA grains
Mouse mutant		
Control	–	Localized to molecular and granule layers
Reeler	Granule cells stay in outer molecular layer	Grains remain in outer molecular layer
Weaver	Granule cells deficient	Grains absent in molecular and granule cell layer
Nervous	90% loss of Purkinje cells	Normal
Lesions		
Unilateral eye removal	Optic nerve terminals degenerate in contralateral superior colliculus	Abolished in contrateral superior colliculus
Cerebral cortex ablation	Cortical afferents to corpus striatum and thalamus degenerate	Normal in corpus striatum and thalamus
Fornix lesion	Pathway connecting hippocampus and thalamus degenerate	Normal in hippocampus and thalamus

Adapted from Goodman et al. (1983)

With other neurotransmitter systems, such as enkephalin, the localization of receptors reflects fairly well the localization of nerve terminals containing the presumed neurotransmitter (Simantov et al. 1977). Thus, conceivably neuronal systems associated with adenosine exist in areas of the brain enriched in adenosine receptors.

The localizations of adenosine receptors can also explain the neurophysiologic presynaptic inhibitory actions of adenosine. To localize the adenosine receptors which are highly concentrated in the molecular layer of the cerebellum, we made use of neurologic mutant mice that lack specific nerve types (Goodman et al. 1983) (Table 2). We found that Weaver mice, which lack granule cells, also lack adenosine receptors. On the other hand, mutants such as Nervous, which lack Purkinje cells but have normal granule cells, have normal patterns of adenosine receptors. In Reeler mice, whose granule cells are transposed to a different layer, there is a similar transposition of adenosine receptors. Accordingly, it is apparent that adenosine receptors in the cerebellum are localized to granule cells, especially their axons and terminals in the molecular layer.

Of the five neuronal subtypes of the cerebellum only the granule cells are excitatory. Thus, the localization of adenosine receptors on granule cell axons and terminals suggests that a function of adenosine in the cerebellum is to inhibit the release of the granule cell excitatory neurotransmitter, which is thought to be glutamic acid (Young et al. 1974). This would explain the presynaptic inhibitory actions of adenosine in this part of the brain.

In the superior colliculus we found adenosine receptors localized to axon terminals of excitatory neurons (Goodman et al. 1983) (Table 2). Unilateral removal of an eye in rats produced a depletion of adenosine receptors in the contralateral superior colliculus coincident with the degeneration of the excitatory optic nerves. Thus, presumably adenosine could act in the superior colliculus by inhibiting release of the excitatory transmitter from optic nerves.

3 Adenosine Receptor Binding Properties

The first biochemical analysis of adenosine receptor activity was by Sattin and Rall (1970), who showed that adenosine can increase the accumulation of cyclic AMP in brain slices by a mechanism that does not involve conversion of adenosine to cyclic AMP, but rather an action on extracellular receptors. They also showed that the effects of adenosine were blocked by theophylline. The effects of adenosine on the enzyme adenylate cyclase, which synthesizes cyclic AMP, reveal two distinct subtypes of adenosine receptors, designated A_1 and A_2 (Burnstock and Brown 1981; Londos et al. 1981; van Calker et al. 1979). In some systems adenosine increases adenylate cyclase activity, while in other systems it decreases adenylate cyclase activity. The enhancing actions of adenosine on adenylate cyclase occur at micromolar concentrations via A_2 receptors. Through A_1 receptors, adenosine at nanomolar concentrations inhibits adenylate cyclase activity. There are structure-activity differences between A_1 and A_2 receptors. The most striking is the marked stereospecificity in the effects of phenylisopropyladenosine (PIA) at A_1 receptors, with L-PIA being much more potent than D-PIA. In contrast, the two isomers have relatively similar effects at A_2 receptors. Most xanthines have similar potencies in blocking both A_1 and A_2 receptors.

As with the major neurotransmitter systems, understanding receptor mechanisms in the adenosine system has been facilitated greatly by direct binding studies with radiolabeled ligands. We have labeled adenosine receptors with [^{3}H]CHA and with the xanthine derivative 1,3-diethyl-8-phenylxanthine ([^{3}H]DPX) (Bruns et al. 1980). Other adenosine ligands can also be employed (Schwabe and Trost 1980; Williams and Risley 1980; Yeung and Green 1981). In all species studied [^{3}H]CHA binding displays properties of adenosine A_1 receptors with nanomolar potency for adenosine derivatives and stereospecificity for PIA isomers. In bovine, rabbit, and rat brain [^{3}H]DPX binding shows a drug specificity essentially the same as that of [^{3}H]CHA, while in guinea pig and human brain [^{3}H]DPX binding has much lower affinity and is inhibited poorly by adenosine derivatives (Bruns et al. 1980; Murphy and Snyder 1982). In guinea pig and human brain [^{3}H]DPX binding may be associated in part with A_2 receptors or some other site. There is some evidence that one can label A_2 receptors with an adenosine derivative, [^{3}H]5'-N-ethylcarboxamidoadenosine ([^{3}H]NECA) (Yeung and Green, 1981).

Our binding studies suggest hereogeneity of adenosine receptors even beyond the A_1, A_2 distinction. There are considerable species differences in [^{3}H]CHA binding (Murphy and Snyder 1982). For instance, DPX is about 250 times more potent in competing for [^{3}H]CHA sites in calf than in guinea pig and human brain. Moreover, PIA and CHA are 20–100 times more potent in calf than in rat and rabbit brain. One strong item indicating heterogeneity is the marked differences in regional variation of [^{3}H]CHA and [^{3}H]DPX binding in several species (Fig. 2). These differences raise the possibility of developing drugs with considerable selectivity for one or another organ.

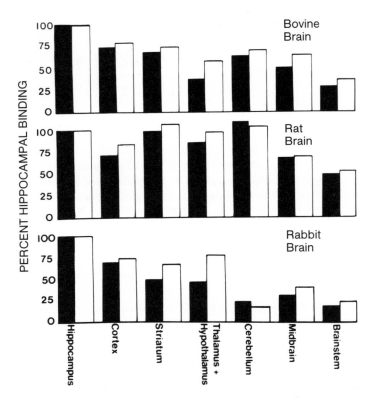

Fig. 2. Brain regional binding of [³H]CHA *(solid bars)* and [³H]DPX *(hollow bars)*. Homogenates of various brain regions pooled from two to five animals each at 10 mg/ml original weight of tissue in a total volume of 2 ml of 50 m*M* Tris HCl buffer, pH 7.7, were incubated with either [³H]CHA (1 n*M*) or [³H]DPX (2.5 n*M*) in parallel in the absence or presence of 10 n*M* L-PIA to determine total and nonspecific binding respectively. Specific binding to each region is defined as the difference between total and nonspecific binding and is expressed as a percentage of the specific binding to the hippocampus. Values presented are the means of two separate experiments performed in triplicate which varied less than 10%. [Adapted from Murphy and Snyder (1982)]

4 Behavioral Effects of Xanthines and Adenosine Derivatives

When adenosine receptors could be labelled by binding techniques we were in a position to ask whether the behavioral effects of xanthines involve actions at adenosine receptors. To monitor these effects we measured locomotor activity in mice, using sensitive, automated detection devices (Snyder et al. 1981; Katims et al. 1983). Our initial studies compared the potencies of various xanthine derivatives in affecting locomotor activity and in blocking adenosine receptors.

Xanthines such as caffeine and theophylline occupy 50% of adenosine receptors at concentrations in the micromolar range, comparable to blood and brain levels of these drugs after ingestion of a few cups of coffee in man or treatment with therapeutic doses of theophylline in asthma (Table 3) (Bruns et al. 1980). Relative poten-

Table 3. Xanthines: behavioral stimulant potencies, effects on adenosine and benzodiazepine receptor binding and brain levels

	Receptor binding		Locomotor stimulation threshold (μmol/kg)	Threshold for reversing L-PIA depression (μmol/kg)
	[^{3}H]flunitrazepam	[^{3}H]CHA IC$_{50}$ (μM)		
7(β-Chloroethyl)theophylline	900	10	2.5	10
Theophylline	2000	20	10	5
1,7-Dimethylxanthine	2000	30	20	10
3-Isobutyl-1-methylxanthine	~1000	50	N/E	2.5
Caffeine	800	50	25	5
7(β-Hydroxyethyl)theophylline	2000	100	30	10
Theobromine	>2000	150	250	250
8-Chlorotheophylline	>2000	500	N/E	N/E
1,9-Dimethylxanthine	>2000	>1000	N/E	N/E
Isocaffeine	1000	>1000	N/E	N/E

Adapted from Snyder et al. (1981) and Katims et al. (1983). The effects of intraperitoneally injected xanthines on locomotor activity of mice were evaluated alone or when administered together with L-PIA (0.15 μmol/kg) as described (Snyder et al. 1981). Threshold doses are minimal doses to alter locomotor activicy significantly from saline controls (Snyder et al. 1981; Katims et al., 1983). Six doses were evaluated for each drug with 10–20 mice at each dose. N/E, no effect with 250 μmol/kg, the highest tested dose.

cies of xanthines in enhancing locomotor activity in general correlate with affinities for adenosine receptors labeled with [^{3}H]CHA (Snyder et al. 1981).

Specificity of these effects is apparent in comparing these actions to those of xanthines at benzodiazepine receptors. It had been speculated that by blocking the sites at which benzodiazepines elicit anxiety reduction and sedation, xanthines might exert stimulant and perhaps anxiogenic effects (Skolnick et al. 1980). However, as with phosphodiesterase activity, millimolar concentrations of xanthines are required to compete for benzodiazepine receptors. Moreover, there is no correlation at all between potencies of xanthines in competing at benzodiazepine receptors and their potencies in causing behavioral effects (Snyder et al. 1981).

These considerations generally support the hypothesis that xanthines act behaviorally by blocking adenosine receptors. There are, however, certain problems. First, some exceptions exist to the correlation between affinities for adenosine receptors and behavioral effects. Thus, 3-isobutyl-1-methylxanthine (IBMX) has about the same affinity as caffeine for adenosine receptors, but does not display locomotor enhancement at any dose examined.

Another problem is the existence of biphasic effects observed with some xanthines. Thus, at lower doses caffeine decreases locomotor activity, but at higher doses enhances it (Snyder et al. 1981). IBMX decreases activity at all doses examined. By contrast, 7-(β-hydroxyethyl)theophylline enhances locomotor activity at all doses evaluated. The fact that the biphasic behavioral effects of xanthines vary with different substances suggests that the enhancing and decreasing effects are me-

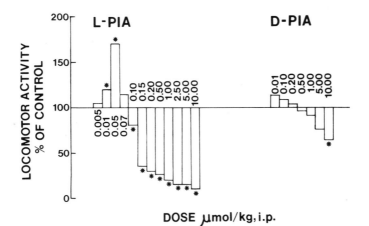

Fig. 3. Effects of L-PIA and D-PIA on locomotor activity of mice. Locomotor activity values are for groups of nine mice at each dose for a selected 10-min period. An overall analysis of variance revealed a significant drug group effect (F=11.6; DF=19,195; $P<.01$), and a significant drug group × time interaction (F=7.4; DF=105.165; $P<.01$). $*P<0.05$ with Duncan's analysis of significance for individual treatment groups from the saline control group. [Adapted from Katims et al. (1983)]

diated by distinct mechanisms. Perhaps xanthines enhance locomotor activity by blocking adenosine receptors and reduce it by some other mechanism. To focus on xanthine actions associated with adenosine effects, we decided to evaluate behavioral actions of adenosine derivatives.

Adenosine itself cannot be employed, since it is very rapidly metabolized by adenosine deaminase and only poorly penetrates the blood-brain barrier. The adenosine derivatives CHA and PIA are metabolically more stable and more lipophilic and thus more likely to enter the brain (Fig. 1), and have dramatic effects on behavior. In low doses L-PIA reduces locomotor activity (Fig. 3). This effect appears to be associated specifically with adenosine A_1 receptors, since L-PIA is substantially more potent than D-PIA.

Certain aspects of the behavioral effects of L-PIA are striking. With many hypnotics, doses slightly higher than those required to reduce locomotor activity produce sleep. By contrast, despite doses of L-PIA increased to levels 500 times greater than the minimum required to lower locomotor activity, mice remained awake (Snyder et al. 1981). Even the righting reflex is intact at doses 100 times those which decrease locomotor behavior. Another striking feature is the absence of lethal effects with L-PIA in doses as great as 800 µmol/kg, about 10000 times the threshold dose for lowering locomotor activity.

This uniquely wide range of behavioral effects has so far not been compared to other psychotropic drugs. If anything, the large safety margin and the decrease of locomotor activity without hypnotic effects tend to resemble the actions of benzodiazepines.

In our initial studies (Snyder et al. 1981) we did not evaluate doses of L-PIA lower than 0.1 µmol/kg at all time points. More recently, when we examined a larger

136

Table 4. Cardiovascular actions of PIA in mice

Dose (μmol/kg)	Mean blood pressure (mm Hg)	Heart rate (beats/min)	Premature ventricular contractions (per min)
Saline			
	107 ± 2	810 ± 74	–
L-PIA			
0.0005	108 ± 2	763 ± 77	–
0.005	107 ± 2	804 ± 72	0.05 ± 0.02*
0.05	105 ± 3	810 ± 62	0.05 ± 0.03*
0.15	106 ± 2	792 ± 59	0.06 ± 0.04*
2.5	92 ± 3*	568 ± 43	3.20 ± 1.2*
5.0	53 ± 12*	244 ± 74*	8.80 ± 3.4*
10.0	26 ± 7*	90 ± 42*	8.40 ± 2.2*
D-PIA			
0.15	105 ± 2	742 ± 65	–
5.0	106 ± 1	755 ± 98	0.06 ± 0.02*
10.0	108 ± 3	676 ± 49	0.07 ± 0.2*
20.0	96 ± 4*	650 ± 41*	0.09 ± 0.3*
50.0	84 ± 5*	368 ± 39*	12.30 ± 3.1*

The effects of L-PIA and D-PIA were examined on mean blood pressure, heart rate, and premature ventricular contractions. Six animals per group were evaluated with each drug dose. Individual cardiac output values were obtained by taking the mean of ten measures of the cardiac output over a 10-min period when the drug exerted its maximal effect. Analysis of variance revealed a significant group effect. Adapted from Katims et al. (1983). Values expressed as mean ± SD. * $P < 0.05$ by Duncan's analysis of significance for individual treatment groups.

range of doses, we were surprised to find that in doses lower than those which depress locomotor activity, substantial enhancement of locomotor activity occurs (Fig. 3) (Katims et al. 1983). Direct visual inspection of the mice indicates that these low doses produce a fairly well coordinated increase of movement. Such apparent stimulatory actions are observed with doses as low as 0.01 μmol/kg intraperitoneally, about 4 μg/kg. To our knowledge such potency exceeds that of any known psychotropic agent in rodents. This potency is even more impressive when one considers that L-PIA has substantially less access to the brain than most potent psychotropic agents. Thus, drugs such as amphetamines, neuroleptics, and tricyclic antidepressants are quite lipophilic and attain brain concentrations up to ten times higher than blood levels. By contrast, brain concentrations of L-PIA at behaviorally effective doses are only one-fifth of the levels one would predict if the drug distributed equally throughout all body compartments (Katims et al., 1983).

Since L-PIA is a potent hypotensive agent, one might wonder whether effects on blood pressure or other cardiovascular features account for its apparent behavioral actions. However, at behaviorally active doses of L-PIA there are no changes in blood pressure or heart rate (Table 4). We observed some intermittent premature ventricular contractions at these doses, with a frequency of one every 10–33 min. However, the premature ventricular contractions occurred at the same rate with both stimulant and depressant doses of L-PIA and thus show no correlation with the behavioral effects. Also, we found that L-PIA doses producing threshold loco-

137

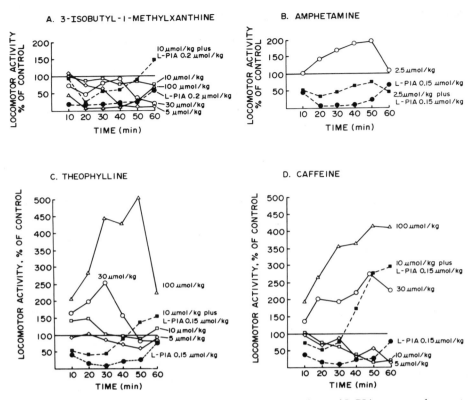

Fig. 4. Interactive effects of alkylxanthines or dextroamphetamine and L-PIA on mouse locomotor activity. Mean values for groups of 10–15 mice at each intraperitoneal dose are expressed as the percentage of values in saline-injected controls. L-PIA and methylxanthines were given i.p. at the same time; 10 min later, the mice were placed in activity-monitoring cages

motor enhancement are associated with brain concentrations sufficient to occupy about 50% of adenosine receptors as monitored by [³H]CHA binding (Katims et al. 1983). Thus, L-PIA's behavioral effects appear to be centrally mediated.

After characterizing the effects of L-PIA alone, we wondered whether xanthines might interact with the behavioral effects of L-PIA. When a low, locomotor-decreasing dose of caffeine is combined with a locomotor-decreasing dose of L-PIA, one sees paradoxically an up to 300% stimulation of locomotor activity (Fig. 4, Table 3). What about other xanthines, such as IBMX, which by itself never produces locomotor enhancement? Combining a locomotor-decreasing dose of IBMX with a dose of L-PIA which alone decreases locomotor activity results in a 250%–300% increase of locomotor activity.

For most of the xanthines reversal of the locomotor decrease caused by PIA is obtained by lower concentrations than those required to increase locomotor activity when administerd alone. 7-(β-Chlorethyl)theophylline is one exception, being more potent in enhancing locomotor activity alone than in reversing L-PIA decrease. The weakest xanthines at adenosine receptors are all either weak or inactive in enhanc-

138

Table 5. Locomotor interactions of caffeine and L-PIA

| | Locomotor activity (% of control) | | |
| | L-PIA dose (µmol/kg i.p.) | | |
	0	*0.05*	*0.15*
Saline	100±3	175±6*	35±2*
Caffeine (10 µmol/kg i.p.)	67±4*	165±4*	266±7*
Caffeine (30 µmol/kg i.p.)	266±5*	263±3*	294±4*
d-Amphetamine sulfate (2.5 µmol/kg i.p.)	190±3*	–	68±3*

Locomotor activity values for groups of 10–20 mice at each dose for a selected 10-min period as in Table 4, expressed as percentage of activity of saline-injected control mice. Values presented (mean ± SEM) are the antilogarithms of logarithmic transformations of this data. An overall analysis of variance revealed a significant drug effect ($F=6.2$; $DF=10, 150$; $P<0.01$), and a significant drug × time interaction ($F=8.4$; $DF=50, 150$; $P<0.01$). * Significantly different from saline ($P<0.01$, $DF=1, 150$) as determined by F-test comparisons. Adapted from Katims et al. (1983)

ing locomotor activity or reversing L-PIA decrease. Unlike the complex joint effects of caffeine and L-PIA, amphetamine and L-PIA add in an arithmetic fashion, emphasizing the selectivity of the synergistic relations of xanthines and L-PIA.

What might account for the behavior increase that occurs when doses of xanthines and L-PIA that individually decrease behavior are combined? Our findings that low doses of L-PIA have enhancing effects may provide an explanation. These actions presumably reflect the existence of sites for which L-PIA has extremely high affinity. Somewhat lower affinity sites, still with relatively high affinity, would mediate the decrease of locomotor activity by L-PIA. We postulate that xanthines block the lower affinity sites, thus unmasking the enhancing effects of L-PIA at the higher affinity sites. Such a formulation would fit with our own observations that caffeine fails to alter the locomotor enhancement associated with extremely low doses of L-PIA (Table 5).

Taken together, the accumulated evidence suggests strongly that xanthines exert their behavior-enhancing effects by blocking adenosine receptors. Research on adenosine mechanisms may have ramifications beyond simply clarifying why caffeine enhances behavior activity. The heterogeneity of adenosine receptors in different tissues identified by binding techniques may afford the possibility of designing potent organ-specific adenosine receptor antagonists. Such agents might have utility as diuretic, cardiac inotropic, or bronchodilating antiasthmatic drugs with reduced side effects. The dramatic behavioral effects of the adenosine derivative L-PIA suggests a therapeutic role for adenosine agonists. Such agents might have utility as sedatives, hypnotics, or antianxietal drugs. Recent electroencephalographic studies indicate that L-PIA in very low doses increases slow-wave sleep with no decrease in REM sleep, thus providing a sleep profile potentially preferable to that obtained with current hypnotics (Radulovacki et al. 1982). Additional therapeutic roles for adenosine agonists may derive from their inhibition of platelet aggregation, inhibition of lipolysis, and dilatation of coronary arteries.

References

Bruns, RF, Daly JW, Snyder SH (1980) Adenosine receptors in brain membranes: binding of N^6-cyclohexyl[^{3}H]adenosine and 1,3-diethyl-8-[^{3}H]-phenylxanthine. Proc Natl Acad Sci USA 77: 5547–5551

Burnstock G, Brown CM (1981) An introduction to purinergic receptors. In: Burnstock G (ed) Purinergic receptors. Chapman and Hall, London New York, pp 1–45

Butcher RW, Sutherland EW (1962) Adenosine 3',5'-phosphate in biological materials. J Biol Chem 237: 1244–1250

Dunwiddie TV, Hoffer BJ (1980) Adenine nucleotides and synaptic transmission in the in vitro rat hippocampus. Br J Pharmacol 69: 59–68

Goodman RR, Snyder SH (1981) The light microscopic in vitro autoradiographic localization of adenosine (A_1) receptors. Neurosci Abstr 7: 613

Goodman RR, Snyder SH (1982) Autoradiographic localization of adenosine receptors in rat brain using [^{3}H]cyclohexyladenosine. J Neurosci 2: 1230–1241

Goodman RR, Kuhar MJ, Hester L, Snyder SH (1983) Adenosine receptors: Autoradiographic evidence for a localization to excitatory neuronal axon terminals. Science 220: 967–969

Harms HH, Wardeh G, Mulder AH (1979) Effects of adenosine on depolarization-induced release of various radiolabeled neurotransmitters from rat corpus striatum. Neuropharmacology 18: 577–580

Hollins C, Stone TW (1980) Adenosine inhibition of GABA release from slices of rat cerebral cortex. Br J Pharmacol 69: 107–112

Jhamandas K, Sawynok J (1976) Methylxanthine antagonism of opiate and purine effects on the release of acetylcholine. In: Kosterlitz HW (ed) Opiates and endogenous opioid peptides, Elsevier/North Holland, Amsterdam, pp 161–168

Katims JJ, Annau Z, Snyder SH (1983) Behavioral interactions between methylxanthines and adenosine derivatives. J Pharmacol Exp Ther 227: 1–7

Lewis ME, Patel J, Edley SM, Marangos PJ (1981) Autoradiographic visualization of rat brain adenosine receptors using N^6-cyclohexyl[^{3}H]adenosine. Eur J Pharmacol 73: 109–110

Londos C, Wolff J, Cooper DMF (1981) Adenosine as a regulator of adenylate cyclase. In: Burnstock G (ed) Purinergic receptors. Chapman and Hall, London New York, pp 287–323

Murphy KMM, Snyder SH (1982) Heterogeneity of A_1 adenosine receptor binding in brain tissue. Mol Pharmacol 22: 250–257

Okada Y, Ozawa S (1980) Inhibitory action of adenosine on synaptic transmission in the hippocampus of the guinea pig in vitro. Eur J Pharmacol 68: 483–492

Phillis JW, Wu PH (1981) The role of adenosine and its nucleotides in central synaptic transmission. Prog Neurobiol 16: 187–239

Radulovacki M, Miletich RS, Green RD (1982) N^6-(L-phenylisopropyl) adenosine (L-PIA) increases slow-wave sleep (S_2) and decreases wakefulness in rats. Brain Res 246: 178–180

Sattin A, Rall TW (1970) The effect of adenosine and adenine nucleotides on the adenosine 3',5'-phosphate content of guinea pig cerebral cortex slices. Mol Pharmacol 6: 13–23

Schwabe U, Trost T (1980) Characterization of adenosine receptors in rat brain by (-)[^{3}H]N^6-phenylisopropyladenosine. Naunyn Schmiedebergs Arch Pharmacol 313: 179–187

Simantov R, Kuhar MJ, Uhl GR, Snyder SH (1977) Opioid peptide enkephalin: immunohistochemical mapping in rat central nervous system. Proc Natl Acad Sci USA 74: 2167–2171

Skolnick P, Paul SM, Marangos PJ (1980) Purines as endogenous ligands of the benzodiazepine receptors. Fed Proc 39: 3050–3055

Snyder SH, Katims JJ, Annau Z, Bruns RF, Daly JW (1981) Adenosine receptors and behavioral actions of methylxanthines. Proc Natl Acad Sci USA 78: 3260–3264

Stone TW (1981) Physiological roles for adenosine and adenosine 5'-triphosphate in the nervous system. Neuroscience 6: 523–555

Sutherland EW, Rall TW (1958) Fractionation and characterization of cyclic adenine ribonucleotide formed by tissue particles. J Biol Chem 232: 1077–1091

van Calker D, Muller M, Hamprecht B (1979) Adenosine regulates via two different types of receptors the accumulation of cyclic AMP in cultured brain cells. J Neurochem 33: 999–1005

Williams M, Risley EA (1980) Biochemical characterization of putative purinergic receptors by using 2-chloro[^{3}H]adenosine, a stable analog of adenosine. Proc Natl Acad Sci USA 77: 6892–6896

Yeung S-M, Green RD (1981) Binding of 5'-*N*-ethylcarboxamide ^{3}H-adenosine (^{3}H-NECA) to adenosine receptors in rat striatum. Pharmacologist 23: 184

Young AB, Oster-Granite ML, Herndon RM, Snyder SH (1974) Glutamic acid: selective depletion by viral induced granule cell loss in hamster cerebellum. Brain Res 73: 1–13

Young WS III, Kuhar MJ (1979) A new method for receptor autoradiography: [^{3}H]opioid receptors in rat brain. Brain Res 179: 255–270

X Caffeine and the Cardiovascular Effects of Physiological Levels of Adenosine*

W. R. von Borstel and R. J. Wurtman

1 Introduction: Caffeine as an Antagonist of Endogenous Adenosine

In spite of the widespread use of the methylxanthines caffeine and theophylline as food constituents and as drugs, the biochemical events mediating their pharmacological actions are not well understood. On the basis of experiments performed mainly upon isolated tissue or organ preprations in vitro, several detailed mechanisms have been proposed which might underlie the effects of methylxanthines on neural, cardiovascular, renal, and respiratory processes; however, the precise actions and potencies of methylxanthines observed in vivo have often been at variance with those observed in in vitro studies (Rall 1980; Neims and von Borstel 1983). Thus the hypothesis, widely held until recently, that caffeine and theophylline act in vivo mainly by inhibiting cyclic AMP (cAMP) phosphodiesterase is untenable given caffeine's relatively low potency as an inhibitor of the enzyme compared with its potency in modulating physiological processes in vivo. Even relatively high doses of methylxanthines fail to increase tissue cAMP levels in intact animals (Burg and Warner 1975). Similarly, differences between the in vivo and in vitro potencies of methylxanthines diminish the likelihood that caffeine acts as a cardiac and CNS stimulant by direct effects upon calcium storage or translocation (Rall 1980).

Over the past decade, considerable evidence has been marshalled suggesting that the most important molecular action for methylxanthines in generating their observed physiological and behavioral effects may involve competitive antagonism at cell surface adenosine receptors (Sattin and Rall 1970; Fredholm 1980; Snyder et al. 1981).

The administration of adenosine to animals can produce sedation, bradycardia, hypotension, hypothermia, and attenuation of the responses of the heart, vasculature, and adipose tissue to sympathetic stimulation (Drury 1936; Fredholm and Hedqvist 1980; Maitre et al. 1974). These effects [apparently mediated through specific adenosine receptors located on the external surfaces of the plasma membranes of cells (Daly et al. 1981)] are generally opposite to those produced by caffeine or theophylline alone. Indeed, methylxanthines competitively antagonize these and other adenosine actions at concentrations similar to those found in plasma after the consumption of one to three cups of coffee (5–30 μM; Rall 1980). No other known

* Some of the studies described in this report were supported by grants from the International Life Sciences Institute and the National Science Foundation

molecular interactions of methylxanthines seem as likely as antagonism at adenosine receptors to account for the multiplicity of caffeine's effects upon biological systems. However, substantial indirect evidence also suggests that adenosine receptor antagonism probably does not fully explain all of caffeine's physiological effects in mammals (Neims and von Borstel 1983).

Cardiovascular responses to peripherally administered adenosine were first reported over 50 years ago (Drury and Szent-Gyorgyi 1929), and since that time, numerous other effects of the nucleoside have been documented. However, in few or no cases has the "physiological significance" (or the magnitude of the influence) of endogenously formed adenosine been unambiguously established. Thus, it is still not known whether the behavioral and physiological responses to adenosine or some of its synthetic congeners reflect a role for adenosine in normal physiological regulation, or whether they have only a pharmacological significance. At present, no plausible molecular mechanisms, other than antagonism at adenosine receptors, that might underlie the biological effects of physiologically relevant concentrations of methylxanthines have been explicitly formulated. Further progress in defining the cellular sites and molecular mechanisms mediating caffeine's effects, as well as the physiological implications of caffeine consumption, may be helped by better characterization of the actions of adenosine in concentrations likely to occur in blood or tissues.

Once this information is available, it should be possible to test the hypothesis that an effect of caffeine upon behavior or on a physiological phenomenon reflects its interference with an action of endogenous adenosine. Such studies should ideally be performed in vivo, since there can sometimes be large differences in the potency of adenosine (and indeed in the nature of the effect) in a given tissue in vivo as compared to the same organ or tissue in vitro (Bianchi et al. 1963; Neims and von Borstel 1983); this is also true for caffeine (Rall 1980; Neims and von Borstel 1983).

A direct approach to the correlation of adenosine levels and effects in vivo might be to monitor, concurrently, adenosine levels in plasma or tissues and selected biochemical, physiological, or behavioral indices before and during administration of exogenous adenosine.

2 Effects of Circulating Adenosine

Reported behavioral and physiological effects of peripherally administered adenosine include suppression of locomotor activity, protection against experimental seizures, hypotension, vasodilatation, bradycardia, and modification of the responses of the heart, vasculature, adipose tissue, and kidney to sympathetic stimulation (Maitre et al. 1974; Drury and Seznt-Gyorgyi 1929; Fredholm and Hedqvist 1980). However, the behavioral effects of adenosine have been assessed only in animals given relatively large doses of adenosine as a bolus injection, which tends to produce pronounced cardiovascular changes (Maitre et al. 1974; Mathieu-Levy 1968). Although there is known to be a facilitated diffusion carrier specific for nucleosides in the blood-brain barrier (Cornford and Oldendorf 1975), it has not yet been established whether behavioral or neurophysiological effects of peripherally administered adenosine reflect a direct influence of circulating adenosine upon the brain or whether they are nonspecific and secondary to peripheral adenosine effects such as hypotension or hypothermia.

Cardiovascular changes are readily produced by administration of adenosine in doses that modify circulating adenosine levels. Adenosine acts as a vasodilator in most tissues (Drury 1936) except the kidney, where it can act as a vasoconstrictor, at least in rabbits and dogs (Fredholm 1980; Osswald 1979). Adenosine also has negative chronotropic and negative inotropic effects upon the heart (Drury 1936).

Adenosine's influences upon excitable tissue can be subdivided into three separable domains or modes of action: it can

1. modify the release of neurotransmitters or hormones,
2. alter the actions of neurotransmitters, drugs, or hormones, or
3. act directly upon a tissue regardless of the presence or absence of a specific neurotransmitter or hormone.

Examples of all three of these modes of action are known, and in some cases all three may be operating simultaneously in the same synaptic ensemble; this is apparently true of the cardiovascular system. The importance of differentiating these three ways in which adenosine can modulate physiological processes is that the direction of adenosine's action upon neurotransmission, whether inhibitory or facilitative, can be different at presynaptic and postsynaptic sites within the same tissue. In rabbit kidney, for example, adenosine potently inhibits the release of norepinephrine from electrically stimulated sympathetic nerves, but a strong enhancement of renal vascular responsiveness to norepinephrine by adenosine overrides the presynaptic effect, so that the net effect of adenosine is potentiation of renal vascular sympathetic nerve stimulation (Hedqvist et al. 1978). Similar examples of opposing pre- and postsynaptic actions of adenosine are known in brain (Taylor and Stone 1980) and sympathetic ganglia (Henon et al. 1980), although in these cases the net influence upon the processes mediated through the affected neurons has not been clearly resolved.

In dogs anesthetized with pentobarbital intravenous infusion of adenosine reduced the responses of heart rate or blood pressure to stimulation of the appropriate sympathetic nerves, while responses to exogenous norepinephrine remained relatively unmodified by the nucleoside (Lokhandwala 1979; Hom and Lokhandwala 1981). This was taken as evidence that the adenosine acts by inhibiting norepinephrine release. The levels of arterial adenosine required to modify responses to nerve stimulation in this study were not determined, although they were high enough to produce a 25% drop in mean arterial pressure. The hypotensive effect of adenosine in this system is not attributable solely to suppression of sympathetic transmission, since adenosine is still a potent vasodilator following sympathetic denervation (Hom and Lokhandwala 1981).

In conscious rats bearing an indwelling arterial catheter for monitoring blood pressure and heart rate and several venous catheters for administering drugs, the controlled infusion of a subhypotensive dose of adenosine can markedly suppress cardiovascular responses to bolus injections of small doses of norepinephrine, the α-adrenergic agonist phenylephrine, and to a lesser extent acetylcholine. This postsynaptic neuromodulatory effect is reversed by a low (3 mg/kg) dose of caffeine (Fig. 1; von Borstel, unpublished results). In rats anesthetized with either pento-

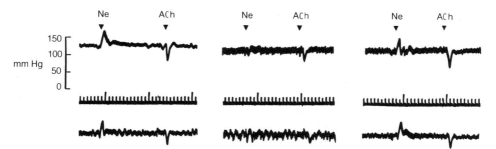

Fig. 1. Suppression of cardiovascular responses to norepinephrine *(Ne)* and acetylcholine *(ACh)* by adenosine, and their restoration by caffeine. Responses of blood pressure to periodic intravenous bolus injections of norepinephrine (50 ng/kg) and acetylcholine (50 ng/kg) were monitored in conscious, unrestrained rats in control conditions *(left)* and during intravenous infusion of adenosine solution (0.15 mg/kg/min) alone *(middle)* and accompanied by intra-arterial injection of 3 mg/kg caffeine *(right)*. Blood pressure traces from two animals are shown

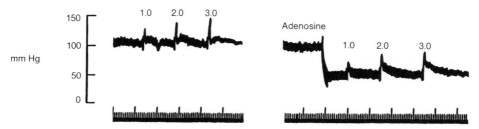

Fig. 2. Failure of adenosine to suppress responses to an α-adrenergic agonist in anesthetized rat. Animals anesthetized with α-chloralose/urethane received phenylephrine via an intravenous catheter in the doses indicated (μg/kg) before *(left)* and during *(right)* adenosine infusion (0.15 mg/kg/min)

barbital or a mixture of chloralose and urethane, adenosine fails to attenuate pressor responses to phenylephrine or norepinephrine; in addition, the hypotensive effect of adenosine appears to be exaggerated in anesthetized rats (Fig. 2; von Borstel, unpublished results). Since most studies on the physiological effects of adenosine in vivo are performed in anesthetized animals, artifacts due to the presence of anesthesia (or possible secondary effects, such as hypoxia) might yield an inaccurate picture of the functions of adenosine in otherwise untreated organisms.

Nicotine produces hypertension and tachycardia by inducing the release of norepinephrine and epinephrine from the sympathoadrenal system (Loffelholz 1979); it is not clear whether nicotine's main site of action is within sympathetic ganglia or at sympathetic terminals (or the adrenal medulla). Surprisingly, subhypotensive doses of adenosine given by intravenous infusion can strongly potentiate the pressor response to low doses of nicotine (Fig. 3) in rats; this effect is also reversed by caffeine (von Borstel, unpublished results). It is not yet known whether this phenomenon reflects a general presynaptic influence of adenosine upon cardiovascular sympathetic neuroeffector transmission (which is, however, opposite to the effects reported in studies on isolated vasculature and hearts in vitro), or whether it is unique to sympathetic activation induced by nicotine. Adenosine potentiates the pressor response to nicotine in conscious as well as anesthetized animals, and also

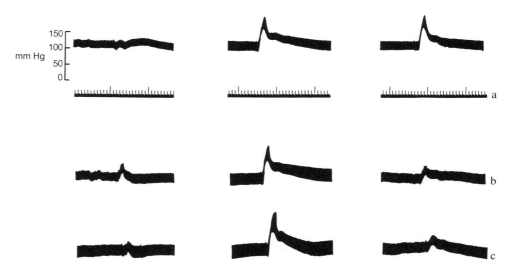

Fig. 3a–c. Potentiation of the pressor response to nicotine by adenosine and its prevention by caffeine. Pressor responses to bolus injections of nicotine (35 μg/kg i.v.) were monitored before *(left)* and during *(middle)* an intravenous infusion of adenosine. Caffeine (5 mg/kg i.a.) was then administered to rats **b** and **c** *(right)*. Animals were anesthetized with pentobarbital (60 mg/kg)

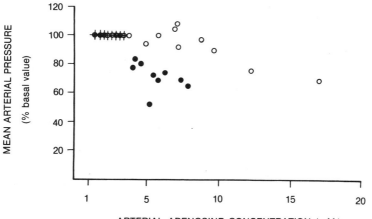

ARTERIAL ADENOSINE CONCENTRATION (μM)

Fig. 4. Inhibitory effect of acute caffeine treatment upon the hypotensive effect of adenosine infusion. Acute caffeine treatment (15 mg/kg i.a. 5 min before adenosine infusion) significantly ($P <$ 0.01) attenuated the hypotension resulting from intravenous adenosine infusion in awake animals. Mean arterial pressure (MAP) and arterial plasma adenosine concentration were measured in control rats (•) and in animals pretreated with 15 mg/kg caffeine (○), and found to be correlated above concentrations of 4–5 μM. After a basal blood sample had been withdrawn (✦ control; ⊕ caffeine-treated), animals received continuous adenosine infusion at a constant flow rate for 3–5 min, by which time blood pressure had stabilized. MAP was then noted and another arterial sample withdrawn. The infusion rate was then increased, and after stabilization, MAP was again noted and another blood sample was withdrawn via the arterial catheter. Each rat was subjected to four or five different rates (between 0.1 and 1 mg/kg/min) of adenosine infusion. Each treatment group contained four rats

146

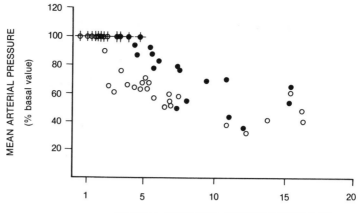

Fig. 5. Enhancement of the hypotensive effect of adenosine infusion by chronic caffeine treatment followed by acute caffeine withdrawal. Rats given drinking water containing caffeine (0.1%) for 3 weeks followed by an abrupt return to plain tap water for 24 h before testing (○) exhibited greater sensitivity to infused adenosine than did control animals (●). Cardiovascular responses to infused adenosine were now seen at arterial plasma adenosine concentrations which were ineffective in control animals and which fell within the control range for basal adenosine concentration. A significant fall ($P < 0.01$) in mean arterial pressure was observed at 2–4 μM adenosine, and the fall at 5–6 μM was significantly greater than that seen in control animals ($P < 0.01$). Adenosine was administered and blood samples collected for adenosine assay as described in the legend to Fig. 4. The control group contained five rats and the caffeine withdrawal group seven

in rats subjected to adrenalectomy and cervical spinal cord transection (von Borstel, unpublished results).

The hypotensive effect of adenosine is significant when arterial plasma adenosine concentrations are at or above approximately 5 μM (Fig. 4.; von Borstel et al. 1983). Since the normal values for plasma adenosine levels in rat arterial blood are typically 1–4 μM (von Borstel et al., 1983), the attenuation of cardiovascular responses to norepinephrine and acetylcholine and the potentiation of pressor responses to nicotine might represent effects that could be responsive to changes in endogenous adenosine levels within the physiological range.

The cardiovascular effects of adenosine can be suppressed by acute caffeine treatment, as is shown in Figs. 1, 3, and 4. However, when rats consume a 0.1% caffeine solution (65 mg/kg/day) as their only source of liquid for 3 weeks, followed by an abrupt return to tap water 24 h before testing, there is a substantial increase in the hypotensive potency of adenosine (Fig. 5; von Borstel et al. 1983). Hypotension in such animals appeared at arterial adenosine levels which were ineffective in control animals and which fell within the control range for basal adenosine concentrations. A significant fall in blood pressure was here observed at 2–4 μM adenosine, and the fall at 5–6 μM was significantly greater than that seen in control animals.

A complementary finding is that chronic caffeine consumption in rats can result in an increase in the density of brain adenosine receptors (Fredholm 1982; Boulenger et al. 1983). The binding of radiolabeled adenosine derivatives to cardiovascular adenosine receptors has not yet been adequately demonstrated, according to the rigorous standards set in the identification of brain adenosine receptors; it is there-

147

fore not yet possible to determine whether chronic caffeine exposure also produces alterations in cardiovascular adenosine receptor density or kinetic properties.

The observations that the long-term blockade of adenosine receptors by caffeine makes the cardiovascular system more sensitive to adenosine and that such treatment also increases brain adenosine receptor density raised the possibility that some of the common sequelae of caffeine withdrawal, such as headache and jitteriness (Goldstein et al. 1969), might reflect enhanced tissue sensitivity to endogenous adenosine. For example, caffeine itself is used to treat several types of headache, where its beneficial effect has been suggested to result from its ability to constrict cerebral arteries (Rall 1980); adenosine is a potent dilator of the cerebral vasculature (Winn et al. 1981).

The effects of endogenous adenosine on cardiovascular tissues have generally been thought to be restricted to the particular tissue in which the adenosine was formed and released (Fredholm 1980; Sollevi et al. 1981). Indeed, adenosine is produced in the heart and vasculature in response to hypoxia or sympathetic stimulation, and may act locally to attenuate effects of these stimuli by inducing vasodilation and by inhibiting further norepinephrine release or postsynaptic effects (Berne 1980). However, the cardiovascular sensitivity to adenosine as determined in the studies described above (particularly in the case of rats withdrawn from chronic caffeine exposure) suggests that circulating adenosine might also be able to function in a hormone-like role, perhaps affecting vascular dynamics in tissues throughout the body.

3 Implications of the Interaction of Caffeine with Endogenous Adenosine

The strategy for determining the actual adenosine levels needed to produce cardiovascular effects in unanesthetized, unrestrained rats might be applicable to other easily monitored physiological functions that peripherally administered adenosine is known to modulate, such as lipolysis (Sollevi et al. 1981), renal function (Hedqvist et al. 1978), and behavior (Maitre et al. 1974). In addition, such studies could be used to test for alterations in tissue sensitivity to adenosine following various hormonal, nutritional, or pharmacological treatments.

The significance of such information in the context of caffeine's effects is that if a given effect of caffeine is indeed due to antagonism at adenosine receptors, then the magnitude of the caffeine effect should be directly related to the magnitude of the influence of endogenous adenosine. Determination of the sensitivity of various physiological processes to modulation by adenosine might help to resolve which of caffeine's effects are indeed mediated through adenosine receptor blockade. This has several implications that might be relevant to the human use of caffeine. It may be possible to identify particular disease states or hormonal imbalances in which either adenosine levels or tissue sensitivity to adenosine is altered, in which case the use of methylxanthines might have predictable therapeutic efficacy or, alternatively, might be particularly inadvisable. That such conditions might exist is suggested by the observation that rats made hypothyroid with dietary propylthiouracil (0.15% in chow for 2 weeks) are more sensitive to adenosine's hypotensive action than are untreated or hyperthyroid (70 mg/kg thyroxine daily for 1 week) animals (Fig. 6; von Borstel, unpublished observations).

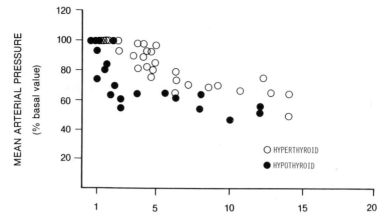

Fig. 6. Correlation between arterial plasma adenosine levels and blood pressure in hyperthyroid and hypothyroid rats. Catheterized rats were made hyperthyroid by daily injections of thyroxine (75 µg/kg s.c.) for 1 week, or hypothyroid with dietary propylthiouracil (0.15% in chow) for 2 weeks. The relationship between circulating arterial adenosine levels and arterial pressure before and during adenosine infusion was tested according to the protocol described in Fig. 4 and 5. Each treatment group contained six animals

If the potentiation of the cardiovascular effects of nicotine by adenosine represents a physiological phenomenon, then it is possible that the prevention of this effect by caffeine may be a relevant aspect of the observation that smokers tend to consume more coffee than nonsmokers (Gilbert 1976).

References

Berne RM (1980) The role of adenosine in the regulation of coronary blood flow. Circ Res 47: 807–813

Bianchi A, DeNatale G, Giaquinto S (1963) The effects of adenosine and its phosphorylated derivatives upon the respiratory apparatus. Arch Int Pharmacodyn Ther 145: 498–517

Boulenger J-P, Patel J, Post RM, Parma AM, Marangos PJ (1983) Chronic caffeine consumption increases the number of brain adenosine receptors. Life Sci 32: 1135–1142

Burg AW, Warner E (1975) Effect of orally administered caffeine and theophylline on tissue concentrations of 3′,5′ cyclic AMP and phosphodiesterase (Abstr). Fed Proc 34: 332

Cornford EM, Oldendorf WH (1975) Independent blood-brain barrier transport systems for nucleic acid precursors. Biochem Biophys Acta 394: 211–219

Daly JW, Bruns RF, Snyder SH (1981) Adenosine receptors in the central nervous system: relationship to the central actions of methylxanthines. Life Sci 28: 2083–2097

Dreisbach RH, Pfeiffer C (1943) Caffeine-withdrawal headache. J Lab Clin Med 28: 1212–1219

Drury AN (1936) The physiological activity of nucleic acid and its derivatives. Physiol Rev 16: 292–325

Drury AN, Szent-Gyorgyi A (1929) The physiological activity of adenine compounds with especial reference to their action on the mammalian heart. J Physiol 68: 213–237

Fredholm BB (1980) Are the actions of methylxanthines due to antagonism of adenosine? Trends Pharmacol Sci 1: 129–132

Fredholm BB, Hedqvist P (1980) Modulation of neurotransmission by purine nucleotides and nucleosides. Biochem Pharmacol 29: 1635–1643

Gilbert RM (1976) Caffeine as a drug of abuse. In: Gibbins RJ, Israel Y, Kalant H (eds) Research advances in alcohol and drug problems, vol. 3. Wiley, New York

Goldstein A, Kaizer S, Whitby O (1969) Psychotropic effects of caffeine in man. IV. Quantitative and qualitative differences associated with habituation to coffee. Clin Pharmacol Ther 10: 489–497

Hedqvist P, Fredholm BB, Olundh S (1978) Antagonistic effect of theophylline and adenosine on adrenergic neuroeffector transmission in the rabbit kidney. Circ Res 43: 592–598

Henon BK, Turner DK, McAfee DA (1980) Adenosine receptors: electrophysiological actions at pre- and postsynaptic sites on mammalian neurons (Abstr 94.24). Society for Neuroscience, 10th annual meeting, Cincinnati

Hom G, Lokhandwala MF (1981) Presynaptic inhibition of vascular sympathetic neurotransmission by adenosine. Eur J Pharmacol 69: 101–106

Loffelholz K (1979) Release induced by nicotinic agonists. In: Paton DM (ed) The release of catecholamines from adrenergic neurons. Pergamon, New York, pp 275–301

Lokhandwala MF (1979) Inhibition of cardiac sympathetic neurotransmission by adenosine. Eur J Pharmacol 60: 353–357

Maitre M, Ciesielski L, Leeman A, Kempf E, Mandel P (1974) Protective effect of adenosine and nicotinamide against audiogenic seizure. Biochem Pharmacol 23: 2807–2816

Mathieu-Levy N (1968) Contribution à l'étude du mécanisme de la potentialisation du sommeil expérimental par l'acide adénosinétriphosphorique (ATP). Sur quelques actions d'ATP au niveau du système nerveux central. Therapie 23: 1157–1173

Neims AH, von Borstel RW (1983) Caffeine: its metabolism and biochemical mechanisms of action. In: Wurtman RJ, Wurtman JJ (eds) Nutrition and the brain, vol 6. Raven, New York, pp 1–30

Osswald H (1979) Renal effects of adenosine and their inhibition by theophylline in dogs. Naunyn-Schmiedebergs Arch Pharmacol 288: 79–86

Rall TW (1980) The xanthines. In: Gilman AG, Goodman LS, Gilman A (eds) The pharmacological basis of therapeutics, 6th edn. Macmillan, New York, pp 592–607

Sattin A, Rall TW (1970) The effect of adenosine and adenine nucleotides on the cyclic adenosine /3-,5-phosphate content of guinea pig cerebral cortex slices. Mol Pharmacol 6: 13–23

Snyder SH, Katims JJ, Annau Z, Bruns RF, Daly JW (1981) Adenosine receptors and behavioral actions of methylxanthines. Proc Natl Acad Sci USA 78: 3260–3264

Sollevi A, Hjemdahl P, Fredholm BB (1981) Endogenous adenosine inhibits lipolysis induced by nerve stimulation without inhibiting noradrenaline release in canine subcutaneous adipose tissue in vivo. Naunyn Schmiedebergs Arch Pharmacol 316: 112–119

Taylor DA, Stone TW (1980) The actions of adenosine on noradrenergic neuronal inhibition induced by stimulation of locus coeruleus. Brain Res 183: 367–376

von Borstel RW, Conlay LC, Wurtman RJ (1983) Chronic caffeine consumption potentiates the hypotensive action of circulating adenosine. Life Sci 32: 1151–1158

Winn HR, Rubio R, Berne RM (1981) The role of adenosine in the regulation of cerebral blood flow. J Cerebral Blood Flow Metab 1: 239–244

Section V

Direct Assessments of Effects on Health

Editor of Section V: W. R. Grice

XI Influence of Ingested Caffeine on Animal Reproduction

W. R. Gomes

1 Introduction

A rather diverse literature exists on the relationship between ingestion of caffeine and reproductive phenomena. The variations in species, dose level, method and duration of administration, control groups analyzed, and end points measured have all contributed to this diversity. In order to better compare results from the various experimental designs, the studies reviewed in this chapter are organized by species and grouped by method of delivery of caffeine.

2 Rats

2.1 Details of Experimental Reports

2.1.1 Caffeine in Drinking Solution

Bachmann et al. (1946) treated rats with caffeine for up to 3.5 years. At weaning age, 25 groups of two male and two female littermates were divided into control and treated male/female pairs. The control rats drank tap water throughout the experiment, the treatment group only a sweetened beverage containing 0.2 mg caffeine/ml. The average consumption of caffeine was calculated to be 40–50 mg/kg body weight/day. When the animals were 100 days old (i. e., about 11 weeks after the start of the experiment) the pairs were caged together for the duration of the experiment. Records were kept on the date of birth of each litter, litter size at birth, and the number of young that survived to weaning (at 21 days). A pair remained in the experiment until the female failed to become pregnant within 3 months after the birth of a litter. The animals were then killed and the testes were removed from the males for histological examination.

In this experiment, caffeine was without effect on growth or reproductive performance of rats. Treated pairs produced a lifetime average of 5.4 litters, compared with 4.2 for controls (N. S.); similarly, litter size and weaning rate were uninfluenced by caffeine administration, as was the average period between pairing the animals and birth of the first litter. Histological examination of the testes from 23 caffeine-treated and 15 control animals revealed no changes that could be related to caffeine ingestion.

153

Three studies have been conducted in which rats were given caffeine solution or coffee dilutions to drink [Kensler 1976 (cited by Collins 1979); Nolen 1981; Palm et al. 1978]. The study by Kensler involved the administration to female Sprague-Dawley rats of 50% coffee as the only source of liquid. Coffee was administered for 21 days prior to mating and throughout the gestation and nursing periods. The offspring were devided into four groups, receiving coffee as their dietary liquid at the following ratios: 0% (control), 25%, 50%, and 100%; measured consumption of caffeine was 0, 14, 35, and 54 mg/kg/day respectively. Ten male rats at each concentration were sacrificed after 1 year and 15–22 more were sacrificed from each group after 2 years survival on treatment. Histological examination of testes was conducted at the 1- and 2-year intervals and on all rats that died prior to the end of the 2-year experiment. Testis weights did not differ between control and caffeine-treated groups at any time. In the 1-year treatment period, no evidence of seminiferous tubular atrophy was seen in any group; two instances of focal mineralization in the seminiferous tubules and two instances of focal mineralization of the intratesticular arteries were noted; these were apparently not dose related. Rats surviving to 2 years included five bearers of interstitial cell tumors, one in a control group, one each at the 25% and 50% coffee levels, and two in the 100% coffee group. Intratestincular arteritis was recorded for 13 of 49 controls and 19 of 51 caffeine-treated rats. No dose-response trend was seen for tubular atrophy, mineralization of seminiferous tubules or intratesticular arteries, medial degeneration of testicular arteries, or sperm granuloma. Variations did exist in some of these micropathological lesions (e.g., two cases of tubular mineralization were seen, both in the 100% coffee group, and 11 cases of arterial mineralization were noted in 67 controls but none in the 45 rats in the 100% coffee group), but these appeared random. Similarly, rats which died prior to termination of the experiment (49 controls, 82 treated rats) did not exhibit lesions which were related to caffeine treatment.

Nolen (1981) examined the effects of brewed and instant coffee on growth and reproduction of Sprague- Dawley rats from weaning through two pregnancies. Seven groups of 20 male and 30 female rats were assigned to the control treatment (distilled water); to 100%, 50%, or 25% brewed coffee; or to 100%, 50%, or 25% instant coffee. Animals were caged individually until they had been in the experiment for 91 days (growth period); at that time ten rats of each sex were killed in each group. The remaining rats were mated (one male to two females), and after gestation and weaning of litters, the females were mated a second time to the same males. Males were killed after the second mating; half the females in each group were killed on day 13 of gestation and the remainder on day 21.

During the 13-week growth period, intake of caffeine ranged from 47 to 178 mg/kg/day (mean 91 mg/kg/day) in males receiving 10% brewed coffee and from 85 to 181 mg/kg/day (mean 106 mg/kg/day) in females on the same treatment. Average daily consumptions were about 91, 54, and 28 mg/kg for all rats consuming 100%, 50%, and 25% coffee respectively, with females slightly higher than males and consumption of caffeine in brewed coffee somewhat higher than that in instant coffee.

After 13 weeks of the experiment, rats consuming coffee had grown at a rate equal to, or greater than, controls. Weights of testes and ovaries did not differ among control and coffee-drinking groups.

By the end of the reproductive period (26–28 weeks) male rats drinking brewed coffee had consumed 50, 30, and 17 mg/kg/day of caffeine in the 100%, 50%, and 25% groups respectively; males drinking instant coffee consumed about 80% as much. Values for females were 80, 45, and 30 mg/kg/day for brewed coffee and 70, 40, and 25 mg/kg/day for instant coffee. No differences existed between control and treated rats in body size, relative gonad weight (testis or ovary weight/kg body weight), pregnancy rates, litter size, or numbers of living or weaned pups.

Palm et al. (1978) administered coffee to Sprague-Dawley rats to examine toxicity and teratogenic potential of the compound (only reproductive data will be reviewed here). Female rats weighing 152 g were given 0%, 12.5%, 25% or 50% coffee as their sole beverage for 5 weeks prior to breeding and throughout gestation. Untreated males were used for mating. Daily caffeine intake averaged about 0, 9, 19, and 38 mg/kg in the 0%, 12.5%, 25%, and 50% coffee groups respectively (LD_{50} in acute studies was 230 and 249 mg/kg for males and females respectively). Weight gains and food consumption were not influenced by treatment. The mean days of pregnancy and (at sacrifice on day 19 of gestation), number of fetuses per litter, live fetuses, sex ratio, and fetal weight did not differ with caffeine treatments (40 control females and 20 animals at each coffee level). Those females allowed to litter (ten controls, five at each coffee level) did not differ in litter size, number of living pups, or weight of pups at birth or at 38 days of age (even though dams continued to receive coffee during lactation).

In another experiment (Palm et al. 1978), groups of 25 mated females were given about 30 mg caffeine/kg/day in the drinking water. Two additional groups of 25 were given tap water (controls). Upon killing of 20 females per group on day 19 of gestation, no effects of caffeine (whether administered in the drinking water or by gavage) were seen in number of fetuses, number of dead fetuses, sex ratio, or mean fetal weight. The mean period until pregnancy was significantly longer in the groups treated with caffeine before caffeine was administered. When five females per caffeine group were allowed to litter, no differences were recorded in litter size or weight of pups at birth. In these groups neither lactating dams nor pups received caffeine. A significantly reduced number of pups survived to 38 days of age from the group in which pregnant females received caffeine in the drinking water, but not in the gavage group. Weight of pups at 38 days was not affected by treatment.

In the coffee- and caffeine-treated groups reported by Palm et al. (1978), fetal body sizes and organ weights (as a percentage of body weights) varied, in some cases, between control and treated groups. Fetuses in coffee-treated rats tended to be larger than controls and tended to have smaller relative organ weights. However, the actual organ weights of fetuses from coffee- and caffeine-treated fetuses tended to be larger than controls. The incidence of partial, unilateral cryptorchidism was increased in caffeine-treated but not coffee-treated groups. Cryptorchidism was not reported in newborn pups.

Reproduction of surviving pups from coffee- and caffeine-treated dams was measured at about 100 days of age, without further caffeine treatment. Females and males were randomly mated and the females were allowed to litter normally. The fertility rates of these groups did not differ with coffee or caffeine treatment. The mean number of days until pregnancy was greater in rats whose dams had received 25% or 50% coffee and especially in rats from dams treated with caffeine during pregnancy – a group of females with longer periods until pregnancy before treatment. Litter size, birth weight, pups dead at birth, survival to 28 days, and weight at 28 days were not different among progeny of rats from control females and those of females treated with coffee or caffeine.

2.1.2 Caffeine in Feed

As reported in a letter to FASEB, Reeves and Zeitlin (SCOGS 1978), in a pilot study, incorporated caffeine into the diet of rats at a concentration of 0.18%, for a consumption rate of approximately 120/mg/kg/day. Unspecified numbers of rats were observed for reproduction for two generations with two litters per generation. Progressive reduction in litter size was observed, birth weights, postnatal survival, and growth rates throughout lactation were decreased postweaning, but growth and development were not affected.

In a series of studies by Friedman and associates (Friedman et al. 1979b; Weinberger et al. 1978) rats were fed diets containing caffeine, theobromine, or theophylline with or without sodium nitrate. In experiment I, 20 male Osborne-Mendel rats served as controls and 20 others were fed a diet containing 1.0% caffeine (specifics of the other diets will not be detailed here); extensive weight loss of the treated animals during the next 3 weeks led to a reduction in caffeine concentration to 0.5% of the diet. Rats surviving for 64 weeks were killed and necropsy examinations were performed. Histopathological examination was made of most glands and organs, including testes, seminal vesicles, prostate glands, pituitary glands, and adrenal glands. In experiment II, groups of 20 Osborne-Mendel rats were fed diets containing 0% or 0.5% caffeine; six rats from each group were killed after 14 weeks of the experiment and those of the remainder that survived were killed after 75 weeks. Samples were collected as in the first experiment, but adrenal and pituitary glands were also weighed.

In experiment III, 35 Holtzman rats were given the control diet and 41 were fed 0.5% caffeine. Rats were killed at 19 weeks after the onset of treatment and necropsied. Only testes were weighed, and testes, epididymides, seminal vesicles, and prostates were examined microscopically. Blood constituents including testosterone were assayed.

Rats fed caffeine lost weight initially in experiment I and gained more slowly than controls in all experiments. Body weights in treated rats were lower than in controls, and where reported, food intake and food efficiency were depressed by caffeine ingestion. Even though some of the other compounds fed in the experiments depressed food intake as much as caffeine, none reduced food efficiency to the same level. Adrenal weight was doubled in treated rats (experiment II, weight reported to only one significant digit), and testis weight was reduced to 30%–50% of control values. Histopathological examination of testes in experiment I showed oligospermatogenesis in one testis of one of 14 control rats; all other testes were normal. Conversely, testes from all 13 caffeine-fed rats were atrophic, showing a complete lack of spermatogenesis. Results in experiment II were similar, with three cases of oligospermatogenesis and five cases of aspermatogenesis among eight rats surviving to 75 weeks; experiment III extended the observation (all 15 controls were normal, all 11 caffeine-treated rats showed testicular atrophy) to a second strain of rat.

It is difficult to determine average consumption of caffeine in the studies by Friedman and associates. Although final weights of rats are given, initial weights are not reported. Weight gain is shown graphically for something less than the entire period of experiments I and II and in tabular form for a portion of experiment I. However, the graph indicates that control and caffeine-treated rats gained about 400 and 280 g, respecitvely in 25 weeks, and the table assigns values of 499 and 308 g for this same interval. Food intake is enumerated for a portion of experiment I and for all of experiment II, so that average daily consumption of caffeine can be crudely assessed, but changes throughout the studies in consumption rate as a function of body size are not reported. In experiment III, treated rats consumed 1426 g diet in 19 weeks, on average of 10.72 g/day. These rats gained 196 g to a final weight of 306 g. Using the simple mean of beginning and ending body weights, i. e., $\frac{306+102}{2}$, the average consumption of diet was 51.54 g feed/kg/day, and the mean consumption of caffeine was 258 mg/kg/day. Collins (1979) estimates caffeine consumption from a 0.5% caffeine diet to be approximately 250 mg/kg/day.

In a preliminary report of an additional study, Friedman et al. (1979a) described experiments in which they fed male Osborne-Mendel rats diets containing 0%, 0.125%, 0.25%, and 0.5% caffeine for up to 6 months. Depressed weight gain and feed intake were observed in a majority (of an unreported number) of rats at 1 month of administration of 0.5% caffeine. This impairment was reported to be severe and irreversible, but details were not given. Slightly impaired spermatogenesis was reported in 27% (of an unreported number) of rats fed 0.25% caffeine for 6 months, and testicular atrophy was seen in adult rats fed 0.5% caffeine for 8 months. None of the effects described was seen in pair-fed controls.

2.2 Summary and Conclusions

No detrimental effects of ingested caffeine on reproductive processes have been reported in most experiments when rats consumed up to 50 mg/kg/day for periods ranging from 13 weeks to 3.5 years (Bachmann et al. 1946; Nolen 1981). Palm et al. (1978) also reported no effect on reproductive parameters of long-term treatment of rats with 30–38 mg/kg/day, with two exceptions. First, offspring of caffeine- or coffee-treated rats needed a significantly higher number of days before achieving pregnancy than offspring from controls. This phenomenon appeared to be related to the group of parents used, however, and not to caffeine treatment. Second, fetuses of rats treated with caffeine exhibited reduced organ:body weight ratios and an increased incidence of partial unilateral cryptorchidism. The reduction in organ:body weight ratios appears to be related to smaller body weights in fetuses from the control rats. The incidence of unilateral cryptorchidism in rats was higher with caffeine treatment, but not with caffeine administered at higher levels in coffee.

Treatment of rats with extremely high doses of caffeine, however, appears to result consistently in reduced weight gains, impaired feed efficiency, and loss of spermatogenic cells in the adult testis. The suppression of spermatogenesis in rats following administration of toxic levels of caffeine is not surprising; indeed toxic or stressful conditions have frequently been associated with testicular atrophy, particularly in rats (Johnson et al. 1970).

3 Mice

3.1 Details of Experimental Reports

3.1.1 Caffeine in Drinking Water

Thayer and Kensler (1973 b) treated CD-1 mice with caffeine and examined reproductive patterns over a four-generation period. Groups of 20 female and 10 male mice were supplied drinking water containing caffeine at the following rates: 0 (control), 0.02, 0.06, and 0.12 mg caffeine/ml water. Each male was mated with two females from the same treatment group, beginning 4 weeks after the onset of treatment. In each subsequent generation, each male was paired with a single female; the pair was allowed to produce two litters. All treated groups received caffeine continuously throughout the duration of the experiment, i.e., throughout mating, pregnancy, lactation, and postweaning growth. Intake of caffeine was determined during the 4-week premating period for the parental generation and during the first week after pairing in the second and third generations. Consumption of caffeine during these measuring periods was 0, 4–5, 12–18, and 29–39 mg/kg/day for groups given 0, 0.02, 0.06, and 0.12 mg caffeine/ml drinking water respectively. Examination of the three-generation reproductive data in this study reveals no consistent dose-response relationships between caffeine and fertility (proportion of females littering), fecundity (litter size), or preweaning normality (apparent decreases in total litter weaning weight in three of 12 treatment groups were attributed by the authors to laboratory accidents and other deaths unrelated to caffeine administration). Weaning weights were not different between control and caffeine-treated groups in any generation, but weights in treated animals were more variable and the data suggest an increased proportion of "runts" in caffeine-treated groups. This effect was confined to the earlier generations and was not dose related. Sex ratios for all generations were 0.84 (males:females) for controls and 1.03 for caffeine-treated rats.

In a shorter-term study, Thayer and Kensler (1973 a) administered caffeine in the drinking water to male CD-1 mice for a period of 8 weeks. Dose levels of caffeine were 0 (control), 0.02, 0.06, 0.2, and 0.6 mg/ml; ingestion of the compound for the 8-week period averaged 0, 3.6, 12.4, 49.2, and 121.6 mg/kg/day respectively. At the end of the treatment period, six males from each group were each mated to five females each week for 8 weeks; no caffeine was administered during the mating period. Females were killed 12–13 days after mating and early and late embryonic deaths were assessed. Treatment of males with caffeine apparently reduced weight gain during the 8-week period, but control mice tended to be smaller at the start of the experiment. Fertility of males, reflected in proportion of pregnant females among those exposed, was apparently decreased in the 0.2 and 0.6 mg/ml groups, but the fecundity of pregnant females (litter size) was not altered. These data suggest changes in mating behavior of males treated with high levels of caffeine. No effects on embryonic mortality could be attributed to caffeine treatment; indeed the proportion of early embryonic deaths appeared lower in females mated to males in the 0.2 and 0.6 mg/ml (49 and 122 mg/kg/day) groups.

Thayer and Kensler (1973a) also administered caffeine in drinking water to male mice at rates of 0, 0.02, and 0.06 mg/ml for 16 weeks, followed either by no further treatment or by treatment with X-rays (100 r) or the mutagen triethylenemelamine (TEM; 0.2 mg/kg). Five males from each of the nine subgroups were mated with five females weekly for 7 weeks after treatment.

Caffeine intake from the 0.02 and 0.06 mg/ml solutions averaged 4.2 and 12.7 mg/kg/day respectively. Caffeine consumption at these rates was without effect on growth of males or pregnancy rates of mated females. Caffeine treatment appeared to improve pregnancy rates in females mated with X-irradiated or TEM-treated males, but this was probably a reflection of experimental variation. In addition, no differences due to caffeine were seen in numbers of implantation sites or in embryonic mortality rates.

Aeschbacher et al. (1978) administered caffeine in drinking water to 150 male SPF Swiss CD-1 mice at an average consumption rate of 112 mg/kg/day for 8 weeks; another 150 males served as untreated controls. Each male was mated with two females during the 1st and 3rd weeks after treatment. Females were killed 13 days after the middle of the mating period. No differences in pregnancy rate, litter size, or embryonic mortality were seen between control and caffeine-treated groups during either mating period.

Epstein et al. (1970) administered caffeine to ten male ICR/Ha Swiss mice at a 1.0 mg/ml (0.1%) solution in the drinking water for 8 weeks. An additional ten males served as controls. At the end of the treatment period, each male was mated with three females weekly for 8 successive weeks. Females were autopsied 13 days after the middle of each weekly mating period. The consumption of caffeine and the weights of the mice were not reported, but interpolation of data from the other studies using mice suggests that caffeine intake was of the order of 200–250 mg/kg/day. The proportion of females impregnated by caffeine-treated males was lower than the control value, but litter size, preimplantation losses, and rates of early embryo death were not affected.

In an additional experiment, Epstein et al. (1970) administered caffeine to male mice for 8 weeks at concentrations of 0% (control), 0.05%, 0.1%, 0.2%, and 0.4% in drinking water (estimated consumption – see above – would be in the range of 0, 110, 200, 275, and >300 mg/kg/day). After caffeine treatment, mice from each group were X-irradiated with a single exposure of 50 or 200 r. Each male was then mated with three females per week for 8 weeks; females were autopsied as above. Mortality of males was not affected by caffeine or X-ray treatment. Pregnancy rates of females were not different between X-irradiated and X-irradiated–caffeine-treated males, nor were total implants or early fetal death rates altered by combined X-ray and caffeine treatment compared with X-irradiation alone.

As reported by the Life Sciences Research Office, FASEB (SCOGS 1978), Lyons et al. (1962) treated male and female mice with a 0.1% solution of caffeine in the drinking water from conception throughout life and reported no noticeable effect on reproduction, and Cattanach obtained negative results in efforts to induce translocations in mouse chromosomes of the type reducing male fertility. Administration of caffeine in drinking water at a 0.3% concentration for 3 months (about 300 mg/kg/day) caused a transient decrease in fertility with no effect on fertility of subsequent generations of male offspring.

Adler and Rohrborn (1969) treated male C3H and 101×3CH mice with 0.002%, 0.01%, or 0.5% caffeine in drinking water; untreated controls were carried with each strain at each caffeine level. Treatment was started at 3 weeks of age and continued for 245–351 days; at the end of the treatment period the spermatogenic cells were examined for chromosomal aberrations. With caffeine intake of 3.5, 14.9, and 305 mg/kg/day, cytogenetic analysis of metaphase I figures indicated no caffeine-related changes in translocations or univalent chromosomes.

3.1.2 Caffeine Administered by Gavage

Aeschbacher et al. (1978) treated 50 male SPF Swiss mice of the CD-1 strain with caffeine at the rate of 90 mg/kg/day for 5 days by gavage. Tap water was administered to another 50 mice during the same period. The mice averaged about 10 weeks of age at the beginning of the experiment. Each male was mated with three virgin females during the 1st, 3rd, and 6th week after treatment. Mice treated with caffeine showed no differences in fertility or fecundity at any time after treatment. Of the 450 females mated with control mice, 412 became pregnant; in the caffeine-treated group 411 females were impregnated. In addition, no differences were seen in average number of living implants (12.7 for both groups) or dead implants (1.1 for both groups) per female.

3.1.3 Caffeine Administered by Injection

Thayer and Kensler (1973a) administered caffeine to male Ha/ICR mice in a single intraperitoneal (i. P.) injection of 15 mg/kg. Five males were treated with caffeine, five were untreated controls, and three groups of five mice each were treated with caffeine plus X-irradiation before, simulatneously with, or after caffeine injection. Each male was then mated with five females weekly for 7 weeks. Caffeine alone had no effect on pregnancy rates, number of implants per female, or embryo deaths, nor did caffeine enhance or ameliorate the deleterious effects of X-irradiation on the parameters.

Epstein et al. (1970) treated male ICR/Ha mice with a single i. p. dose of caffeine (0, 168, 192, 200, 214, or 240 mg/kg) or with two injections (175 mg/kg/day) on successive days. Between five and ten mice were treated at each level, with a total of 40 mice used as vehicle (Tricaprylin or water)-treated controls. Following injection, each male was caged with three females weekly for 3–8 weeks. Females were killed 13 days after mid-week of exposure to males. An additional group of male mice was

160

treated with 186–200 mg caffeine/kg in a single i.p. dose or with 175 mg/kg given twice; these mice were also treated with the mutagens methyl methanesulfonate (50 mg/kg), triethylenephosphoramide (TEPA; 0.312 or 1.250 mg/kg), or X-irradiation (50, 200, or 250 r).

Mortality of males was not releated to caffeine treatment, but mean pregnancy rates for females mated to caffeine-treated males were lower than control values. In females which became pregnant, there were no differences due to caffeine treatment in implantation rates, embryonic loss, or number of living implants. In addition, there appeared to be no influence of caffeine on implantation or embryo loss rates in females mated with mutagen-treated males.

Adler (1968) administered caffeine to 10-week-old mice in a single i.p. injection of 250 mg/kg in two replicate experiments 1 year apart. In the first experiment, 15 males were treated with caffeine and five were injected with isotonic saline (controls); the second group consisted of 14 caffeine-treated males and five controls. Each male was mated with three females weekly for 8 weeks. Females were autopsied on days 14.5–16.5 of pregnancy.

Although the dose of caffeine administered by Adler (1969) was reported to be at the LD_{50} for mice, no mortality was seen in this experiment. (At a dose of 330 mg/kg, Adler found 75% rapid mortality in eight mice.) Extensive analysis of the data led Adler to the conclusion that copulation frequency was significantly reduced in caffeine-treated males, but implantation rate and embryonic mortality in pregnant females were not affected by caffeine treatment.

To study further the effects of caffeine on the spermatogenic process, Wyrobeck and Bruce (1975) treated C57BLXCH3/Anf mice with caffeine, using five consecutive daily intraperitoneal doses. Sperm suspensions were made from cauda epididymides taken 1, 4, and 10 weeks after the end of treatment: these were stained and examined for morphological normality. The daily doses of caffeine administered, reported only in graphic form, were estimated to be 100 and 250 mg/kg. At these levels, sperm abnormalities were less than 3% throughout the experimental period, a value well within the control range.

3.2 Summary and Conclusions

Several studies utilizing the serial mating technique demonstrated no effects of caffeine on fecundity or embryonic mortality (Thayer and Kensler 1973a; Epstein et al. 1970; Aeschbacher at al. 1970; Adler 1969). Wyrobeck and Bruce (1975) found no effect of caffeine on epididymal sperm of treated males, and Adler and Rohrborn (1969) found no caffeine-related chromosomal aberrations after treatment with caffeine. Lifelong (Lyon et al. 1962; cited in SCOES 1978) or multigeneration (Thayer and Kensler 1973b) studies also failed to reveal detrimental effects of caffeine on reproduction.

Doses of caffeine above 100 mg/kg/day tended to reduce mating in mice, but the general toxic effects of high levels could lead to reduced libido.

Data available from studies on mice lead to the firm conviction that caffeine is without effect on reproduction in this species except at very high doses; even then, there is uncertainty about the mechanisms involved.

4 Domestic Chickens

Ax and his co-workers (Ax et al. 1974a, b, 1976) conducted a series of experiments in which caffeine was incorporated into the diet of chickens and various reproductive phenomena were observed.

In an initial series of experiments, Ax et al. (1974a) administered caffeine to groups of White Leghorn hens and artificially inseminated the hens with semen from untreated roosters. Groups of 20 White Leghorn pullet of unspecified age and weight were fed diets containing 0%, 0.1%, 0.5%, and 1.0% caffeine. The pullets were each inseminated with 10^8 motile sperm from a semen pool collected from three White Leghorn and three Columbian roosters. From the day of first fertile eggs, eggs were collected for 14 days. Eggs were incubated at 37.8 °C and candled at 7 days of incubation; those considered fertile were allowed to incubate to hatching or subsequent death.

Pullets fed 0.5% or 1.0% caffeine in the diet laid numerous soft-shelled eggs, and egg production essentially ceased within 3 days. Whether cessation of laying was due to interference with ovarian function and ovulation or whether it represented malfunction of the shell membrane–shell producing functions was apparently not investigated.

The hens fed caffeine at the 0.1% rate "showed higher embryonic mortality for the 14 days when compared ... to the controls" according to Ax et al. (1974a), but the data supporting this statement and the level of significance, if any, were not shown. The authors fed 40 more pullets 0.1% dietary caffeine without concurrent controls. For their statistical analyses, the authors compared the pooled 0.1% treatment groups with the controls from their preliminary study and with a group of control females examined 3 years earlier. Fertility rates in the pooled group of treated females (58.2%) were not different from the controls carried in this study (56.8%), but embryonic mortality was significantly higher.

In a second study, Ax et al. (1974b) fed White Leghorn pullets diets containing 0%, 0.05%, or 0.1% caffeine. Each pullet was inseminated with 0.05 ml semen pooled from ten New Hampshire Red roosters. Eggs were collected for 14 days starting on the first day of fertile eggs. Fertility of hens was uninfluenced by caffeine treatment: fertilization rates were 41.7%, 41.7%, and 43.5% for the 0%, 0.05%, and 0.1% caffeine groups respectively.

A later publication by Ax et al. (1976) reported studies in which eight roosters were fed a diet containing 0.1% caffeine. Semen was collected twice weekly and sperm concentrations were recorded. Untreated White Leghorn pullets were inseminated with semen pooled from four of the roosters and fertility and embryonic mortality were assessed (Ax et al. 1974a).

Fertility of semen from four roosters (single pool/insemination) was 30.8% at the onset of the experiment. No change in fertility or embryonic mortality was observed with semen collected after 7 days of caffeine feeding, but fertility decreased significantly (to 3.3%; $P < 0.01$) after the roosters had been fed caffeine for 14 days.

Pooled semen volume for the eight roosters totaled 5.6–6.4 ml at each collection for a period beginning 3 days prior to caffeine treatment and extending 17 days into the treatment period; concentration of sperm in the pooled semen samples did not vary outside a range of 5.8×10^9 to 6.0×10^9 sperm/ml during this period. The sample collected at 21 days of treatment contained only 3.2 ml semen with 9.6×10^7 sperm; both semen volume and sperm concentration declined in samples collected at 25 and 29 days. Single roosters killed after 31, 38, and 63 days of caffeine treatment and single roosters killed after 31 days of caffeine in the diet and 7 or 14 days of caffeine-free diet ejaculated no semen prior to death. One rooster was reported to be killed without caffeine treatment, but whether he was one of the eight described above is not clear. Two roosters were treated with caffeine for 35 days, then fed a caffeine-free diet for 28 days. These roosters resumed semen production at 11 days after withdrawal of caffeine and produced semen of normal volume and sperm concentration by 21 days after removal of caffeine treatment. Semen collected 28 days after withdrawal exhibited pretreatment fertility levels when inseminated into untreated females; embryonic mortality was also at pretreatment rates.

Histological examination of testes suggested oligospermatogenesis after 31 or 63 days of treatment. Testes from roosters treated for 35 days with caffeine and fed a caffeine-free diet for 28 days appeared normal. Evaluation of testes from birds withdrawn from treatment for 7 or 14 days was not reported, nor was testis weight at any time.

The series of experiments at Ax et al. (1974a, b, 1976) were all conducted with chickens of unspecified age and weight. Feed intake and body weight changes were not reported. Therefore, it is extremely difficult to calculate the caffeine consumption by the birds. The SCOGS report (1978) and the FDA proposal (1980) assign values of 80 and 160 mg/kg/day to the 0.05%, and 0.1% groups respectively, but these values were apparently developed on a totally arbitrary basis.

5 General Observations

Recent actions by the FDA have prompted renewed scrutiny of the influence of caffeine on reproductive processes in humans and laboratory animals. Epidemiological studies with women have generally failed to demonstrate cause-and-effect relationships between caffeine consumption and altered reproductive function (see Dews 1982 for discussion) or have suffered from such serious flaws in design and controls (Weathersbee et al. 1977) that results cannot be accurately interpreted.

Use of very high sublethal doses in rodents and chickens suggests that caffeine can have detrimental effects on reproduction if sufficiently high doses are administered. The etiology of these effects cannot be determined from the data collected, but it is likely that the reproductive deficiencies were secondary to the generally toxic action of the massive doses of caffeine, and not to a direct action of caffeine on the gonads.

When caffeine was administered to animals at doses that may reflect high levels of human consumption, no effects on reproduction were found in rats or mice. Indeed, the consumption of caffeine at levels up to 100 mg/kg/day was without effect on reproduction except in the study by Palm et al. (1978); in that case, differences noted appeared to be attributable to pretreatment variability in rats and to small fetuses in the control group, rather than to direct effects of caffeine.

In sum, the data evaluated in this review lead to the conclusion that levels of caffeine consumed by the general public pose no hazard to the human reproductive process.

References

Adler ID (1969) Does caffeine induce dominant lethal mutations in mice? Humangenetik 7: 137–148

Adler ID, Rohrborn G (1969) Cytogenetic investigation of meiotic chromosomes of male mice after chronic caffeine treatment. Humangenetik 8: 81–85

Aeschbacher HU, Milon H, Wurzner HP (1978) Caffeine concentrations in mice plasma and testicular tissue and the effect of caffeine on the dominant lethal test. Mutat Res 57: 193–200

Ax RL, Bray DJ, Lodge JR (1974a) Effects of dietary caffeine on fertility and embryonic loss in chickens. Poult Sci 53: 428–429

Ax RL, Lodge JR, Bray DJ (1974b) Increased embryonic loss in chickens from 0.05% dietary caffeine. Poult Sci 53: 830–831

Ax RL, Collier RJ, Lodge JR (1976) Effects of dietary caffeine on the testis of the domestic fowl, *Gallus domesticus*. J Reprod Fertil 47: 235–238

Bachmann G, Haldi J, Wynn W, Ensor C (1946) Reproductivity and growth of albino rats on a prolonged daily intake of caffeine. J Nutr 32: 239–247

Burg AW (1977) Comments on the health aspects of caffeine, especially the contribution of soft drinks, with particular reference to the report of the Select Committee on GRAS Substances. (Cited by SCOGS, 1978)

Collins TFX (1979) Review of reproduction and teratology. Studies of caffeine. FDA Bylines 9: 352–373

Dews PB (1982) Caffeine. Annu Rev Nutr 2: 323–341

Epstein EE, Bass W, Arnold W, Bishop Y (1970) The failure of caffeine to induce mutagenic effects or to synergize the effects of known mutagens in mice. Food Cosmet Toxicol 8: 381–401

Food and Drug Administration (1980) Soda water; standard of identity, and caffeine; detection of GRAS status, proposed delcaration that no prior sanction exists, and use on an interim basis pending additional study; proposed regulations. Fed Reg 45: 69816–69838

Friedman L, Weinberger MS, Farber TM, Moreland FM, Kahn MA, Keys JE, Stone CS (1979a) Some effects of short-term chronic feeding of caffeine to rats (Abstr). Toxicol Appl Pharmacol 48: A122

Friedman L, Weinberger MA, Farber TM, Moreland FM, Peters EL, Gilmore CE, Kahn MA (1979b) Testicular atrophy and impaired spermatogenesis in rats fed high levels of the methylxanthines caffeine, theobromine, or theophylline. J Environ Pathol Toxicol 2: 687–706

Johnson AD, Gomes WR, VanDemark NL (eds) 1970) The testis, vol 3. Influencing factors. Academic, New York

Nolen GA (1981) The effect of brewed and instant coffee on reproduction and teratogenesis in the rat. Toxicol Appl Pharmacol 58: 171–183

Palm PE, Arnold EP, Rachwell PC, Leyczek JC, Teague KW, Kensler CJ (1978) Evaluation of the teratogenic potential of fresh-brewed coffee and caffeine in the rat. Toxicol Appl Pharmacol 44: 1–16

Select Committee on GRAS Substances (1978) Evaluation of the health aspects of caffeine as a food ingredient. SCOGS-89 Federation of American Societies for Experimental Biology, Bethesda/MD (Available from the National Technical Information Service, Order No. PB 283-441/AS)

Thayer PS, Kensler CJ (1973a) Genetic tests in mice of caffeine alone and in combination with mutagens. Toxicol Appl Pharmacol 25: 157–168

Thayer PS, Kensler CJ (1973b) Exposure of four generations of mice to caffeine in drinking water. Toxicol Appl Pharmacol 25: 169–179

Weathersbee PS, Olsen LK, Lodge JR (1977) Caffeine and pregnancy: A retrospective study. Postgrad Med 62: 64–69

Weinberger MA, Friedman L, Farber TM, Moreland FM, Peters EL, Gilmore CE, Kahn MA (1978) Testicular atrophy and impaired spermatogenesis in rats fed high levels of the methylxanthines caffeine, theobromine, or theophylline. J Environ Pathol Toxicol 1: 569–688

Wyrobek AJ, Bruce WR (1975) Chemical induction of sperm abnormalities in mice. Proc Natl Acad Sci USA 72: 4425–4429

XII The Teratogenic Potential of Caffeine in Laboratory Animals

J. G. Wilson and W. J. Scott Jr.

1 Introduction

Interest in or concern about a teratogenic potential for caffeine is of relatively recent origin. The first publication on the subject seems to have been that by Nishimura and Nakai (1960), who injected pregnant mice with a single dose of 250 mg/kg caffeine between gestation days 9 and 14 and observed some offspring with cleft palate and digital defects. Since then there have been more than 30 reports of animal studies in which caffeine was given to pregnant animals either by injection or stomach tube or in food or drinking water. It is now established that a high doses, at or near those which cause maternal toxicity, caffeine treatment during the period of organ formation may result in developmental defects in a low to moderate percentage of the offspring. Such results have been reported mainly for mice and rats, although one limited study indicates that similar results may be obtainable also in rabbits.

2 Results of Previous Animal Studies

A substantial amount of experimental research in laboratory animals has already been devoted to evaluating the teratogenic potential of caffeine. Significant research is still in progress and doubtless will continue indefinitely into the future, owing to the several issues of both theoretical as well as practical import raised by caffeine studies to date. Research to date has reached some level of consensus on several important points, but has produced little agreement on other questions, either because of disparate results from different investigators using different animals or simply because that particular line of research has not been pursued to a logical conclusion.

2.1 Concordant Results

A degree of concordance seems to have been reached on several important points pertaining to the teratogenic potential of caffeine.

Caffeine has a variable but low level of teratogenicity in some laboratory animals, demonstrated mainly in rats and mice. One rabbit study reported six of 64 pups with ectrodactyly after daily treatment of the pregnant does at 100 mg/kg (Bertrand et al.

165

1970). Mice may be more sensitive to the teratogenic effects of caffeine than rats, since doses as low as 50 mg/kg/day have been reported to cause craniofacial malformations in seven of 745 fetuses (0.9%), but this result is of dubious significance (Knoche and König 1964), since the incidence of defects is scarcely greater than are usually seen in control mice. One laboratory has obtained a low (2%–7%) incidence of head malformations in mice at 75 mg/kg/day (Group d'Etude des Risques Teratogènes 1969), but other laboratories failed to find any malformations at this or higher doses (Cannon Laboratories, see Collins 1979). The lowest dose to produce malformations in rats – ectrodactyly in about 6% – was 80 mg/kg/day (Collins et al. 1981), but other authors failed to observe any malformations until dosage reached or exceeded 125 mg/kg/day (Bertrand et al. 1965, 1970; Leuschner and Schwerdtfeger 1969; Leuschner and Czok 1973). No other species have been tested except hamsters, and there the dosage (30 mg/kg/day) was too low to represent a valid test, since it is apparent from the above that a teratogenic response is unlikely in laboratory animals at less than 75–80 mg/kg/day and is not seen with any regularity until dosage is well above 100 mg/kg/day.

The high dosage required, as well as the generally low percentage of individuals actually showing teratogenic responses at high doses, is indicative of a low teratogenic potential. The best explanation for low-level and variable teratogenicity is that the effect results from the interaction of many factors. In other words, no one causative agent but a combination of two or more causes acting together is responsible for the observed effect. Unless all of the presumed causative agents are present simultaneously, the effect in question will not be seen or will be only sporadically or incompletely expressed. There is no direct evidence in support of this hypothesis from the animal studies reviewed; however, the results of Bertrand et al. (1970), discussed near the end of Sect. 3.3 below, are consistent with a genetic factor which must be present before caffeine is able to produce ectrodactyly in certain strains of Wistar rats.

Teratogenic effects from caffeine depend upon high dosage, as in single daily gavage or injection. In other words, when doses known to be teratogenic, such as the 80 mg/kg dose given via gavage once per day by Collins et al., are divided and given as multiple treatments amounting to equal – or even greater – total daily intake, no malformations are observed. Gilbert and Pistey (1973) injected total daily amounts as high as 80 mg/kg in four divided doses and obtained no malformations in rats. Sullivan (1982) gave total daily amounts of 100 mg/kg in four divided oral doses and failed to produce ectrodactyly in Charles River rats known to exhibit this defect when this amount is given in once-daily treatments. Fujii and Nishimura (1972) fed Sprague-Dawley rats with diets containing 180 or 330 mg/kg/day caffeine throughout pregnancy and observed no malformations after the lower regimen but reported significantly increased internal and skeletal anomalies after the higher dosage. Leuschner and Schwerdtfeger (1969) produced teratogenic effects by intubation of Wistar rats with 130 mg/kg of caffeine once daily, but when the equivalent dosage was incorporated into the diets, no increase in malformations above control levels were seen. Nolen (1981) gave pregnant Sprague-Dawley rats various concentrations of brewed coffee as the only source of fluid, including 100% coffee, equivalent to approximately 85 mg/kg/day caffeine, but observed no malformations in excess of those seen in controls.

Thus, the rate of caffeine dosage is a factor in determining teratogenicity. In rats of some strains approximately 80 mg/kg given in a single daily dose, by gavage or injection appears to be sufficient to produce a low but significant increase in malformations. When caffeine is given in divided doses, whether by multiple daily gavage, in food, or as the only source of drinking water, the stated threshold of 80 mg/kg/day total dose may be considerably exceeded without inducing malformations. In a second study Collins et al. (personal communication) gave caffeine in drinking water at concentrations equivalent to total daily dosages as high as 100 and 144 mg/kg and observed no increase in malformations. At least one study (Fujii and Nishimura 1972) indicated that divided or widely distributed dosage, as in food, can attain teratogenic levels if the total daily intake is raised to a sufficient level (330 mg/kg). Sullivan (1982) has shown that maternal plasma levels of caffeine in rats rise to about 80 µg/ml after single daily doses of 100 mg/kg but are maintained at levels around 25 µg/ml after the same total doses in four parts at 6-h intervals. Similarly, Ikeda et al. (1982) have shown that peak maternal blood levels and fetal concentration are about tenfold higher when 80 mg/kg caffeine is administered by gavage than when it is administered in the drinking water. In this study 7% of the fetuses from gavaged mothers had ectrodactyly, whereas none of the fetuses from mothers receiving caffeine in their drinking water were so affected.

The malformations produced at high doses of caffeine tend to be limited in type, and until dosage is raised to very high levels, are not seen in association with high levels of intrauterine or postnatal death of offspring. The most prevalent types of malformations reported, regardless of species, were digital reduction defects and cleft palate. In rabbits the one study reporting malformations found only ectrodactyly. The majority of positive rat studies have also found mostly or only ectrodactyly, although one study (Leuschner and Schwerdtfeger 1969) observed mainly cleft palate at 180 mg/kg/day. Palm et al. (1978) observed statistically significant cleft palate in rats only at the lowest dosage level in a reproduction study but the lack of dose relatedness makes this result of doubtful validity. Mice have also generally shown some digital reduction defects after caffeine treatment of pregnant females, but not to the exclusive degree seen in rats. In mice, facial defects, largely cleft palate, were seen approximately as often as digital defects, and defects of the cranium, eyes, and tail were also noted but were less frequent.

With notable regularity, malformations of the head and extremities (feet and tail) were observed at doses of caffeine which were also noted to produce hemorrhages in these regions of some offspring. Although hemorrhages are not themselves malformations, their presence suggests a mechanism whereby the observed malformations could have been initiated during fetal life. An association between the occurrence of hemorrhages in the head and extremities and subsequent malformation in these parts after treatment during pregnancy with hormonal substances such as epinephrine ACTH, and vasopressin has been known since the classic studies of Jost and associates (Jost 1953 a, b; Jost et al. 1964, 1973). To review briefly, treatment of rats with these substances at appropriate stages of development, e.g., days 15–17 of gestation, caused swelling and hemorrhages at the tips of the extremities in the embryos. The affected areas later died and underwent sloughing, finally leaving the appearance of amputated toes and feet. Although the frequency and degree of malformation seen in these earlier studies were generally greater than those seen in the

167

caffeine studies, the doses of hormones used by Jost were quite large. It is noteworthy that hormones given prior to the 18th day of gestation in rats tended to result at term in amputation of feet and toes, whereas treatment at later times was more frequently associated with persistent hemorrhages and swelling.

The distribution and frequency of ectrodactyly and hemorrhages in the caffeine studies was such as to suggest that caffeine at 80 mg/kg/day and higher doses had effects equivalent to low doses of the hormones used in the Jost studies. Nishimura and Nakai (1960) observed superficial hemorrhages and subsequent toe malformations in the offspring of mice treated with large doses of caffeine, and Fujii and Nishimura (1974) proposed that catecholamines released by the action of caffeine induced circulatory disturbances which later led to hemorrhages. In fact it has been reported (Berkowitz and Spector 1971) that concentrations of epinephrine and other catecholamines are increased in the blood plasma of rats treated with large doses of caffeine. Thus, a plausible explanation of the observed low incidence of ectrodactyly after the high doses of caffeine is that elevated epinephrine or other catecholamines during early limb formation could cause hemorrhages of sufficient severity to interfere with development of toes, since ectrodactyly has been observed after treatment of pregnant rats and rabbits with these hormones (see Jost et al. 1973). To the best of our knowledge such a mechanism has not been involved in human teratology in relation to either caffeine or epinephrine. The possible mechanism of teratogenic action of caffeine in rodents will be discussed further in Sect. 4.

Delayed ossification of fetal skeletons has often been observed after caffeine exposure in utero. In fact virtually all studies which have employed adequate methodology, e.g., soft tissue clearing and alizarin staining, have found some degree of slowed maturation of bone after a wide range of dosage. Various interpretations and fetopathic prognostications have been given to this developmental variable by investigators of the teratogeneticity of many agents other than caffeine. In recent years there has been a growing realization that the underlying process in delayed ossification is one of the slowing of a natural developmental parameter, not the intervention of a divergent or aberrant process, as is the case in teratogenesis. Most experienced teratologists and some regulatory agencies now accept the views that slowed ossification as seen in this context is transitory and without adverse consequence for the animal's future well-being and longevity. It was, therefore, surprising that Collins et al. (1981) went to some lengths to place delayed deposition of bone minerals in a few small skeletal elements in the context of adverse fetopathic effects. The fallacy of regarding delayed ossification as a fetopathic manifestation has recently been demonstrated. At the Fourth International Caffeine Workshop, Holick et al. (1982) reported that sternebral seen to have various ossification deficiencies in 21-day rat fetuses exposed to caffeine in utero were essentially indistinguishable from controls when such animals were allowed to live until the 4th postnatal day before evaluation of the degree of mineralization.

2.2 Discordant Results

The most conspicuous point of disagreement among the several investigators who have studied the teratogenic potential of caffeine has been whether teratogenesis occurs in a given species at a particular range of dosage. There is general consensus

168

among most authors that caffeine has low teratogenic potential in rats and mice and probably also in rabbits. There is less agreement about the lowest dosage level that is associated with malformations and/or other embryotoxicity, but it may be noted that 50 mg/kg/day approximated the lowest teratogenic dose in mice and that 80 mg/kg/day is about the dosage level at which rats began to respond, assuming in both cases that the caffeine is given in a single daily dose by injection or gavage. Some strains of both species do not respond to doses well in excess of these lower levels, and it is not possible in all cases to attribute the negative result to methodological or strain differences. As already noted, variability of results may be characteristic of low-potency teratogens.

Thus, the area of greatest discord appears to relate to what criterion should be accepted in in defining the no-effect level of dosage in the production of true embryotoxic-fetotoxic effects. Specifically, should delayed ossification and the minor skeletal variants be used in making regulatory decisions? At present the weight of existing evidence and the opinions of experienced teratologists favor regarding these productive variables as reflections of temporary maternal physiologic stress without lasting effect on the conceptus, therefore of no regulatory significance.

Otherwise, it is difficult to cite well-defined issues over which there is pointed disagreement. Questions have been raised about such matters as whether the teratogenic effects of caffeine in rodents is the result of direct action by caffeine or one of its metabolites, or indirectly the result of some maternal metabolic imbalance attendant on instantaneous and massive dosage with caffeine. These questions have been studied too little to warrant discussion here, although preliminary information has recently been reported (Sullivan 1982; Kimmel 1982).

3 Previous Reviews of Animal Studies

Earlier published animal studies dealing with the teratogenic potential of caffeine have already been reviewed in some detail in various connections and therefore need no exhaustive discussion here (FASEB Report 1978; Citizens Petition to FDA 1979; Collins 1979). It is of interest, however, to examine the conclusions arrived at by the respective reviewers all of whom had somewhat different objectives in view and doubtless also varying degrees of bias. Furthermore, one of the recent studies, that of Collins et al. (1981), is deserving of critical review because of the unusual regulatory significance assigned to it.

3.1 Federation of American Societies of Biology Report

In May, 1978, a select committee of qualified scientists, set up by the Federation of American Societies of Experimental Biology (FASEB) to evaluate available information on the GRAS (generally regarded as safe) status of caffeine, made its report, "Evaluation of the Health Aspects of Caffeine as a Food Ingredient." The committee did not regard teratogenesis as a major health hazard from caffeine. Of many pages devoted to various aspects of chronic toxicity in animals, relatively little space was devoted to teratogenesis in rats and mice. After considering all animal studies available at that time, including all rates and routes of treatment, this conclusion was expressed:

... many animal tests showed that teratogenic effects are generally absent at caffeine doses up to 50 mg per kg body weight. At doses up to 75 mg per kg of body weight, teratogenic effects of caffeine are neither striking nor consistently demonstrated. At bolus doses greater than 75 mg per kg teratogenic effects are apparent ... Teratogenic effects in oral studies varied with the time period over which the dose was administered, the strain of animal, and the method of oral administration (intubation or feeding).

Noted but not emphasized were the facts that even in animal studies at doses of 100 mg/kg and higher, birth defects were not always observed, or were observed with low to moderate frequency and often in association with signs of maternal toxicity. Also not emphasized was the fact that amounts of caffeine which produced true teratogenic effects were usually administered in instantaneous, massive doses, as by daily injections or via a stomach tube, rather than in a more protracted manner such as would approximate human consumption.

In summarizing the meager human data, it was noted that "two retrospective studies of more than 14,000 mothers on whom caffeine consumption histories were obtained, revealed no association between caffeine intakes and abnormalities in offspring." On the contrary, the Select Committee's attention regarding the health aspects of caffeine as a commercially-added food ingredient seemed to focus particularly on questions of supposed behavioral effects in children, not on teratogenic effects.

3.2 Citizens' Petition to the Food and Drug Administration

In November 1979, a public advocacy group, Center for Science in the Public Interest, submitted a petition to the FDA requesting:

1. that tea and coffee packaging bear a warning label indicating that caffeine might be harmful to unborn children, and
2. that an educational campaign be initiated to inform pregnant women "about the ability of caffeine to interfere with reproduction."

Based on a review of 14 animal studies, 12 of which had been reviewed in the FASEB Report, the author of the Citizens' Petition concluded that caffeine had been shown to be a teratogen in three strains of mice, two strains of rats, and one strain of rabbit, and thus that the consumption of caffeine at any dose during pregnancy should be avoided.

The latter admonition was reminiscent of the Delaney Clause, promulgated several years ago for the regulation of food additives with respect to their carcinogenic potential, which stated that a chemical could not be an artificial ingredient of human food if it were found to cause cancer in laboratory animals at any dose tested. The basis for the rule was the assumption that there was no safe dose, however small, for man as regards the potential to cause cancer once a substance had been shown to cause cancer in a test animal, regardless of the animal's comparability to man. The literal application of this principle is now questioned by most toxicologists, but there is still a lingering tendency for some to apply the Delaney Clause to teratogenesis as well as carcinogenesis.

To forestall such inappropriate application the Teratology Society (1974) unanimously passed a resolution to the effect that since most biologically active substances could be shown to be teratogenic at some dose, application of the Delaney Clause to teratogenesis would be meaningless, impractical, and altogether ill-advised.

The Citizens' Petition based its evaluation on essentially the same published literature as had the FASEB Report, but arrived at a much different conclusion. The Select Committee of the FASEB did not identify teratogenesis as a major concern in its consideration of the health aspects of caffeine, but the Citizens' Petition had identified the teratogenic potential of caffeine as its major concern. When the reasons for these divergent views are sought by reexamining the original literature, it becomes evident that the FASEB Committee gave the data a more critical and expert evaluation than did the writers of the Citizens' Petition.

Without going into too much detail, it can be noted that the Citizens' Petition was somewhat selective in what it emphasized in the reported animal studies. For example, little attention was given to the dose-response aspects of the collective data base, namely that true teratogenesis occurred only at relatively high doses in each species and that even at extremely high dosage several strains of animals only responded minimally or not at all. Although only experiments involving oral administration were considered, the physiologic differences between bolus treatment by gavage, on one hand, and protracted gradual consumption such as by drinking caffeine-containing beverages, on the other, were not emphasized.

Undue emphasis was placed on one experiment (Palm et al. 1978) in which cleft palate in rats was reported to be statistically significantly increased above control value at only the lowest of three doses in fetuses removed before term on day 19 of gestation. Other presumed malformations such as hydrocephalus and delayed ossification, were not observed postnatally and must be assumed to have been the result of a transitory developmental delay in these fetuses examined 1 day earlier than is customary in teratogenicity studies.

In addition to such inappropriate interpretations of animal data, the Citizens' Petition seems to assume that rodent results can be readily extrapolated to human risk assessment without due consideration of 1. differences in route and rate of dosage, and 2. species differences in metabolism and pharmacokinetics of caffeine. It need only be said in conclusion that the author of the Citizens' Petition used inadequate animal data to make inappropriate extrapolations of animal studies as evidence of human teratogenic risk from caffeine.

3.3 Food and Drug Administration Review of Reproduction and Teratology Studies on Caffeine

In September 1979 the FDA over the name of Thomas F. X. Collins, published in its *FDA By-Lines* No. 7 a moderately detailed review of most animal studies to date on the effects of caffeine on the outcome of pregnancy. In January 1981 this was supplemented and updated so that in sum it represents the most comprehensive effort to document the results of caffeine on mammalian reproduction up to that time. A total of 35 publications dealing with the effects on the offspring of caffeine given by various routes, mainly to pregnant mice and rats, were examined. Results generally were reported accurately but negative findings were given less emphasis than positive results, and the final interpretation presented a bias toward greater teratogenic potential for caffeine. For example, the introductory statement notes that "... caffeine is one of the compounds known to cross the placental barrier," as if it were one of only a few compounds with this capacity. Actually, it is now accepted that some fraction of every compound which enters the maternal bloodstream, except those of very large molecular size or extreme electrical charge, does in fact cross the placenta, and caffeine is not exceptional in this regard.

The most unfortunate aspect of this literature review, however, was that it concluded that little valid information relative to the teratogenicity of caffeine could be gleaned from any or all collectively of the 35 earlier studies in which this compound had been administered to pregnant animals. It was stated that "Many studies were performed before 1970 when the state of the art in teratology was not as well developed as it is currently," and particular concern was expressed about the "small number of animals" used in several of the studies. It was true that some of the studies did not conform to modern standards for teratogenicity tests in laboratory animals, but that does not justify regarding the lot as valueless. The basic facts concerning the teratogenic potential of caffeine were already contained in the accumulated literature as of 1979.

Nevertheless, on 21 October 1980 the FDA published in the *Federal Register* its proposal to delete caffeine from the GRAS list pending completion of studies considered necessary to resolve questions about its safety as a food additive. Drawing on the Collins review, the FDA characterized the animals studies prior to 1979 as follows:

... many of the studies had deficiencies (e. g., lack of proper control animals, small number of animals, lack of concurrent control animals, insufficient information on procedures). Moreover, many of them were conducted a decade or more ago when teratology study techniques were less developed. Despite these deficiencies, the animal studies available at the time the review was published taken together demonstrate clearly that, at sufficiently high levels of exposure, well above what humans are exposed to in the diet, caffeine can cause birth defects in animals. The studies were not adequate, however, to determine with eny confidence a no-effect level for the teratogenic effects of caffeine in animals, i.e., the level of exposure at which no teratogenic effects are observed.

No real issue can be taken with the first two sentences of this summary: some prior studies did indeed have the deficiencies stipulated. It is not correct, however, to attribute these methodological problems to the presumption that the deficient studies antedated some striking advance in teratological technology. In fact many were done after January 1966, when the FDA issued its *Guidelines for Reproduction Studies for Safety Evaluation of Drugs for Human Use*. Admittedly the prior studies might have been better experiments had all followed the guidelines, but the simple fact is that caffeine had been known to be a weak teratogen, i. e., one producing inconsistent and/or low incidence of terata at high dosage, in rodents since 1960 (Nishimura and Nakai 1960).

The last sentence in the above quote, regarding a no-effect level, is not correct. Earlier research had with surprising consistency shown that no teratogenic effect occurred in mice at doses lower than 50 mg/kg/day. Mice are notorious for intraspecies variability, and the fact that no strains showed teratogenic responses at lower doses is further indication that caffeine is indeed a weak teratogen. Rats had not in any reasonably well-conducted studies been shown to react teratogenically to caffeine at doses lower than 75 mg/kg/day, as was emphasized in the FASEB Report, a fact which was actually confirmed in the Collins gavage study, which found no terata in rats at doses below 80 mg/kg, with a low incidence of one malformation at this dose.

The low incidence of malformations in all caffeine studies is deserving of special note, although it was overlooked in both the Collins review (1979) and the *Federal Register* document (1980). Several strains of mice and rats have been shown to be teratogenically unresponsive to caffeine at the levels mentioned above, which appears to constitute no-effect levels, but in other instances no effects were observed at appreciably higher doses (see Leuschner and Schwerdtfeger 1969; Bertrand et al. 1970; Fujii and Nishimura 1972). Even when malformations were induced by treatment at higher doses, the percentage of offspring responding rarely exceeded 20% and was usually much lower. Some authors reported a significant teratogenic response after caffeine treatment during pregnancy even when the percentage of affected offspring was lower than seen by most other workers in controls. For example, Knoche and König (1964) considered seven of 745 instances of external abnormality to be significant, although modern investigators expect about 1% of controls to be abnormals. Finally, *little mention was made of the frequent finding that dosages around 100 mg/kg began to be associated with maternal toxicity,* the embryotoxic significance of which will be discussed later.

Caffeine may be considered to be a weak or low-potency teratogen for two reasons:

1. it produces few terata at high dosage in susceptible species, and
2. there is uncertain likelihood of teratogenesis in some stocks and strains of animals, despite a demonstrated potential in others of the same species (see Fraser 1977).

This suggests that caffeine, when causally associated with malformations, may be interacting with other unknown factors present in the experimental situation. This was in fact demonstrated by Bertrand et al. (1970), who treated pregnant female rats of four different stocks of the Wistar strain with the same level (125 mg/kg) of caffeine. None of the stocks regularly displayed ectrodactyly (missing toes) when untreated, but after caffeine treatment during pregnancy females of two stocks delivered offspring with a moderate incidence of ectrodactyly, a third reacted minimally, and the fourth showed no teratogenic effect. These authors attributed the observed differences in teratogenic sensitivity among the four stocks to a genetically determined predisposition in some stocks not possessed by others. This experiment probably exemplified interaction between a genetic factor and an environmental factor, caffeine. Similar teratogenic interactions are known to occur between two or more environmental factors in rats and mice (Fraser 1977). When one such factor is known and the other(s) not, the presence of the latter would determine whether a teratogenic response occurred, and thus would account for variable responses. Whatever the mechanism, caffeine is clearly a low-potency teratogen of variable expressivity. The existence of a similar mechanism or potential in man cannot be presumed from its having been shown to occur in rodents at extremely high doses.

3.4 National Soft Drink Association's Critique of the Collins Gavage Study

The Collins gavage study was accorded pivotal importance by the FDA in its proposal to change the GRAS status of caffeine. The FDA agreed with a panel of appropriately qualified experts, the Interagency Epidemiology Working Group (1980), that there was no acceptable epidemiologic evidence of teratogenic risk to human users of caffeine during pregnancy, and furthermore, rejected all previous animal studies on caffeine exposure during pregnancy as a starting point for estimating teratogenic risk. It was, therefore, determined that additional animal studies "... should be made to resolve whether caffeine is indeed a teratogen, and if so, whether a no-effect level can be established." The Collins gavage study, to be discussed here, was the first of two studies conducted in the Bureau of Foods of the FDA and it has now been published (Collins et al. 1981); the second has not.

The stated objectives of determining teratogenicity and establishing a no-effect level had in essence been attained by earlier investigators, whose observations were in reality only confirmed by the Collins gavage study. Whether the much larger goal, that of providing a scientific basis for changing the GRAS status of caffeine by demonstrating reasonable grounds to suspect adverse health effects in man, was achieved by the gavage study alone will be critically analyzed in this discussion.

The general design of the Collins gavage study conformed to current standards for conducting teratogenicity tests, although there were a number of minor deviations from Good Laboratory Practice rules, in addition to two major problems.

Other studies have shown a tendency for large dosage of caffeine in rodents to be associated with some delays in skeletal ossification and increases in the incidence of developmental variants, particularly in the skeleton (Palm et al. 1978; Nolen 1981). The emphasis and interpretations placed on the skeletal variants by Collins et al. (1981) has aroused considerable disagreement. As will be discussed in greater detail in Sect. 3.4.3, most experienced teratologists regard these skeletal variants either as transitory or as having no adverse connotation except perhaps reflecting mild metabolic stress on the part of the pregnant female. Since undue emphasis was placed on these minor variants, it would have been appropriate to show that contrary to prevailing views among teratologists, these variations in skeletal development were adverse to the animals affected, as intimated in the study and by the FDA.

Also in connection with skeletal issues, the process of ossification in the albino rat is known to undergo very rapid change on day 20, the time at which fetuses in the Collins study were removed for examination. Only a few hours of fluctuation in the stage when fetuses were removed can make considerable difference in the state of ossification of certain bones such as sternebrae, vertebrae, and small bones of the skull and limbs (Aliverti et al. 1979; Khera 1980; Fritz and Hess 1970). Whether the fluctuations were occasioned by a slight developmental delay or by actual variation in the time at which mothers were killed, the result would be similar, namely an increase in the number of fetal skeletons in which ossification appeared to have been delayed. Such artifactual variations in ossification could have been avoided by delaying the killing of the mothers until day 21 of pregnancy, a practice which has been recommended for precisely the reasons noted here. The undue emphasis placed by Collins et al. (1981) on skeletal variations would certainly have justified the taking of such precautions.

3.4.1 Procedural Criticisms

The present reviewers we were struck by two procedural matters which may have significantly affected the results as well as their interpretations. *First,* in the section on procedure in the paper by Collins et al. it was stated:

One half of fetuses, randomly selected, were fixed in Bouin's solution and were submitted to visceral examination by Wilson's razor-blade section method ... The remaining fetuses were fixed in alcohol, stained with Alizarin Red S ... and submitted to skeletal examination. Fetuses with grossly apparent anomalies were not subjected to the randomizing procedure but were assigned to that method which better defined the anomaly ...

The last sentence of this quote means in fact that all fetuses which had ectrodactyly, an externally "apparent anomaly," were prepared for skeletal study. Since ectrodactyly was the only malformation recognized by these authors, all fetuses with a known malformation were subjected to intensive skeletal examination and received no visceral examination. Thus the animals selected for skeletal study contained all animals known to have any malformation, in addition to those selected by the randomization process. Not only was this study group heavily weighted with the animals known to have been affected teratogenically, it also received the animals most likely to have skeletal variations, because ectrodactyly is in part a skeletal defect, although it is a true malformation and not merely a minor developmental variation. It is quite likely that some of the excess of skeletal variation reported by these authors can be attributed to the *nonrandom selection of the animals for skeletal evaluation.*

A *second* major procedural criticism concerns failure of the Collins paper to define in advance such terms as "enlarged kidney/ureter" and "ectrodactyly." The second of these terms is of importance for more than one reason. As noted above, it was the basis of nonrandom selection of disproportionate numbers of animals with likely skeletal variations for intensive skeletal examination. Perhaps of even greater inportance, ectrodactyly was *incorrectly defined:* "Any limb which had incomplete digits was considered ectrodactylous, the condition ranged in severity from a single hypoplastic nail to the absence of one or more digits, according to the definition of Bertrand et al. (1965)." In standard biological and medical usage ectrodactyly is defined as congenital absence of one or more digits and does not include incomplete digits (brachydactyly, aphalangia, etc.) or hypoplastic or absent nails. The error in definition meant that all cases of brachydactyly, true ectrodactyly, or incomplete digits, as well as many of underdeveloped nails, the last not universally recognized as a malformation, were lumped together as a single malformation. The effect was to increase the apparent incidence of the single malformation ectrodactyly, which even then was not excessive considering the high dosage via gavage after which it was reported.

Table 1. Corrected incidence of ectrodactyly reported by Collins et al. (1981) at high doses of caffeine

| Dose (mg/kg) | FDA data (Ectrodactyly with missing and reduced nails included) | | Corrections after removing missing and reduced nails from ectrodactyly | | | |
| | | | Missing and reduced nails only | | True ectrodactyly[a] of one or more digits | |
	Fetuses affected/total	%	Fetuses affected/total	%	Fetuses affected/total	%
80	62/544	11.4	30/544	5.5	32/544	5.9
125	113/396	28.5	48/396	12.1	65/396	16.4

[a] Actually this designation still includes a few instances of brachydactyly

   Not only is there no recognized precedent for enlarging the definition of this malformation to include the nails, there are logical and scientific reasons for not confusing ectrodactyly and incomplete development of nails. In the first place, true ectrodactyly is one of the most easily produced limb malformations by experimental means in rats (Warkany and Schraffenberger 1944, 1947; Layton and Hallesy 1965; Jost et al. 1973; Wilson et al. 1977). The numerous authors who have produced ectrodactyly experimentally with various drugs and chemicals have found no reason to associate it with variations in development of the nail. Furthermore, there is no biochemical or embryological basis for associating the two in development. In embryology the digits are developed around skeletal elements composed largely of cartilage and bone, while nails are formed somewhat later as keratinous appendages of the skin. Since the range of developmental variations of nails has not been extensively studied, it is not known to what extent underdevelopment of nails may be compensated for after birth. When the Collins data are corrected by removing from the ectrodactyly classification all fetuses which had missing or reduced nails as the only toe malformation, as is done in Table 1, the incidence of true ectrodactyly is appreciably reduced. There remains a modest, but statistically significant and dose-related, incidence of ectrodactyly in the two highest dosage groups. There is no basis whatever for regarding this level of teratogenesis as more serious or more meaningful than that reported in several earlier papers on caffeine effects in rodent pregnancy (Nishimura and Nakai 1960; Bertrand et al. 1965, 1970).

3.4.2 Maternal Toxicity

One of the unquestionably valid observations to come out of the Collins et al. (1981) study was that the two highest doses, 80 and 125 mg/kg, produced unmistakable signs of maternal toxicity. This was evidenced by maternal mortality (one of 56 and six of 49 females, or 1.8% and 12.2% respectively); by significant and/or persistent failure to gain weight throughout pregnancy (final weight deficiency of 35% and 44% respectively below controls); by reduced food consumption, particularly during the 1st and probably well into the 2nd week; and by the number of whole-litter resorptions (two and four respectively, compared to none in controls). Whole-litter resorption is included here because it is often associated with other known signs of maternal toxicity. Only when associated with high mortality among individual embryos and fetuses and low maternal toxicity can it be assumed that the primary effect is on the conceptus. The importance of maternal toxicity in relation to teratogenicity test results will be discussed more fully in Sect. 4.2. For present purposes it is sufficient to note that teratogenic effects obtained at doses causing appreciable maternal toxicity are not a valid basis for setting margins of safety and other regulatory purposes because of possible confounding of maternal with direct fetal effects. Some of the above-noted signs of maternal toxicity were also produced at the 40 mg/kg dose, but were only of transitory nature. Reduced weight gain and food consumption at other dosages were either statistically marginal or observed only in the first few days of pregnancy before acclimatization to unaccustomed handling and to the anorectic effects of caffeine.

True embryotoxic and fetotoxic effects were manifested by significantly increased levels of individual resorptions, reduced fetal weight, and the occurrence of malformations of the digits. These effects were consistently seen only at doses of 80 and 125 mg/kg, the same doses associated with unquestioned maternal toxicity. These criteria of direct effects on the conceptus, namely resorptions, reduced growth, and malformations, usually occur together at similar levels of dosage and tend to increase in dose-related fashion as dosage is increased. However, one or more of the three is sometimes seen irregularly at lower doses, as was noted in this experiment at 40 mg/kg, but such sporadic occurrences are rarely of more than questionable statistical significance.

3.4.3 Skeletal Variants

The present authors disagree with the interpretations placed on the skeletal variants and on delayed ossification as reported in the Collins gavage study. The *Federal Register* statement (1980) sets the tone of these interpretations as follows:

The FDA gavage study raises serious concerns about caffeine because it is the first large, well-designed and controlled teratology study on caffeine to show irreversible terata (e. g., missing digits) at levels as low as 80 mg/kg and *other adverse* [italics added], but probably reversible effects at levels as low as 6 mg/kg. The levels of caffeine exposure at which these effects occurred in the rats are not significantly greater than those humans might be exposed to in the food supply . . .

The "other adverse" effects seen at 6 mg/kg deserve special comment. This refers to the skeletal variants and delayed ossification which were strongly emphasized in the Collins paper and elsewhere. No evidence has been cited that these minor skeletal deviations have any adverse connotation. Nevertheless, the strong implication of toxicity continues in the Collins et al. paper. "Fetotoxicity was manifested by the many types and large numbers of ossification problems found in the fetuses." Not only are they called fetotoxic but they are listed in the same table with generally accepted skeletal malformations such as missing phalanges and fused ribs. Careful examination, however, reveals that aside from those associated with ectrodactyly and the several manifestations of reduced ossification, very few of the 52 items listed in

Table 9 in Collins et al. (1981) attain statistical significance compared with control values. Even at the two highest doses (80 and 125 mg/kg) only 16 of the 52 items are significantly different from controls. The most consistent site of statistical significance was the sternum, where three of five types of variations attained significance at the two highest doses. The sternum as a whole has often been found to be developmentally one of the most variable bones in the rat skeleton (Khera 1980; Fritz and Hess 1970; Aliverti et al. 1979; Kimmel and Wilson 1973). As if to capitalize on this innate variability of the sternum, various combinations and permutations are used in Tables 10 and 11 in Collins et al. (1981) to achieve statistical significance by compounding the variations seen in separate sternebrae or sternal features. For example, many of the sternebral variations on which these tables are based represent different degrees of a single parameter, delayed ossification, but Collins et al. list litters and fetuses with one, two, and three sternebral variations separately, as if they were separate entities. This is logically the equivalent of counting a foot with five toes missing as having five malformations, which fortunately these authors did not do. In any event, these are questionable statistical procedures.

The emphasis placed on minor skeletal variations, including varying degrees of ossification, becomes all the more questionable when the time of preservation of these fetuses in relation to the timetable of ossification in rats is taken into consideration. Aliverti et al. (1979) undertook a detailed study of the process of ossification in the skeleton of rat fetuses on days 19, 20, and 21. Although these investigators used Wistar rats instead of the Osborne-Mendel strain used by Collins et al., and the timing of pregnancy differed by about 12 h, information critical to the present discussion was nonetheless presented. Pregnant females were killed and their fetuses prepared for skeletal study as in the Collins study, but on three different days, 19, 20, and 21, rather than only on day 20, as was the case in the Collins study. The authors found that most of the ossification of the six sternal segments occurs between days 19 and 20, as noted in the following:

"Over 90% of day 19 fetuses presented no or only one center of ossification. In contrast, nearly all day 20 fetuses presented four to six ossified sternebrae and nearly all day 21 fetuses presented six ossified sternebrae."

Thus, the fetuses in the Collins study were taken at a time of rapid change in the number of ossified sernal centers. At this time variations equivalent to a few hours delay in development, such as might have been caused by reduced maternal food intake, could have appreciably altered the number as well as the degree of ossification of separate centers, and other bones in offspring of caffeine-treated rats were also undergoing rapid changes in ossification on day 20. To avoid the possibility that such rapid changes in fetal ossification might coincide with maternal factors which could result in developmental delay and thereby exacerbate fluctuations in the numbers of centers and the degrees of ossification, Aliverti et al., have proposed:

"... have gestating rats in teratogenic studies be sacrificed on day 21 of gestation when ossification of the fetus is sufficiently advanced, homogeneous and uniform to permit meaningful observations."

3.4.4 No-Effect Levels

One of the stated objectives of the Collins gavage study was to define a no-effect level for terata and for skeletal variants. Accordingly, in the Discussion of the published paper it is stated that "In this study a clear no-effect level for frank terata was found, namely, 40 mg/kg/day." This statement could be questioned on certain grounds. Although it is customary in toxicology to define a no-effect level as the highest dose producing no observed effect, in the present context it must also be considered in relation to maternal toxicity, as well as to the full range of embryotoxicity. The lowest dose which produced low but statistically valid embryotoxicity, i.e., increased intrauterine death, decreased intrauterine growth, and increased malformations, was 80 mg/kg/day, which also produced signs of maternal toxicity. Thus, it was not demonstrated that a dose devoid of maternal toxic effects will produce any embryotoxicity. It is an accepted principle in teratology that a test dose which causes maternal toxic effects should not be used in setting safety standards because of the possible compounding or interaction of primary fetal and secondary maternal effects.

Furthermore, other studies cited in both the FASEB report (1978) and the Collins (1979) literature review, as well as the more recent results of Nolen (1981), clearly indicate that doses higher than 40 mg/kg/day are no-effect doses in rats. Finally, an increment of 100% from the no-effect dose (assuming 40 mg/kg) to the lowest effect dose (assuming 80 mg/kg) is hardly reasonable in constructing a meaningful dose-response curve. One or more intermediate doses would be indicated.

4 Remaining Unresolved Issues

4.1 Mechanism(s) of Teratogenic Action in Rodents

Very few studies have been concerned with the mechanism by which caffeine induces congenital malformations. This dearth of investigation is probably due in part to the fact that caffeine is a weak teratogen, making mechanistic studies more difficult than usual.

Most of the information so far produced leads to the suggestion that caffeine-induced malformations have a vascular basis via secretion of catecholamines, a hypothesis which will be discussed shortly. However, it is important to point out first that two significant facts necessary to the understanding of the mechanism of teratogenic action of any agent, the site of action and the proximate teratogen, remain unknown with regard to caffeine. Thus we do not know whether the primary action of caffeine which initiates abnormal development occurs in the mother, the placenta, or directly within the embryo itself. This question is of added significance here because teratogenic doses of caffeine produce toxic effects in the mother. Likewise, we have no idea whether caffeine or one of its many metabolites is the actual or proximate teratogen.

There is no doubt that caffeine and its major metabolites do reach the rodent (Sieber and Fabro 1971; Tanimura and Terada 1968; Ikeda et al. 1982; Scott, to be published) and human (Goldstein and Warren 1962) conceptus. Concentration of caffeine within the embryo is very similar to that in maternal plasma, in keeping with the view that caffeine distributes uniformly in a variety of tissues in proportion to their water content (Soyka 1981). The demethylated metabolites (theophylline, paraxanthine, and theobromine) can also be found in embryonic tissue, but their concentraions are an order of magnitude less than that of caffeine (Scott, to be published). On the other hand, uric acid metabolites, although present in maternal serum, were undetectable in the embryo (Scott, to be published).

The idea that vascular disruption might be the basis of caffeine-induced malformations sprang from the observation of hematomas associated with caffeine-induced malformations, especially in the limbs of mouse embryos (Nishimura and Nakai 1960). Hematomas were found within 12 h of caffeine injection, and many were present at the usual time of killing near term. These results were confirmed and extended by Bartel and Gnacikowska (1972), who also showed that outside the hematoma the limb tissues appeared healthy, suggesting that caffeine does not cause cell death within the embryo.

Fujii and Nishimura (1974) were the first to suggest that the vascular effects of caffeine within the embryo might be due to release of catecholamines into the circulation. They supported this hypothesis by showing that propranolol, a β-adrenergic antagonist, reduced the embryotoxic effects of caffeine. It is important to note that these workers were unable to completely ameliorate the teratogenic effects of caffeine with propranolol, and appeared to reach a maximum protective effect with 5 mg/kg, since 10 mg/kg gave the same amount of protection. Even the much more potent β-adrenergic blocker, timolol, was unable to prevent caffeine embryotoxicity completely (Fujii 1976). Hayasaka and Fujii (1977) took the opposite approach and showed a potentiation of caffeine embryotoxicity in mice by pargyline or cocaine. Pargyline inhibits monoamine oxidase, the major catabolic enzyme of catecholamine degradation, whereas cocaine enhances catecholamine action by blocking neuronal norepinephrine uptake.

Supportive of the hypothesis are results from intrafetal injection of catecholamines (Davies and Robson 1970; Jost 1953 a). Within a few hours of the injection, edema, hemorrhage, and hematomas are evident in the limb. A portion of the distal extremity is often cast off, some time later, resulting in ectro- and adactyly. It is not difficult to imagine that caffeine-induced limb malformations follow a similar pathogenesis.

Also supporting the general hypothesis is the developmental age when caffeine or other methylated xanthines cause limb deformity. In studies which utilized drug administration on a single day of pregnancy, Nishimura and Nakai (1960) demonstrated that mouse embryos most often had digital deformities following caffeine administration on day 12. Snigorska and Bartel (1970) suggest that day 12 and day 13 mouse embryos were most susceptible to the limb-deforming activity of caffeine; however, the tabular form of their results does not support such a conclusion. In fact there seems to be little difference in the frequency of limb defects in mouse embryos whose mothers received caffeine at any time between days 9 and 13. Tucci and Skalko (1978) administered theophylline in single, intraperitoneal injections to mice on days 10–13 of gestation and found day 11 to be the most sensitive for induction of limb deformities.

This relatively late sensitivity to digital deformity has an important bearing on the possible mechanisms by which caffeine could initiate pathogenesis. On day 12 of mouse development, which often coincides with maximal sensitivity to caffeine-induced digital deformity, the fore- and hindlimb buds are in an advances stage of differentiation (Rugh 1968). The anlagen of forelimb digits are clearly visible as digital rays. The fact that caffeine can cause ectrodactyly in such a limb indicates that the drug acts to cause removal of performed tissue. Most agents are thought to produce ectrodactyly by preventing the formation of digital tissue, since most are given well before digit morphogenesis. Exceptions to this rule include uterine vascular clamping (Leist and Grauwiler 1974), oligohydramnios induced by amniotic sac puncture (Singh and Singh 1973), and administration of epinephrine, norepinephrine, or vasopressin by direct fetal injection (Davies and Robson 1970; Jost 1953a).

The idea that caffeine acts to induce malformations by causing release of catecholamines is attractive, but by no means established. Other possibilities have, of course, been suggested and are worthy of mention here.

Elmazar et al. (1981) showed that a nonteratogenic dose of caffeine (100 mg/kg) produced an increased level of corticosterone in mouse maternal plasma which reached a peak that was ten times greater than control levels and which stayed well above control levels for at least 8 h. The well-known sensitivity of mice to glucocorticoid-induced cleft palate makes corticosterone release an attractive hypothesis to explain the mechanism by which caffeine induces this defect.

A recently discovered action of caffeine and other methylated xanthines is related to their ability to act as adenosine antagonists by blockade of adenosine receptors (see Snyder this volume Cap. 9). Clark et al. (1982) have shown that coadministration of adenosine agonists and caffeine in some cases potentiated the teratogenic effects of caffeine. These studies are still in a preliminary state but suggest another possible avenue by which caffeine could act to cause malformations.

One of the most publicized effects of caffeine is its ability to raise cAMP through inhibition of phosphodiesterase. cAMP has been shown to be important in development of both limb and palate, the two anatomical sites most often affected by caffeine, but no studies have yet been conducted which have measured the level of this second messenger in embryos from caffeine-treated mothers. In fact the caffeine levels within mice embryos exposed to a teratogenic dose of caffeine (Scott, to be published) are in the range (1 mM) necessary to inhibit many phosphodiesterases. One could also expect cAMP levels to be increased through catecholamine secretion or adenosine receptor blockade, so measurement of cAMP would seem to be a project worthy of pursuit.

In summary, there is curcumstantial evidence which suggests that caffeine induces abnormal development via stimulation of catecholamine secretion. The inability totally to prevent the teratogenic effects of caffeine with beta-blocking agents hints at involvement of a second biochemical effect of caffeine. Perhaps the well-known ability of caffeine to raise levels of cAMP is responsible. The increased level of corticosterone induced by caffeine is an enticing explanation for cleft palate induction, and it is not inconceivable that abnormal palate and limb development could be the result of different mechanisms.

This subject has already been discussed in some detail in the critique of the Collins et al. (1981) gavage study (Sect. 3.4.3). However, additional points are appropriately addressed here. One concerns the interpretation to be placed on a seemingly dose-related increase in the incidence of delayed ossification and other skeletal variants, in either the presence or the absence of maternal toxicity.

It is well known that these developmental variants are often seen to increase above control levels in instances involving overt maternal toxicity (weight loss, diarrhea, increased mortality, etc.). There is also some consensus among teratologists that such increases in these developmental features may be secondary to physiologic stresses which are associated with the maternal toxicity. Regulatory scientists and toxicologists tend to agree that increased occurrence of delayed ossification or skeletal variants should not be assigned fetotoxic or other adverse significance, and consequently not used in safety evaluations, when seen in the presence of maternal toxicity. The rationale is simply that toxic effects in the mother may introduce another set of unknowns into the procedure intended only to measure the effects of the test compound on the conceptus.

Less frequently seen, but by no means unknown among experienced teratologists, is a statistically significant increase above control levels of these developmental variants in the absence of maternal toxicity and of true malformations or other fetotoxicity. Examples were seen in the caffeine studies by Collins et al. (1981) and Nolen (1981).

Both delayed ossification and other skeletal variants are thought sometimes to show increased incidence under some conditions which involve transitory stress to the mother, whether physiologic or emotional, even when true toxicity or pathology is absent. Such stress may be transitory bur recurrent at regular intervals, as after daily gavage or subcutaneous injection of irritating chemicals, although not sufficiently stressful to cause recognizable maternal toxicity. The subject has not been experimentally examined, but a possible example might be a surge of catecholamines into the maternal bloodstream which would be directly transferred, or secondarily reflected by biochemical changes in fetal blood. In other words, it is suggested that metabolic or endocrine changes occurred in the maternal organism of sufficient magnitude to be transmitted across the placenta to secondarily affect the rapidly growing fetus, but insufficient to cause overt maternal toxicity. To test this hypothesis would require the application of various chemically or mechanically induced stresses in nondamaging doses during the latter part of rodent pregnancy, followed by routine examination of the skeletons of perinatal offspring.

Metabolic or endocrine changes in fetal blood, as suggested above, could quite conceivably slow or otherwise disrupt the mobilization and desposition of mineral salts during the rapid ossification which occurs in fetal life, thus resulting in identifiable delay in the schedule of bone formation observed several days later at the time of killing.

These postulated metabolic and endocrine changes are not as readily visualized as causative factors in the increase in incidence of skeletal variants such as bifid sternebrae and vertebral centra or accessory ribs. However, it has been assumed for some time by geneticists that the developmental variants of this type, which occur in all mammalian species, show variable morphological expression because they are determined by multiple genes which are in a state of precarious balance. It is thought that when less than optimal conditions exist, whether due to endogenous, maternal, or external influences, the usual balance of these unstable genetic loci is upset and some genetic expression other than the usual one occurs (Fraser 1977). If this expression occurs at a low incidence and results in no impairment of the individual's well-being or longevity, it is usually considered a developmental variant. Thus an infrequent happenstance is postulated to become a more frequent, induced occurrence under as yet undefined conditions of maternal stress.

There is little scientific evidence to support the contention that increased incidence of developmental variants at a nonteratogenic range of dosage in a teratogenicity study is predictive of a teratogenic outcome at the next higher range of dosage. On the contrary, several research papers have provided substantial support for the view that these are not developmental defects in the sense of malformations, although no single study has addressed all of the issues and opinions discussed above (see Aliverti et al. 1979; Benya et al. 1981; Fritz and Hess 1970; Jones and Chernoff 1978; Kimmel and Wilson 1973; Khera 1980).

4.3 Interaction of Caffeine with Known Teratogens

A potentially serious problem associated with caffeine is its ability to interact with other agents and induce a teratogenic response. Three reports (Fujii et al. 1978; Ritter et al. 1982; Yielding et al. 1976) have shown that caffeine enhances the teratogenic potential of cytotoxic agents. Caffeine and other methylated xanthines are well known to potentiate cytotoxicity due to X-rays, alkylating agents, and various other cytotoxic agents (see Ritter et al. 1982 for references). Since the teratogens used in these studies probably produce their effect by killing embryonic cells, enhancement of cytotoxicity by caffeine provides a reasonable explanation for the teratogenic potentiation observed. Ritter et al. (1982) reported that caffeine potentiated the unusual teratogenic effects of the diuretic agent acetazolamide. This agent clearly does not produce teratogenesis by killing embryonic cells (Holmes and Trelstad 1979), suggesting that caffeine can interact with other agents in a variety of ways. Skalko and Kwasigroch (1983) have recently shown that caffeine interacts with phenytoin and 5-bromodeoxyuridine, resulting in synergistic embryotoxic responses, and demonstrated that the timing of administration of the interacting agents is crucial in determining the extent of the synergism. Further attesting to multiple mechanisms of interaction, Runner (1983) has shown that caffeine can prevent some of the teratogenic effects of retinoic acid, and Nomura (1983) reported that caffeine can prevent the embryotoxic effects of urethan.

From these few investigations we are assured that caffeine can interact with a wide variety of agents probably through different mechanisms. The doses of caffeine used in most of these studies were well below teratogenic levels, but still represent higher levels than most people would be exposed to. Thus we can say only that interaction of caffeine with other chemical agents represent a potential hazard which needs a great deal of further study before meaningful conclusions can be reached.

The question of complications secondary to emotional stress after gavage has often been raised. Indeed, it is reasonable to suppose that the insertion of a rigid or semi-rigid tube through the mouth and into the stomach of a rat or mouse under forceful restraint, together with the introduction by this means of a relatively large bolus of test material plus vehicle, would constitute considerable emotional if not physical stress. After examining all available animal studies involving caffeine dosage during pregnancy, however, there is no clear evidence that gavage alone added appreciably to the teratogenic responses reported. The same malformations in approximately similar low incidence were observed after intraperitoneal or intravenous injection as after intubation. The critical point seems to have been that the total daily dosage was administered at one time rather than at intervals, as in divided doses given in four or more treatments per day, or more or less continuously, as when caffeine was incorporated into food or drinking water. Several workers have shown that divided dosage was much less effective than equivalent total dosage given as a single daily treatment. Continuous dosage via food or water may be even less effective than divided dosage by gavage, but data are not sufficient to establish this point conclusively. In any event, Kimmel (1982), Sullivan (1982), and Ikeda et al. (1982) have presented data indicating that a high peak concentration of caffeine in maternal plasma is stronly correlated with the occurrence of a teratogenic response.

The above does not rule out the possibility that maternal stress resulting from gavage did not contribute to the high incidence of skeletal variants in the Collins et al. (1981) gavage study. Control incidence of such variants seemed higher than that reported by other authors for other strains of rats. The few instances in which there were statistically significant, dose-related increases of variables in caffeine-treated animals compared with vehicle-treated controls could be attributed to interaction between the caffeine and a postulated maternal stress factor secondary to gavage.

5 Summary and Conclusions

The original study by Nishimura and Nakai (1960) indicated that caffeine is a mammalian teratogen. Subsequent studies have confirmed this and refined understanding of the conditions necessary for caffeine to act as a teratogen. In acute studies utilizing one or two injections of caffeine, as much as 200 mg/kg is needed to induce a reproducible teratogenic response. When the dosage regimen is more chronic (e.g., throughout pregnancy) and administration is by bolus once per day, somewhat more than 50 mg/kg is required. However, when daily dosage is divided (e.g., multiple injections, incorporation in food or drinking water), more than 100 mg/kg is necessary to produce an embryotoxic response with regularity. A teratogenic response is characterized by a low frequency of affected survivors usually having only facial or limb defects, often with accompanying hematomas and a variety of skeletal variants, most notably in the sternum. A true teratogenic response has usually been associated with doses that produce maternal toxicity, including reduced food intake, reduced body weight gain, convulsions, and death. As expected, caffeine and its major metabolites pass from the mother into the embryo, but it is impossible at present to state with any certainty whether caffeine or one of its metabolites is responsible for the teratogenic effects or where the proximate teratogen has its initial action leading to subsequent abnormal development. Prevailing opinion suggests that the teratogenic mechanism of caffeine-induced malformations is related to the vasoactive effects of catecholamines released in response to caffeine injection. However, the information supporting this idea is not unequivocal, and other possibilities, such as corticosterone release and adenosine receptor antagonism, have been envisaged.

Overall, the information accumulated from animal studies suggests that caffeine consumed in moderate amounts, especially by protracted intake, poses little hazard to the developing mammalian embryo. A possible reservation to this comforting statement concerns the ability of caffeine to interact with a number of known teratogens. Doses of caffeine used to induce teratogenic synergism have been lower than embryotoxic doses of caffeine alone, but still significantly higher than usual human levels of intake.

References

Aliverti V, Bonanomi L, Giavine E, Leone G, Mariani L (1979) Extent of fetal ossification as an index of delayed development in teratogenic studies on the rat. Teratology 20: 237–242

Bartel H, Gnacikowska M (1972) Histological studies on the influence of caffeine on embryonic development of the limbs in mice. Folia Morphol (Warsz) 31: 178–184

Benya TJ, TerHaar G, Goldenthal EI, Rodwell DE (1981)Teratogenic evaluation of methyl cyclopentadienyl manganese tricarbonyl (MMT) in rats. Toxicologist 1: 148

Berkowitz B, Spector S (1971) Effects of caffeine and theophylline on peripheral catecholamines. Eur J Pharmacol 13: 195–196

Bertrand M, Schwan E, Fandom A, Vagne A, Alarg J (1965) Sur un effet tératogène systématique et spécifique de la caféine chez les Rongeurs. C R Soc Biol (Paris 159: 2199–2201

Bertrand M, Girod J, Rigaud MF (1970) Ectrodactylie provoquée par le caféine chez les Rongeurs. Rôle des facteurs spécifique et génétiques. C R Soc Biol (Paris) 164: 1488–1489

Citizens Petition to FDA (1979) Center for Science in the Public Interest, Washington, D.C.

Clark RL, Fox KE, Cusick W (1982) Interactions of caffeine and adenosine agonists in mouse embryotoxicity and teratogenicity. Teratology 25: 35A

Collins TFX (1979) Review of reproduction and teratology studies of caffeine. FDA By-Lines 7, September

Collins TFX, Welsh J, Black T, Collins E (1981) A comprehensive study of the teratogenic potential of caffeine in rats when given by oral intubation. Regul Toxicol Pharmacol 1: 355–378

Davies J, Robson J (1970) The effects of vasopressin, adrenaline and noradrenaline on the mouse fetus. Br J Pharmacol 38: 446P

Elmazar M, McElhatton P, Sullivan F (1981) Acute studies to investigate the mechanism of action of caffeine as a teratogen in mice. Hum Toxicol 1: 53–63

FASEB (1978) Evaluation of the health aspects of caffeine as a food ingredient. Federation of American Societies of Experimental Biology, Bethesda/MD

Federal Register (1980) 45: 69817–69823

Fraser FC (1977) Interactions and multiple causes. In: Wilson JG, Fraser FC (eds) Handbook of teratology, vol 1. Plenum, New York

Fritz H, Hess R (1970) Ossification of the rat and mouse skeleton in the perinatal period. Teratology 3: 331–338

Fujii T (1976) Mitigation of caffeine-induced fetopathy in mice by pretreatment with β-adrenergic blocking agents. Jpn J Pharmacol 26: 751–756

Fujii T, Nishimura H (1972) Adverse effects of prolonged administration of caffeine on rat fetus. Toxicol Appl Pharmacol 22: 449–457

Fujii T, Nishimura H (1974) Reduction in frequency of fetopathic effects of caffeine in mice by pretreatment with propanolol. Teratology 10: 149–152

Fujii T, Inoue M, Shoji R (1978) Caffeine enhancement of the teratogenic action of mitomycin C in the mouse. Mutat Res 54: 210

Gilbert EF, Pistey WR (1973) Effects on the offspring of repeated caffeine administration to pregnant rats. J Reprod Fertil 34: 495–499

Goldstein A, Warren R (1962) Passage of caffeine into human gonadal and fetal tissue. Biochem Pharmacol 11: 166–168

Groupe d'Etude des Risques Teratogènes (1969) Tératogènese expérimentale: étude de la caféine chez la souris, Therapie 24: 575–580

Hayasaka I, Fujii T (1977) Potentiation of the fetopathic effects of caffeine in mice by pargyline or cocaine. Congen Anom 17: 487–492

Holick MF, Schunior A, Tassinari M, Holtrop M (1982) Effects of caffeine on rat sternebrae development and ossification. Fourth International Caffeine Workshop, Oct. 17–21, Athens, Greece. Sponsored by International Life Sciences Institute

Holmes L, Trelstad R (1979) The early limb deformity caused by acetazolamide. Teratology 20: 289–296

Ikeda G, Sapienja P, McGinnis M, Bragg L, Walsh J, Collins T (1982) Blood levels of caffeine and results of fetal examination after oral administration of caffeine to pregnant rats. J Appl Toxicol 2: 307–314

Interagency Epidemiology Working Group (1980) Findings and Recommendations. An assessment of human epidemiological data concerned with caffeine consumption and problems of pregnancy. Submitted to the Commissioner of the FDA, August

Jones KL, Chernoff GF (1978) Drugs and chemicals associated with intrauterine growth deficiency. J Reprod Med 21: 365–370

Jost A (1953a) Dégénérescence des extrémétés du fétus du rat provoquée par l'adrénaline. C R Seances Acad Sci 236: 1510–1512

Jost A (1953b) La dégénérescence des extrémetés du fétus du rat sans des actions hormonale (acroblapsie expérimentelle) et la théoree des bulles myelencephalique de Bonnevie. Arch Fr Pediatr 10: 855–860

Jost A, Petter C, Duval G, Maltier JP, Roffi J (1964) Action de l'adrénaline sur le partage du sang entre le fétus et al placenta. Facteur hémodynamique de certain lésion congénitales des extrémetés. C R Seances Acad Sci 259: 3086–3088

Jost A, Maltier JP, Petter C (1973) Some effects of adrenaline on the vessels of the 17-day old rat fetus. In: Boreus LO (ed) Fetal pharmacology. Raven, New York

Khera KS (1980) Embryological deviations or teratological effects. Third International Caffeine Workshop, Hunt Valley/MD October 26–28

Kimmel C (1982) Pharmacokinetic parameters and teratogenic end-points following prenatal caffeine exposure. Fourth International Caffeine Workshop, Oct. 17–21, Athens, Greece. Sponsored by International Life Sciences Institute

Kimmel CA, Wilson JG (1973) Skeletal deviations in rats: malformations or variants? Teratology 8: 309–316

Knoche C, König J (1964) Zur pränatalen Toxizität von Diphenylpyralin-8-chlortheophyllinat unter Berücksichtigung von Erfahrungen mit Thalidomid und Coffein. Arzneimittelforsch 14: 415–424

Layton MM, Hallesy DW (1965) Deformity of forelimb in rats associated with high doses of acetazolamide. Science 149: 306–308

Leist K, Grauwiler J (1974) Fetal pathology in rats following uterine vessel clamping on day 14 of gestation. Teratology 10: 55–68

Leuschner F, Czok FG (1973) Reversibilität pränataler Coffeinschäden bei Ratten. Colloq Int Chim Cafes [CR] 5: 388–391

Leuschner F, Schwerdtfeger W (1969) Über den Einfluß von Coffein und anderen Methylxanthinen auf die Fortpflanzung von Wistar-Ratten. In: Heim F, Ammon HPT (eds), Coffein und andere Methylxanthine. Schattauer Verlag, Stuttgart New York, pp 209–215

Nishimura H, Nakai K (1960) Congenital malformations in offspring of mice treated with caffeine. Proc Soc Exp Biol Med 104: 140–142

Nolen GA (1981) The effects of brewed and instand coffee on reproduction and teratogenesis in the rat. Toxicol Appl Pharmacol 58: 171–183

Nomura T (1983) Comparative inhibiting effects of methylxanthines on urethan-induced tumors, malformations and presumed somatic mutations in mice. Cancer Res 43: 1342–1346

Palm PE, Arnold EP, Rachwall PC, Leyczek JC, Teague KW, Kensler CJ (1978) Evaluation of the teratogenic potential of fresh-brewed coffee and caffeine in the rat. Toxicol Appl Pharmacol 44: 1–16

Ritter EJ, Scott WJ, Wilson JG, Mathinos PR, Randall JL (1982) Potentiative interactions between caffeine and various teratogenic agents. Teratology 25: 95–100

Rugh R (1968) The mouse. Burgess, Minneapolis

Runner M (1983) Rescue from disproportionate dwarfism in mice by means of caffeine modulation of the 4-hour early effect of excessive vitamin A. In: Fallon J, Caplan A (eds) Limb development and regeneration, part A. Liss, New York, pp 345–353

Scott WJ (to be published). Caffeine-induced limb malformations: description of malformations and quantitation of placental transfer. Teratology

Sieber S, Fabro S (1971) Identification of drugs in the preimplantation blastocyst and in the plasma, uterine secretions and urine of the pregnant rabbit. J Pharmacol Exp Ther 176: 65–75

Singh S, Singh G (1973) Hemorrhages in the limbs of fetal rats after amniocentesis and their role in limb malformations. Teratology 8: 11–18

Skalko R, Kwasigroch T (1983) The interaction of chemicals during pregnancy: an update. Biol Res Preg Perinatol 4: 26–35

Snigorska B, Bartel H (1970) Studies on the teratogenic influence of caffeine on white mouse fetuses. Folia Morphol (Warsz) 29: 353–363

Soyka L (1981) Caffeine ingestion during pregnancy: in utero exposure and possible effects. Semin Perinatol 5: 305–309

Sullivan FM (1982) Effects of different dosing regimens on the teratogenicity of caffeine in rats. Fourth International Caffeine Workshop, Oct. 17–21, Athens, Greece. Sponsored by International Life Sciences Institute

Tanimura T, Terada M (1968) Transplacental passage of C^{14}-caffeine into the mouse embryo. Proc Congr Anom Res Assoc Jpn 8: 39–40

Teratology Society (1974) Teratogens and the Delaney clause. Teratology 10: 106

Tucci S, Skalko R (1978) The teratogenic effects of theophylline in mice. Toxicol Lett 1: 337–341

Warkany J, Schraffenberger E (1944) Congenital malformations induced in rats by maternal nutritional deficiency. VI. Preventive factor. J Nutr 27: 477–484

Warkany J, Schraffenberger E (1947) Congeintal malformations induced in rats by roentgen rays. AJR 57: 455–463

Wilson JG, Scott WJ, Ritter EJ (1977) Digital abnormalities in monkeys and rats. In: Bergsma D, Lenz W (eds) Morphogenesis and malformation of the limbs. Liss, New York, pp 203–217

Yielding LW, Riley TL, Yielding KL (1976) Preliminary study of caffeine and chloroquine enhancement of x-ray induced birth defects. Biochem Biophys Res Commun 68: 1356–1361

XIII Epidemiologic Studies of Birth Defects*

A. Leviton

1 What Is Epidemiology?

The term "epidemiology" was originally used to describe the study of epidemics. At first the word "epidemic" was confined to acute illnesses that appeared to "spread" within hours or days to afflict large numbers of people, but over the last half century the definition has broadened. Shortly after the Second World War it became apparent that some diseases, which probably had "incubation periods" of months or years, had become much more frequent than previously, and they began to be viewed as epidemics. Lung cancer and heart disease were the two conditions that appeared to prompt a dichotomy of epidemiology into infectious disease epidemiology (e. g., cholera, whooping cough, smallpox), and chronic disease epidemiology (e. g., lung cancer, heart attack). That dichotomy has been eliminated for many reasons, one of which is that epidemics of a number of chronic infections are now appreciated (e. g., kuru; Nathanson 1980).

A commonly-accepted definition of epidemiology is that it is the study of the distribution and determinants of disease in populations (MacMahon and Pugh 1970; Lilienfeld and Lilienfeld 1980). The basic task of epidemiology is to seek the causes of a disease by finding out how people who develop the disease differ from people who do not.

2 Why the Need for Epidemiology?

Pharmacologists and teratologists can give pregnant laboratory animals high doses of an agent such as caffeine to see what happens to their offspring compared to the offspring of control animals. If some abnormality is found, they can then design experiments to investigate the mechanisms by which the agent exerts its effects.

---

* This chapter is not intended to be a comprehensive historical review. Rather it is intended to focus on the state of the art in order to illustrate the difficulties encountered in conducting epidemiologic studies of substances like caffeine that are consumed by a large segment of the population, in the case of caffeine in a wide variety of beverages. The chapter begins with a general overview of problems encountered in conducting epidemiologic studies and continues (Sect. 5) with discussion of recent epidemiologic studies of caffeine and birth defects in the light of the problems each study poses

For many obvious reasons this approach is not acceptable in the study of human subjects. How then shall we determine whether caffeine consumption by pregnant women adversely affects their offspring? By taking advantage of a range of different intakes, of course. Women have distributed themselves along the range of caffeine consumptions, from 0 mg/day to more than 1 g/day. Thus, without any investigator asking some women to ingest no caffeine and other women to consume large amounts, a range of intakes exists. The people who have assumed responsibility for collecting and analyzing these data are called epidemiologists. This then is epidemiology's major strength; it is able to assess directly whether the usual levels of caffeine consumption by pregnant women adversely affect the human fetus.

3 Limitations of Epidemiology

3.1 Associations, Not Causes

The object of epidemiology is to reduce the occurrence of disease by identifying "risk factors" whose presence or effects can be eliminated or reduced. To a large extent this is achieved by observation of what is happening rather than by intervening to create an experiment. In its being an observational science, the major limitation of epidemiology is that causal inferences can be based only on observed associations. Unlike experiments in which variables can be controlled and manipulated, epidemiologic studies are based on observations of people who make their own decisions about the innumerable factors that might influence the disease under study. What constitutes epidemiologic evidence of causality is a philosophic issue (Buck 1975; Davies 1975). Epidemiologic findings, however, are now being used to justify changes in public health policy (White and Henderson 1976; Knox 1979).

3.2 Quality of Data

Further limitations of epidemiology arise from the imperfect quality of the data on the exposure to the putative agent, the assessment of the outcome of interest, and the knowledge of other characteristics (i.e., covariates) that might be associated with both exposure and outcome (Feinstein and Horwitz 1982).

3.2.1 Measures of Exposure

Questionnaires to assess caffeine consumption are of uncertain validity. Validity is shown by agreement between information obtained by questioning people and some independent assessment of the true state of affairs (e.g., cans of coffee purchased each month, blood caffeine levels).

Reliability, on the other hand, is a measure of the agreement between a person's answer given on one day to a question, and the answer to the same question given on another day. Obviously, day-to-day variation is expected in a person's activities. Thus variation in the answers to the question "How many cups of coffee did you drink yesterday?" is expected, but variation in the answers to "How many cups of coffee do you usually drink each weekday?" indicates limited reliability.

To date no questionnaire about hot beverage consumption has had its reliability and validity assessed. Unlike alcohol consumption, where answers to questions are known to be biased (Lucas et al. 1977), consumption of moderate to large amounts of coffee, tea, and cola should pose no problem of bias based on social undesirability. Thus valid, reliable questionnaires about caffeine consumption may be possible.

3.2.2 Outcome Data

Even the best observers vary in their ability to make a judgment about the presence or absence of a finding of interest (Koran 1975; Spodick 1975; Lindsay et al. 1983). Those who study sensory perceptions are concerned about "signal-to-noise ratio" in the systems. Whether it is in identifying blips on a radar screen or in interpreting X-rays, electrocardiograms, electroencephalograms, or histologic slides of tumors, observers are not completely consistent in their judgments. Thus, intraobserver variability needs to be taken into account, though it tends to be less than interobserver variability.

A separate problem concerning "outcome" data is "Where should the line be drawn between normal and abnormal?" How high is high? This question applies to blood pressure when the outcome of concern is hypertension, and to blood sugar levels when diabetes is the outcome. Should the people whose physicians diagnose a "touch" of diabetes be considered as part of the group with unquestioned diabetes, or as part of the group considered free of diabetes? One approach is to eliminate entirely from an epidemiologic study those people whose status is questionable, whose measurements or characteristics fall into the gray zone between black and white (Zadeh 1969; DuBois and Prade 1980). Another is to see whether people of questionable status are more like people with the disease or people without the disease and then combine them with the more similar group.

These issues of uncertainty apply to birth defects. When is a minor deviation a variant of normal, and when is it an anomaly? Are all anomalies of equivalent weight in identifying a teratogen? Should all birth defects be lumped together? Does webbing between fingers or toes have the same implications as a hole in the heart?

These questions raise the issue of etiologic heterogeneity (Weiss and Liff 1983). Some of us accept the proposition, "The more biologically homogeneous and unique the disorder, the greater the likelihood its risk factors will be identified." For example, thalidomide was identified as a teratogen in man because ingestion of it resulted in the characteristic, biologically unique deformity of phocomelia. The teratogenic potential of thalidomide would have been considerably less evident if it had increased the risk of a diverse group of unrelated birth defects.

It is possible, therefore, that some substances have not yet been identified as teratogens in humans because they produce a nonspecific teratogenic enhancing effect involving a variety of organs. Thus, it seems reasonable that investigators should want to search for associations both between caffeine and birth defects in general (Linn et al. 1982) and between caffeine and specific birth defects (Rosenberg et al. 1982).

190

3.2.3 Covariates

Epidemiologists apply the word "confounders" to variables related both to the exposure and to the outcome (Miettinen 1974; Schlesselman 1978; Greenland and Neutra 1980). For example, women who tend to consume four or more cups of coffee per day are more likely than abstainers to smoke cigarettes (Table 1). This is important because it appears that cigarette smoking may contribute much more than coffee consumption to fetal adversity (Linn et al. 1982; Kuzma and Sokol 1982). Thus, unless the effects of cigarette smoking can be separated from the effects of coffee, it will appear that coffee drinkers are at increased risk of bearing a low-birth-weight or deformed baby. Several strategies exist for identifying the contribution of each covariate.

The conceptually simplest strategy is to exclude all women with the confounder. However, in eliminating all women who smoke, for example, the number of subjects in the study may be reduced considerably – perhaps too much.

The strategy of stratification avoids discarding a large component of any sample. Stratification allows evaluation of the relationship between coffee consumption and birth defects separately in women who smoke and in those who do not. The stratification approach loses its attractiveness when the number of potential confounders is large. Based on previously reported studies, it appears that the risk of birth defects is influenced by many maternal characteristics, including alcohol consumption, age, number of previous pregnancies, illnesses, toxin exposure, and drug ingestion during pregnancy. The distribution of coffee consumption in women with one of these characteristics may differ from the distribution in women without that characteristic. Thus, it would be prudent to view each of these as potential confounders and to stratify accordingly. If these six groups of characteristics were to be dichotomized (alcohol consumption: yes/no; maternal age: above/below X years; etc.) then 64 separate strata would result. Thus, the greater the number of confounders and the greater the number of levels of each category, then the greater the number of strata. Unfortunately, because the available sample has to be divided up among the strata, the greater the number of strata the fewer the subjects in each stratum and the greater the variability due to sampling errors.

Since the risk of birth defect is influenced by a number of risk factors, it seems plausible that each risk factor adds to the probability of the birth defect. The more risk factors, or the greater the intensity of magnitude of each risk factor, the greater

Table 1. Covariates of coffee consumption in pregnant women (from Linn et al. 1982)

Characteristic	Cups of coffee per day				
	0	1	2	3	4+
Age ⩾ 35 years (%)	7.1	9.5	11.9	12.9	14.8
Alcohol in the first trimester (%)	17.3	26.0	33.9	32.5	32.6
Smoking ⩾ 3 cigarettes/day at delivery (%)	17.8	17.8	26.8	37.4	53.6

the total risk. Considering multiple variables (or *multi*ple *variates*) results in a multivariate model. Such models have the basic form:

Risk of birth defect = sum of products of value assigned to presence (or magnitude) of each exposure × weight for that exposure

Multivariate models not only assess the contribution of each risk factor in the light of the contribution of other risk factors, they can also evaluate the interaction of multiple variables. In essence, this answers the question, "Do two or more variables magnify the risk above and beyond the expected sum of the risks conveyed by each?" Interaction is especially important when the possibility exists that a subset of the population is relatively or uniquely susceptible to the effects of an exposure.

The problem with multivariate models is that they may have poor reproducibility, according to the number of parameters estimated from the data (Gordon 1974). The more complex a model, the greater the probability that quite different values will be obtained from another data set.

3.3 Biases

Epidemiologists are very much concerned that their data may be biased (i.e., consistently tending to understate or overstate values of interest). Indeed, a list has been published of most of the identified biases (Sackett 1979). Potential biases are not discussed here, but rather when describing the appropriate studies in Sect. V.

4 The Past

The laboratory studies that contributed to the concern about the relationship between caffeine and birth defects are reviewed by Wilson and Scott in Chap. 12 of this volume. Most of the relevant epidemiologic studies published prior to 1982 have been reviewed elsewhere (Interagency Epidemiological Working Group 1980; Dews 1982). Although relatively complete, these reviews have not always included every relevant study (Tennes and Blackard 1980).

5 Recent Publications

5.1 Harvard Study

The Harvard study (Linn et al. 1982), supported by the National Foundation – March of Dimes, was designed to evaluate to what extent family planning practices (including induced abortions and contraceptive use) influenced the risk of undesirable birth outcomes. More than 12 000 women who gave birth to single babies at Brigham and Women's Hospital, a Harvard University teaching hospital, between August 1977 and March 1980 participated. Shortly after delivery, information was collected routinely about a wide variety of demographic variables, habits, obstetric

192

history, pregnancy events, delivery characteristics, and infant outcomes. One of the questionnaire items concerned the number of cups of coffee and tea consumed on a daily basis during the first trimester of pregnancy.

The issue of confounding (see Sect. III.4.3) is pertinent to this study. A number of potentially confounding variables were identified that were related to both coffee consumption and the risk of adverse birth outcomes. For example, the proportion of women aged 35 years or over increased consistently with coffee consumption, from 7.1% in women who did not drink any coffee to 14.8% in women who consumed four or more cups every day (Table 1).

The proportion of women who smoked three or more cigarettes a day at the time of delivery increased from 17.8% in women who consumed no coffee or at most one cup per day to 53.6% among women who consumed four or more cups per day. Alcohol consumption showed a less consistent trend. Since greater age, cigarette smoking, and alcohol consumption are related to coffee consumption, as well as to low birthweight and congenital anomalies, the investigators viewed them as potential confounders in evaluating a relationship between caffeine consumption and birth outcomes.

Linn and his associates assessed coffee and tea consumption in relation to two general undesirable outcomes. First, they directed their attention to low birthweight. In confirmation of previous reports, cigarette smoking was one of the more prominent risk factors for a birthweight of less than 2.5 kg. When their cigarette smoking was taken into consideration, women were not at increased risk of delivering a low-birthweight baby if they consumed three, four to six, or even seven or more cups of coffee each day (Fig. 1). Multivariate analysis was used to assess the contribution of each of 11 variables to the risk of low birthweight; only four were associated with a significantly increased risk (Table 2), and consumption of four or more cups a day of coffee was not one of them. This analysis compared the 4105 women who did not consume any coffee or tea during the first trimester to 595 women who consumed four or more cups of coffee each day. Although the point estimate of the risk ratio suggests that women who consume four or more cups of coffee a day may be 17% more likely than women who consume no coffee to bear

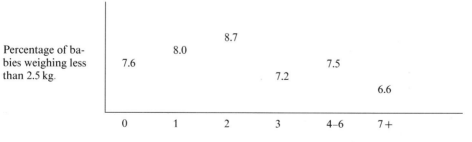

Cups of coffee/day (standardized for smoking)

Fig. 1. Low birthweight and maternal coffee consumption ($n=12\,000$). The risk of delivering a baby of low birthweight does not appear to be associated with the level of maternal coffee consumption during pregnancy. (From Linn et al. 1982)

Table 2. Results of logistic regression for birthweight less than 2.5 kg (from Linn et al. 1982)

Variable	Risk ratio	95% Confidence interval
Smoking 3+ cigarettes/day	1.83	1.42–2.36
Previous stillbirth	3.03	1.93–4.77
Previous induced abortion	1.41	1.08–1.84
Previous spontaneous abortion	1.35	1.02–1.79
Coffee consumption 4+ cups/day	1.17	0.85–1.61

Table 3. Percentage of babies with malformation born to women in "high" and "low" coffee consumption groups (from Linn et al. 1982)

	No coffee or tea	4+ Cups coffee/day
Major nonskeletal malformation	2.5	2.0
Major skeletal malformation	0.8	0.5
Minor malformation	6.7	5.4
Any malformation	9.2	7.4

a baby of less than 2.5 kg, this difference does not achieve nominal statistical significance even in this sample of 4700 women.

The second outcome of interest was the full range of birth defects. Linn and his associates employed a coding scheme developed for the congenital malformations surveillance program at the Centers for Disease Control of the U.S. Public Health Service in Atlanta, Georgia. This allowed every child to be classified into one of four categories: major nonskeletal malformation, major skeletal malformation, minor malformation, and no malformation. Women who consumed four or more cups of coffee per day were not at increased risk of delivering a child with any malformation (Table 3). Indeed, on univariate analysis (i.e., not controlling for the numerous potential confounders) it appears that women who consumed four or more cups of coffee per day were 20% less likely to bear a child with any malformation than were women who consumed no coffee.

One of the major attractions of this study is its "power." Statisticians and epidemiologists are concerned with two kinds of errors. The alpha or type 1 error occurs when a difference is seen between two samples even though there is in fact no difference between the populations from which the samples were drawn. The P value assigned to a statistical analysis usually refers to the probability that such an observation occurred randomly in the sampling process. The beta or type 2 error occurs when no difference is shown between two samples, and yet there really is a difference. For example, women are on the average shorter than men, but it is easy to see that a random sample of half a dozen men and half a dozen women may average about the same height. Power is defined as 1 minus the beta error. Most epidemiologists aim for a power of 0.8–0.9, i.e., beta errors of 0.1–0.2; if there were a significant biological difference it would be missed only 10%–20% of the time. Linn and his colleagues conducted a study that had a power of 0.93 to find whether consuming

194

more than four cups of coffee per day was statistically significantly associated with a true 1.5-fold increase in the risk of all malformations. The study also had a 0.85 chance of finding a threefold increase in skeletal malformations and a twofold risk of major malformations. By standards of what can usually be achieved these were high levels of power.

The major limitation of this study was the less than ideal measure of caffeine consumption. Indeed, caffeine consumption was only indirectly assessed from estimates of coffee and tea consumption. Investigators at Yale University have emphasized this point with their own data from 1860 interviews of pregnant women (Bracken et al. 1982). A third of women who drank neither tea nor coffee did drink cola, and a third of this group were estimated to ingest more than 70 mg caffeine daily. Thus, the Yale study raised the possibility that a number of women in the Linn study who were labeled as not drinking tea or coffee may nevertheless have been exposed to caffeine.

5.2 Boston University Study

A study from the Drug Epidemiology Unit of Boston University (Rosenberg et al. 1982) was designed to evaluate the risk of congenital anomalies that might be attributed to maternal drug consumption during the first trimester of pregnancy. It complemented the Harvard study by its emphasis on total caffeine consumption and by its examination of specific congenital anomalies.

During a 4.5-year period, babies who had a congenital malformation were identified in participating institutions in the metropolitan areas of Boston, Philadelphia, and Toronto. Two of the congenital anomalies that had been seen in rodents given high doses of caffeine were the focus of this study. Cleft lip (with or without cleft palate) occurred in 299 babies, and isolated cleft palate was identified in another 120 babies. Neither mothers who consumed more than 200 mg caffeine per day nor those who consumed more than 400 mg of caffeine per day were at significantly increased risk of delivering a baby with either of these clefts (Table 4). While the risk ratios associated with cleft lip are minimally elevated, the risk ratios associated with isolated cleft palate are minimally reduced.

Other than facial clefts, the anomaly seen in the offspring of rodents given high doses of caffeine during pregnancy was ectrodactyly ("missing digits," "split hand"). This anomaly is so rare in humans that no case-control study has yet been mounted. The authors of the Boston University study looked at the somewhat broader group of limb-reduction defects. Among the more than 2000 malformed infants in their study, only 22 had a limb-reduction defect – not enough for a valid case-control study. Nevertheless, in an exploratory evaluation of the data, mothers of these babies did not differ in their caffeine consumption from the mothers of babies with other defects.

Preferential recall of "exposures" can occur when mothers of children with anomalies tend to ruminate more about what they consumed during pregnancy than mothers of controls. This bias was avoided in this study by virtue of temporal sequence of events and design. First, most of the women were interviewed before the widespread publicity given to reports of anomalies in the offspring of rodents

Table 4. Estimated *risk* of selected birth defects in caffeine consumers relative to the risk in women who consumed no caffeine (from Rosenberg et al. 1982)

Defect	Mean daily caffeine consumption	
	⩾ 200 mg	⩾ 400 mg
Cleft lip	1.3 (0.7–2.5)	1.4 (0.7–2.9)
Isolated cleft palate	0.8 (0.3–1.7)	0.5 (0.2–1.4)

given high doses of caffeine. Second, the investigators chose as controls babies who had a wide assortment of other birth defects. This strategy has the drawback that some of the controls may have had anomalies that could conceivably have been associated with maternal consumption of high levels of caffeine.

5.3 Loma Linda Study

Kuzma and Kissinger (1981) conducted a 4-year study of more than 12000 pregnant women who sought prenatal care at four hospitals in one metropolitan area of Southern California. Kuzma and Sokol (1982) described their sample as consisting of only 5000 pregnant women who appear to have been included in the earlier study. This study poses a number of problems. First, the sample is not well described; from a reading of the two papers I was not able to identify the differences between the two samples or ascertain why some women were the subjects of one report but not of the other.

Another concern is with the nature and quality of the data obtained. Although most women completed their questionnaire about "health related habits ... relative to her life *prior* to the pregnancy" (Kuzma and Kissinger 1981) at the time of the first prenatal visits, 37% first completed the questionnaire after delivery. The authors provide no assurance that women who completed the questionnaire early in pregnancy did not differ from women who completed it after pregnancy in either caffeine consumption or their babies' birthweight.

A third concern, that the data obtained in the study may not be generalizable to the universe of all pregnant women, is prompted by the observation that 29% of women in the sample consumed the equivalent of six or more cups of coffee per day. This is considerably higher than that seen in other series (Graham 1978; Linn et al. 1982; Rosenberg et al. 1982; Berkowitz et al. 1982), indicating an unrepresentative sample.

It appears that the authors evaluated the relationship of birthweight to maternal caffeine consumption *before* pregnancy. Nowhere in the report is there a statement about caffeine consumption during pregnancy. Women decrease their consumption of caffeine during pregnancy (Hook 1976), possibly in response to a prolongation of the half-life of caffeine that occurs in the third trimester. The relationship of caffeine consumption prior to pregnancy to caffeine consumption during different parts of the pregnancy is unclear. Without this information, and without information about caffeine consumption during pregnancy in the subjects, no inference can

Table 5. Birthweight variance "explained": percentage of variance of birthweight explained by the stepwise regression model utilizing 13 variables for 5093 mother-infant pairs in the Loma Linda study (from Kuzma and Sokol 1982)

Variable	% Variance explained
Duration of gestation	19.8
Weight gain	5.3
Prepregnancy weight	3.5
Cigarette use	2.1
Caffeine use	0.2
Other eight variables	1.6
All 13 variables	32.5

be made from the Loma Linda data about caffeine consumption during pregnancy and birthweight.

Kuzma and Sokol (1982) set out to test ten hypotheses about alcohol consumption and birthweight, not to evaluate the relationship between caffeine consumption prior to pregnancy and birthweight. Their finding of a weak relationship was unexpected. This distinction between hypothesis generation and hypothesis testing has been discussed elsewhere (Feinstein et al. 1981).

With all these caveats the findings of Kuzma and Sokol can now be examined. They created a stepwise multiple regression model of birthweight as a "function" of 13 variables. Caffeine consumption added only 0.2% to the amount of variance of birthweight "explained" by this model (Table 5). This contrasts with 32.3% of the variance "explained" by the other 12 variables, and 67.5% of the variance not "explained" by any of these variables. In more concrete terms, the authors' findings may be summarized as suggesting that women who consume the caffeine equivalent of six cups of coffee per day prior to delivery gave birth to babies weighing 1.5 oz less than babies born to women who consumed virtually no caffeine. This contrasts with the birthweight reduction of 3.7 oz for consumption of two-thirds of a can of beer per day, and a reduction of 6.4 oz for smoking one or more packs of cigarettes per day.

5.4 Yale Study

The Yale study (Berkowitz et al. 1982) appears to be another study by investigators who did not originally intend to evaluate the contribution of coffee and tea consumption to an undesirable pregnancy outcome. Unlike the other three studies published in 1982, it is a case-control study of preterm birth. A total of 175 women who delivered a baby at Yale–New Haven Hospital before the 37th week of gestation were compared to 313 who delivered during or after the 37th week. The authors did not base their definition of prematurity on the mother's or obstetrician's estimation of the due date, but rather on examination of the baby. The implications of this choice of definition are discussed in the preceding report of this study (Berkowitz 1981).

Table 6. Preterm birth and maternal coffee and tea consumption during the third trimester (from Berkowitz et al. 1982)

Cups per day	Tea		Coffee	
	Point estimate	95% Confidence interval	Point estimate	95% Confidence interval
0	1.0		1.0	
1	0.6	(0.4–1.1)	1.2	(0.7–1.9)
2	1.1	(0.6–2.0)	1.2	(0.7–2.0)
3	1.5	(0.7–3.0)	0.7	(0.3–1.5)
4+	0.5	(0.2–1.1)	1.5	(0.8–3.1)

The estimates are not adjusted for the most obvious exposures and characteristics that might be expected to be associated with preterm birth and beverage choice. Statistically, none of these individual values is significantly different from 1. In addition, the data do not suggest a dose-response effect.

This study is unique among the four presented here in asking about coffee and tea consumption during each trimester. The value of this extra information, however, is uncertain, because all the participants were interviewed *once* only – *after* delivery. Women were classified by daily coffee consumption and by daily tea consumption, but not by total daily caffeine consumption.

When only coffee and tea consumption are considered, no relationship is seen between these "exposures" and the risk of preterm birth (Table 6). The relationship between tea (but not coffee) and preterm birth was then evaluated with a logistic regression model that allowed adjustment for the contribution of the other risk factors of preterm birth. Here again, the estimated risk ratio of preterm birth associated with the daily consumption of four or more cups of tea was not significantly greater than 1.

This study has a power of 90% to appreciate an estimated risk ratio of 3 and a power of 80% to appreciate a risk ratio of 2.5. Thus, the investigators are able to say with confidence that consumption of four or more cups of coffee (or tea) per day during pregnancy does not triple the risk of preterm birth. Less confidence can be attached to statements based on these data that consumption of four or more cups of coffee (or tea) per day during pregnancy does not double the risk of preterm birth.

5.5 Overview

These four studies published in 1982 vary considerably. Cumulatively, they provide rather impressive evidence that caffeine consumption by pregnant women does not materially increase the risk of low birthweight, preterm birth, congenital malformations in general, or the particular congenital malformations produced in laboratory animals by the administration of high doses of caffeine.

6 The Future

None of the four studies discussed in this chapter were specifically designed to study the effect of caffeine consumption. The investigators took advantage of opportunities created by studies undertaken to evaluate other exposures. In light of their essentially "negative" findings and the limited resources available for future studies, it is unlikely that epidemiologists will mount new studies of caffeine consumption and reproductive adversities.

References

Berkowitz GS (1981) An epidemiologic study of preterm delivery. Am J Epidemiol 113: 81–92
Berkowitz GS, Holford TR, Berkowitz RL (1982) Effects of cigarette smoking, alcohol, coffee and tea consumption on preterm delivery. Early Hum Dev 7: 239–250
Bracken MB, Bryce-Buchanan C, Silten R, Srisuphan W (1982) Coffee consumption during pregnancy. N Engl J Med 306: 1548–1549
Buck C (1975) Popper's philosophy for epidemiologists. Int J Epidemiol 4: 159–168
Davies AM (1975) Comments on "Popper's philosophy for epidemiologists" by Carol Buck. Int J Epidemiol 4: 169–171
Dews P (1982) Caffeine. Annu Rev Nutr 2: 323–341
DuBois D, Prade H (1980) Fuzzy sets and systems. Theory and applications. Academic, New York
Feinstein AR, Horwitz RA (1982) Double standards, scientific methods, and epidemiologic research. N Engl J Med 307: 1611–1617
Feinstein AR, Horwitz R, Spitzer WD, Battista RN (1981) Coffee and pancreatic cancer. The problems of etiologic science and epidemiologic case-control research. JAMA 246: 957–961
Gordon T (1974) Hazards in the use of the logistic function with reference to data from prospective cardiovascular studies. J Chronic Dis 27: 97–102
Graham DM (1978) Caffeine: its identity, dietary sources, intake and biologic effects. Nutr Rev 36: 97–102
Greenland S, Neutra R (1980) Control of confounding in the assessment of medical technology. Int J Epidemiol 9: 361–367
Hook EB (1976) Changes in tobacco smoking and ingestion of alcohol and caffeinated beverages during early pregnancy: Are these consequences, in part, of feto-protective mechanisms diminishing maternal exposure to embryotoxins? In: Kelly S, Hook EB, Janerich DT, Portar H (eds) Birth defects: Risks and consequences. Academic, New York, pp 173–183
Interagency Epidemiological Working Group on Special Problems in Cancer Epidemiology (1980) An assessment of human epidemiological data concerned with caffeine consumption and problems of pregnancy. In: Report on caffeine, Food and Drug Administration, Washington
Knox EG (1979) Epidemiology in health care planning. Oxford University Press, New York
Koran LM (1975) The reliability of clinical methods, data and judgments. N Engl J Med 293: 642–646, 695–701
Kuzma J, Kissinger D (1981) Patterns of alcohol and cigarette use in pregnancy. Neurobehav Toxicol Teratol 32: 211–221
Kuzma J, Sokol R (1982) Maternal drinking and decreased intrauterine growth. Alcoholism (NY) Clin Exp Res 6: 396–402
Lilienfeld A, Lilienfeld D (1980) Foundations of epidemiology. Oxford University Press, New York
Lindsay KW, Teasdale GM, Knill-Jones RP (1983) Observer variability in assessing the clinical features of subarachnoid hemorrhage. J Neurosurg 58: 57–62
Linn S, Schoenbaum SC, Monson RR, Rosner B, Stubblefield PG, Ryan KJ (1982) No association between coffee consumption and adverse outcomes of pregnancy. N Engl J Med 306: 141–145
Lucas RW, Mullin PJ, Luna CB, McInroy DC (1977) Psychiatrists and a computer as interrogators of patients with alcohol-related illnesses: a comparison. Br J Psychiatry 131: 160–167
MacMahon B, Pugh TF (1970) Epidemiology: principles and methods. Little Brown, Boston

Miettinen O (1974) Confounding and effect modification. Am J Epidemiol 100: 350–353

Nathanson N (1980) Slow viruses and chronic disease: the contribution of epidemiology. Public Health Rep 95: 436–443

Rosenberg L, Mitchell AA, Shapiro S, Slone D (1982) Selected birth defects in relation to caffeine-containing beverages. JAMA 247: 1429–1432

Sackett D (1979) Bias in analytic research. J Chronic Dis 32: 51–63

Schlesselman J (1978) Assessing effects of confounding variables. Am J Epidemiol 108: 3–8

Spodick DH (1975) On experts and expertise: the effect of variability in observer performance. Am J Cardiol 36: 592–596

Tennes K, Blackard C (1980) Maternal alcohol consumption, birthweight and minor physical anomalies. Am J Obstet Gynecol 138: 774–780

Weiss N, Liff J (1983) Accounting for the multicausal nature of disease in the design and analysis of epidemiologic studies. Am J Epidemiol 117: 14–18

White KL, Henderson MM (1976) Epidemiology as a fundamental science. Its use in health services planning, administration and evaluation. Oxford University Press, New York

Zadeh LA (1969) Biologic application of the theory of fuzzy sets and systems. In: Proctor LD (ed) Biocybernetics of the central nervous system. Little Brown, Boston, pp 199–206

XIV The Carcinogenic Potential of Caffeine

H. C. Grice

1 Animal Studies

1.1 Published

Bauer et al. (1977) administered freshly brewed standard commercial regular ground coffee (5.2 g/100 ml water) to C57BL/6J mice to provide a dose of approximately 120 mg/kg body weight/day. Standard rodent chow was fed ad libitum. One study involved 25 males in the coffee test group and 25 control males (receiving only water), a second study involved 27 animals in the coffee test group and 25 controls. The animals were kept on experiment for over 130 weeks in the case of the second test group. Gross and microscopic examinations were conducted on a wide variety of tissues and no unusual occurrence of tumors or cancer was found.

Macklin and Szot (1980) fed caffeine in the diet to male and female C57BL/6 mice. A total of 106 males and females received 55 mg/kg/day alone or in combination with phenacetin and aspirin for 75–80 weeks. On postmortem examination there were no remarkable findings that could be attributed to administration of these agents. Detailed histological examination of bladder, kidney and liver did not reveal any carcinogenic effect of the test chemical. The authors concluded that no evidence of carcinogenesis was demonstrated for any of the drugs, alone or in combination.

Wurzner et al. (1977) incorporated regular and decaffeinated instant coffees at a 6% level into a commercial standard diet. The coffee samples, extracted at different rates, were obtained from regular and decaffeinated coffees which were either freeze- or spray-dried. Outbred, specific-pathogen-free Sprague-Dawley rats were randomly distributed into 14 groups, each with 40 males and 40 females. A total of 240 males and 240 females received regular coffee and 120 males and 120 females received decaffeinated coffee with caffeine added. After experimental periods of 3 and 12 months, ten rats of each sex were chosen randomly from each group for interim examinations. The study was terminated at 24 months. Detailed gross and microscopic examinations were conducted on all animals. The authors concluded that "the data from our 2 year feeding study of regular and decaffeinated coffees in rats, using maximum tolerated dose levels, indicate no increased risk formation for neoplasms, and treatments providing high caffeine levels even decreased the evidence of neoplasm in both males and females".

Zeitlin (1972) administered instant coffee solids to male and female Sprague-Dawley rats at a concentration of 5.0% in the diet from the weanling stage to 2 years of age. The coffee content of the diet was 3.6%, providing a dietary concentration of 0.18% caffeine. Necropsies and histopathological examinations were conducted on all animals that died during the study and in survivors killed after 2 years. Particular attention was paid to the urinary bladder, which failed to show any evidence of abnormalities.

In a recent study in male Sprague-Dawley rats that was concerned with the potential carcinogenicity of analgesics, caffeine was included in one of the experimental diets at a level of 0.102% (Johansson 1981). Thirty rats were treated for 117 weeks, each receiving a total dose of 21.4 g caffeine. Control rats received the diet alone. The mean survival time for rats receiving caffeine was 78 weeks, with a range of 41–107 weeks. For control animals mean survival was 94 weeks, with a range of 67–116 weeks. There was no significant difference in the incidence of tumors between control and caffeine-treated animals. A total of six tumors were seen in control animals and eight in the caffeine group, all of types known to occur spontaneously in this strain of rat. The results of this study lend further support to the evidence that chronic exposure to very high doses of caffeine is without carcinogenic effect in laboratory animals.

Takayama and Kubawara (1982) reported a long-term study on the effect of caffeine in rats. Wistar rats of both sexes were given synthetic caffeine in their drinking water continuously for 78 weeks. Three hundred rats were divided into three groups of 50 males and 50 females each. Group 1 was given normal tap water without caffeine as a control, group 2 received 0.1% caffeine solution and group 3 was given 0.2% caffeine solution for 78 weeks. All the animals were killed after 104 weeks. Various tumors were found in both experimental and control groups, but their incidences were not higher in the experimental groups.

1.2 Unpublished

The results of unpublished studies are consistent with those of published studies; the findings after long-term administration uniformly indicate an absence of carcinogenic action.

Ito (1978) administered caffeine to groups of 50 ICR mice of each sex at levels of 0.2%, 0.1%, 0.05% or 0% in the drinking water. Male mice were killed after 60 weeks on test and females after 104 weeks. Gross and histological examinations were conducted on all organs. The incidence of neoplastic change was not significantly different in experimental animals and controls. The males were terminated prematurely on this study because of problems associated with fighting. The author concluded that this study provided no evidence for carcinogenic activity of caffeine.

In a National Cancer Institute study (1978), a mixture of aspirin, phenacetin and caffeine (APC) was administered in the feed at either of two concentrations to Fisher 344 rats and B6C3F$_1$ mice. The high dose used in the chronic studies for the male and female rats and mice was 1.4% and the low dose was 0.7%. Fifty males and 49 or 50 females of each species were put on test materials and 50 animals of each sex were used as controls. After a 78 weeks of administration, observation of the rats continued for up to an additional 35 weeks and observation of the mice continued for an additional 16 weeks. No significant association was established between administration of APC and mortality in rats or female mice; however, there was a significant positive association between treatment and mortality in male mice. From the necropsy examinations of the animals in this study, caffeine was not carcinogenic.

1.3 Cited at Scientific Meetings and in Various Stages of Completion

In a study by Palm et al. (1983), young, adult, virgin Sprague-Dawley CD rats (90 males and 90 females) were divided by random selection into two groups, one of 40 males and 40 females, one of 50 males and 50 females, designated the F_0 or parent generation control and treated groups respectively. All males and the control females received tap water; the treated females were provided with fresh-brewed coffee at a dilution of 50% with tap water as the sole beverage for 5–6 weeks prior to copulation and throughout gestation. Forty male and 40 female offspring of the control group and 60 male and 60 female offspring from the treated group were randomly selected and designated the F_1 generation control and treated groups respectively. Dilutions of fresh-brewed coffee resulting in caffeine intakes of approximately 14, 32 and 54 mg/kg/day respectively in males and 27, 56 and 101 mg/kg/day in females were fed to the F_1 treated group from about 6 weeks of age to 24 months of age. All male and female control rats received tap water. This represents a long-term study beginning with in utero exposure and continuing for a major portion of the animal's life span. With the exception of the total number of tumors observed in the skin of male rats at the 25% coffee level (14 mg caffeine/kg/day), neither the incidence of tumors in a particular organ nor the total incidence in all organs appeared to be significantly increased in the coffee-treated rats compared to the water-drinking controls. Therefore, under these conditions there was no evidence of carcinogenic action by caffeine.

Brune et al. (1981), in a lifetime experiment, administered benzo[a]pyrene to Sprague-Dawley rats either as an admixture to the diet or by gavage in 1.5% caffeine solution. There were 32 males and 32 females per group, and the median survival time for the control group (1.5% caffeine given alone) was 102 weeks. The 1.5% caffeine solution (annual dose 27 g/kg) did not exert any carcinogenic activity under the conditions of the bioassay.

Mohr et al. (1982) recently completed a study in albino rats which was initiated as an investigation parallel to that by Takayama et al. (1978) but was expanded to include a greater range of doses and contained a double control group. SPF (barrier-maintained) Wistar-derived albino rats were given caffeine in the drinking water at 2000, 930, 430, and 200 mg/liter. Groups of 50 males and 50 females were used. Three satellite groups (10 rats per sex per treatment) were killed at 3, 6 and 12 months to provide data on hematological and clinical chemical parameters as well as gross and microscopic pathology. The study was terminated at 24 months. It was observed from the inception of the study that the highest dose group (2000 mg/liter) exhibited a depressed growth rate for both sexes. Throughout the study, food consumption remained essentially constant in proportion to body weight and was unaffected by treatment. Water intake was clearly affected by caffeine concentration. Maximum water intake was consistently observed at the 200 mg/liter dose level. Rats in this study drank about the same volume of water daily regardless of body weight, which resulted in an unbalanced dosage between the two sexes, the females receiving nearly twice as much caffeine as the males in relation to unit weight. At the 2000 mg/liter dose level the caffeine intakes for females were 196 mg/kg/day and for males 108 mg/kg/day.

In terms of tumor incidence, there was an inverse (negative) dose response with respect to both frequency and multiplicity. Compared to controls, the number of benign tumors in the highest caffeine group was decreased significantly in both sexes. At the same time, the highest incidence of malignant tumors occurred in the two lower dosage groups (200 and 430 mg/liter).

These differences in the incidence of benign tumors were due mainly to reduced rates of pituitary adenomas (both sexes), adrenal cortical adenomas, adrenal pheochromocytomas and hemangioendotheliomas (males) and fibromas of the mammary gland (females). The distribution of malignant neoplasms among the two lower treatment groups did not appear to favor any particular organ or site and were not dose-related. Although several of these intergroup differences in tumor incidence appeared to be statistically significant, the biological implication of these so-called negative dose responses remain unclear at present. At any rate, the frequency and distribution of neoplasms found in this study were consistent with the pattern usually found in the aging Sprague-Dawley (Wiga) rat. The authors concluded that under the experimental conditions prevailing, the results obtained show that exposure to caffeine at levels including the maximum tolerated dose (MTD) did not enhance, promote or cause neoplasms.

Takayama et al. (1978) reported a statistically significant increase in benign and malignant tumors of the mammary gland and benign tumors of the pituitary gland. The incidence of adenomas and carcinomas of the thyroid was increased and there was a high incidence of uterine adenomas and carcinomas in caffeine-treated females.

However, the results could not be properly assessed because of the early deaths due to disease, especially in the control group. Accordingly, the second study already mentioned in Sect. 1.1 (Takayama and Kuwabara 1982) was undertaken.

1.4 General Conclusions

The carcinogenic potential of caffeine has been examined in a variety of animal studies conducted under a variety of conditions. The following conclusions can be drawn from a review of these studies:

1. There was a common outcome, namely that caffeine was without carcinogenic effect in laboratory animals.
2. The neoplasms that were observed are those that occur spontaneously in the strains of animals used.
3. Caffeine did not accelerate the induction or increase the incidence of these tumors.

In considering the results of long-term studies in animals it is important to establish that the lack of carcinogenicity is not the consequence of the use of inadequate doses. In the studies that have been reviewed above, extremely high doses were employed, including, in some instances, doses that provoked toxic reactions. In spite of this, none of the studies gave any indication that caffeine possesses carcinogenic potential.

In making safety assessments of chemicals, if studies in two species show no evidence of carcinogenic effect, the chemical is regarded as acceptable for human use. The collective evidence from four studies conducted in mice and eight studies conducted in rats (Table 1) indicates that caffeine is not carcinogenic in these species; this exceeds the amount of animal data normally available for substances consumed by humans.

2 Chemical and Metabolic Studies

The question of carcinogenic potential of caffeine may be examined indirectly, seeking insights on the basis of available knowledge of comparative metabolism, metabolic activation, covalent binding, structure-activity relationships and relevant associated biological activities demonstrated in animal models.

2.1 Metabolic Evidence

Miller and Miller (1971) showed that although some chemical carcinogens, such as direct alkylating agents and some metal ions, are electrophiles (that is, electron-deficient molecules), the majority of carcinogens are not. Most carcinogens are converted into electrophilic reactants by the metabolic machinery of the body, a process termed "metabolic activation". Such electrophiles react (undergo "covalent binding") with cellular nucleophiles (electron-sharing molecules), including critical macromolecules such as DNA, RNA and protein. Of these macromolecular targets, DNA plays a major part in the process of mutagenesis and carcinogenesis. More or less simultaneously with metabolic activation, reactions are in progress to bring about detoxication. It is often the balance between activation and detoxication that determines the outcome of exposure to the compound in question.

This concept is important in the present context because it points to a number of criteria by which the likelihood of carcinogenic or mutagenic potential of caffeine may be judged:

1. Is caffeine a direct alkylating agent?
2. Does caffeine undergo metabolic activation to an electrophile?
3. Does caffeine undergo covalent binding with macromolecules?

The evidence concerning each of these issues is presented below, but in brief, caffeine fulfills none of these requirements to be expected of a putative carcinogen or mutagen.

Under the heading of metabolic evidence, consideration should also be given to comparative metabolism, as indicating whether or not animal models are suitable for testing the carcinogenic potential of caffeine. The comparative metabolism of

Table 1. Summary of studies on the carcinogenicity of caffeine in animals

Investigator (year)[a]	Test material	Route	Dose (mg/kg/day)	Species/strain
A. Bauer et al. (1977)	Brewed coffee	Drinking water	120	Mice C57BL/6J
A. Macklin and Szot (1980)	1. Caffeine 2. Caffeine + phenacetin + aspirin 3. Caffeine + phenacetin 4. Caffeine + aspirin	Diet Diet	55 55 55 55	C57BL/6
A. Wurzner et al. (1977)	"Instant" coffee 1. Regular 2. Decaffeinated	Diet	6% level	Rats SPF Sprague-Dawley
A. Zeitlin (1972)	Instant coffee solids	Diet	5% level (coffee content of diet 3%–6% to give dietary concentration of 0.18%)	Rats Sprague-Dawley
A. Brune et al. (1981)	Caffeine	Gavage	102	Rats Sprague-Dawley
A. Johansson (1981)	Caffeine	Diet	0.102% (total dose 21.4 g)	Rats Sprague-Dawley
A. Takayama and Kuwabara (1982)	Caffeine	Drinking water	0.0%, 1%, 0.2%	Rats SPF Wistar derived
B. Ito (1978)	Caffeine	Drinking water	0.2%, 0.1%, 0.04%, 0%	Mice ICR
B. National Cancer Inst. (1978)	Aspirin, phenacetin, caffeine	Feed	1.4%, 0.7%	Mice B6 C3 F1 Rats Fisher
C. Palm et al. (1983)	Brewed coffee	In utero, exposure drinking water	Male: 14, 32, 54 Female: 27, 56, 101	Rats Sprague-Dawley CD
C. Mohr et al. (1982)	Caffeine	Drinking water	Male: 0, 12.2, 27.0, 49.7, 108.9 Female: 0, 18.7, 31.4, 87.0, 196.7	Rats SPF Wistar derived

[a] A., published studies; B., unpublished studies; C., studies cited at scientific meetings

Number of animals/group/sex[b]	Duration of test	Remarks
1. *C 25M **T 25M 2. C 25M T 27M	1. 103 weeks 2. 105 weeks	No unusual occurrence of tumors or cancer in test animals.
1. 2. 40M 40F 3. 4.	75–80 weeks	Gross examination, no remarkable findings. Detailed histological examination of bladder, liver and kidney did not reveal any carcinogenic effect of the test chemical.
1. 240M 240F 2. 120M 120F (40/group)	Interim kill 3–12 months, 10M 10F each group. 24 months remainder	No increased risk of neoplasm formation. Treatments providing high caffeine levels decrease the incidence of neoplasms in males and females.
C 41M 41F T 144M 144F	24 months	Bladders of 94M and 94F (T) and 29M and 29F (C) examined – no abnormalities related to caffeine.
T 32M T 32F	Lifetime	Caffeine did not exert any carcinogenic activity.
T 30M C 30M	117 weeks	No significant difference in the incidence of tumors between treated rats and controls.
C 50M 50F T 50M 50F	24 months	No evidence of carcinogenic action by caffeine.
C 50M 50F T 50M 50F	M 60 weeks F 104 weeks	Incidence of neoplastic change was not significantly different in experimental animals and controls.
C 50M 50F T 49 or 50 M or F C 50M 50F	Administered for 75 weeks. Rats observed additional 35 weeks	From the necropsy examinations, caffeine was not carcinogenic.
C 80M 80F T 80M 80F	Interim kill at 3, 6, 12 months, 10 animals each sex, 24 months	No evidence of carcinogenic action by caffeine.
C 50M 50F T 50M 50F	24 months	No evidence of carcinogenic action by caffeine.

[b] C, control; T, treated

caffeine has been reviewed (Fed. Reg. 1980 pp. 69824–69825) and is dealt with in Chaps. I and III in this book.

There is undoubtedly great variation in metabolism from one species to another, so that no animal species is identical to man with respect to the metabolism of caffeine. Even among the non-human primates, *Macaca cynomolgus* is different from man (Fed. Reg. 1980 p. 69825), and the chimpanzee, rhesus monkey and galago demonstrate substantial differences from one another (Caldwell et al. 1981).

Some of the metabolites reported by Arnaud (1976) as present in rat urine probably do not occur in man. By and large, however, the animal metabolites are also formed in man but a different rates and in different relative proportions. The physiological and pharmacological actions of caffeine being similar in man and animals, the latter may be considered as reasonably representative models for studying the potential carcinogenicity of caffeine in man. Moreover, there is no evidence of the formation of any "unique metabolites" (Fed. Reg. 1980 p. 69834) in man that would be the basis of a failure of animal models to be accurate predictors of carcinogenic risk in human subjects.

2.1.1 Direct Alkylation of DNA or Incorporation into DNA

The standard test of alkylating capacity utilizes 4-(*p*-nitrobenzyl) pyridine (PNBP). Archer and Eng (1981) optimized the reaction conditions for a chemical activation detection system that yielded positive results with PNBP, using about 10 µmol nitrosodiethylamine. Under these conditions, caffeine gave completely negative results, with or without the chemical activation system.

A substantial body of literature attests to the interaction of caffeine and other xanthines with DNA (Kihlman 1977). These are weak physical interactions (Richardson et al. 1981; Pohle and Fritzsche 1981). As regards incorporation into DNA, while Goth and Cleaver (1976) observed that methyl groups from caffeine were used in synthesis of thymine, guanine and adenine in human fibroblasts in culture, caffeine itself was not incorporated. Goldstein et al. (1974) suggested that the presence of a substituent in the 7 position prevents conversion of caffeine to a deoxyribonucleotide.

2.1.2 Does Caffeine Undergo Metabolic Activation?

One test for metabolic activation to a mutagenic metabolite is the *Salmonella*/microsome test, in which caffeine was found to be non-mutagenic (McCann et al. 1975). Among the various reviews on the subject of mutagenicity of caffeine (Timson 1977; Thayer and Palm 1975; Kihlman 1977) the majority conclusion is that in mammals, and particularly in man, there is no evidence of mutagenic or chromosome-damaging effects of caffeine at the levels of human consumption of caffeine-containing beverages and medicinal preparations (SCOGS, 1978).

2.1.3 Does Caffeine Undergo Covalent Binding?

In a study of covalent binding of caffeine to liver microsomal protein of mice, rats and rabbits, Szczawinska et al. (1981) reached the conclusion that such binding does not occur. To overcome the lack of metabolism by microsomes, the authors used the rat liver perfusion technique. Despite extensive metabolism of caffeine under these conditions, no appreciable irreversible binding of caffeine or its metabolites to either microsomal proteins or DNA was found.

Schlatter (1979) and his colleague Meier-Bratschi (1980) studied alkylation of DNA by tritium-labeled caffeine. In their first report, rat liver, kidney and bladder DNA yielded negative results. In the second report, mice were studied in an effort to achieve as large a dose of radioactivity (and hence as high a degree of sensitivity) as possible. Again, covalent binding of caffeine radioactivity to DNA was minimal. The authors reached the conclusion that further study of caffeine binding to DNA was pointless. On the basis of the extremely low covalent binding indices, they considered that caffeine "most probably does not act as an initiator in carcinogenesis".

2.2 Structure-Activity Relationships

Only one class of compounds analogous to the xanthines has been found to be carcinogenic in animal tests. These substances are the hydroxypurines, which on testing by repeated subcutaneous injection have been found to induce local sarcomas in rats. While this outcome by this route of administration may in some instances result from non-specific physicochemical actions of the test material (Grasso and Goldberg 1966), there is adequate evidence that 3-hydroxyxanthine, 3-hydroxyguanine and their 1-methyl derivatives are true animal carcinogens (reviewed by Clayson and Garner 1976). These compounds undergo metabolic activation to reactive metabolites forming 8-mercapto derivatives with thiols.

Substitution of methyl groups in the 7, 8 or 9 positions of the 3-hydroxypurines prevents activation at the 8 position and thus provides compounds that are not carcinogens.

Because it is not a 3-hydroxyxanthine and because it has a methyl substituent in position 7 of the xanthine nucleus, caffeine would be expected to be a non-carcinogenic compound. The metabolite formed by hydroxylation (8-hydroxycaffeine or 1,3,7-trimethyluric acid) would equally be excluded from the class of animal carcinogens described here.

2.3 Associated Biological Activities of Caffeine

The following types of biological activity are relevant to a consideration of the carcinogenic potential of caffeine, insofar as they assess its capacity to modulate the tumorigenic effect of other agents:

1. Activity as a promoter of carcinogenesis or as a cocarcinogen
2. Antineoplastic action

209

The potential for caffeine to function in these capacities is discussed in detail by Roberts in Chap. 16 of this book. Included in his review are the studies by Nakanishi et al. (1978, 1980) which demonstrate that caffeine exercises no promoting or cocarcinogenic action in urinary bladder carcinogenesis. Studies that suggest caffeine actually has antineoplastic action include the work of Weil-Malherbe (1946), Booth and Boyland (1953), Leitner and Shear (1943), Cohen (1973), Reddi and Constantinides (1972), Rothwell (1974), Kakunaga (1975), Nomura (1976, 1980), Denda et al. (1979) and Nakanishi (1978, 1980).

Roberts concludes that the considerable number of studies investigating the carcinogenic effects of caffeine, either alone or in combination with a variety of chemical agents, do not suggest that caffeine can in general potentiate the carcinogenic effect of chemical carcinogens. In fact a majority of the observations seem to indicate that caffeine can often have an inhibitory effect on tumor induction. There is some evidence that caffeine can potentiate chemically-induced cell killing in vivo, and this could be due to an increase in DNA damage following inhibition of cellular DNA repair processes. However, concentrations of caffeine required to produce these effects in vitro are far in excess of those which could be tolerated in vivo. It is unlikely that amounts of caffeine consumed in the normal course of events are able to modify damage induced in DNA by genotoxic chemicals.

Armuth and Berenblum (1981) studied the effect of caffeine on two-stage skin carcinogenesis and on complete systemic carcinogenesis. These studies were undertaken to examine the gene-modulating effects of caffeine after initiation with urethan. A single large dose of caffeine (100 µg/g body weight) was injected at different times in relation to subcutaneous urethan initiation for skin tumorigenesis followed by topical anthranil, which served as a promoter. Caffeine increased papilloma incidence significantly when given 6 h before initiation and to an insignificant extent at 9 h prior to initiation. A tendency for inhibition was evident when caffeine was administered 6 h after treatment. Because papilloma development levelled off almost simultaneously in the three groups, the authors suggest that caffeine acted during the initiation phase and determined the number of dormant cells available for subsequent promotion.

Lung adenoma induction by urethan was unaffected. When caffeine was administered at different times after urethan injection and in the absence of topical anthranil there was no effect on skin papilloma incidence.

2.4 Nitrosation Reactions

The interaction of nitrite with drugs and other nitrogen-containing compounds has been studied extensively with respect to the formation of nitrosamines or other mutagenic and carcinogenic products (Andrews et al. 1980; Takeda and Kanaya 1981). Caffeine and other xanthines do not appear to have been tested in this way in vitro. In an effort to explore the possibility of nitrosation in vivo, Weinberger et al. (1978) fed each of the three methylxanthines (caffeine, theobromine, theophylline) to weanling rats, initially at 1% in the diet and then at 0.5% (about 500 mg/kg). Some groups of rats received an additional 0.5% sodium nitrite in the diet for periods ranging from 14 to 75 weeks. No evidence of neoplastic or preneoplastic activity was forthcoming; had nitrosamines or nitrosamides been formed in significant amounts, it is safe to say that by 75 weeks they would have made their presence known. (Severe testicular injury seen in almost all treated rats was probably a toxic effect compounded by inanition and failure to grow.)

The paper by Weinberger et al. (1978) is also of interest in the light of the report by Arnaud (1976) that in the course of 48 h after a dose of 0.5–10 mg/kg caffeine by stomach tube, rats excreted in their urine amounts of N-methylurea and $N,-N^1$-dimethylurea corresponding to 0.3% and 0.2% respectively of the caffeine administered. These metabolites may be breakdown products of trimethylallantoin formed in the intestine. There is no evidence of the formation of such products in man.

Nitrosation of phenolic compounds, such as chlorogenic acid in coffee, has been emphasized by Challis (1973) and Challis and Bartlett (1975) – not because there is any evidence of mutagenic or any other hazard arising from nitrosophenols, but on the grounds that readily oxidized phenolic materials may catalyze the formation of N-nitrosamines in the digestive tract. This hypothesis was based entirely on an experiment carried out in vitro with buffered aqueous solutions. By the time of writing, no data in any biological system, in vitro or in vivo, have been forthcoming to support alarmist claims by Challis of "health hazards" and "cocarcinogenic effects".

Nevertheless, Challis' work could be viewed as raising the possibility that caffeine might serve in the same capacity as phenols. Caffeine, however, does not undergo ready oxidation to quinones or quinoneimines or to any other compound that could conceivably act as a "transport form" for nitrite that nitrosates amines in the digestive tract.

Taking the evidence as a whole, therefore, the issue of nitrosation of caffeine should be regarded as purely hypothetical and speculative.

2.5 Summary and Conclusions

This section has addressed a variety of issues pertaining to the possible carcinogenicity of caffeine. While no animal model is exactly comparable to man with respect to the qualitative and quantitative aspects of metabolism of caffeine, there are sufficient reasons for accepting such animal models as indicators of the oncogenic potential of caffeine in humans. The conclusion that caffeine does not have carcinogenic potential rests on consideration of its lack of alkylating activity, failure to undergo metabolic activation, inability to bind covalently with DNA, and absence of structural features suggesting a relationship to established purine carcinogens. It is not a mutagen in mammals or humans. It acts neither as a promoter of carcinogenesis nor as a cocarcinogen; in fact, much evidence exists that it has antineoplastic properties. Incorporation of huge levels of caffeine in the diet of rats, with or without a comparable level of sodium nitrite, yields no evidence of carcinogenicity. Caffeine is unlikely to be nitrosated itself, or to act as an enhancer of spontaneous nitrosamine formation in the gut. Review of all these data leads to the conclusion that there exists no ground whatever on which to anticipate or suggest a carcinogenic action of caffeine.

3 Epidemiological Evidence

3.1 Cancer of the Urinary Bladder

While there are no epidemiological studies with caffeine as such, there have been a number of studies that have considered relationships between coffee drinking and cancer in humans. Studies by Cole (1971) suggested an association between coffee drinking and cancer of the lower urinary tract. However, Fraumeni et al. (1971) presented evidence that the association made by Cole (1971) was probably indirect or non-causal in nature. In a second study, conducted by Schmauz and Cole (1974), it was suggested that some environmental exposures associated with bladder cancer, i. e. cigarette smoking, coffee drinking and work with leather, are also related to cancer of the renal pelvis or ureter. Because the Schmauz and Cole (1974) study lacked information on lifetime coffee or tea drinking habits, the same team (Simon et al. 1975) conducted a third study investigating these factors in white women, the group with the greatest association in the earlier study.

In the Simon et al. (1975) study, there was an absence of dose-response relationship between the development of lower urinary tract cancer and coffee drinking as it related to daily intake or duration of habit. These observations support the view that the association was non-causal.

Bross and Tidings (1973) observed an absence of persons drinking little or no coffee among bladder cancer patients compared with controls, but also found no clear dose-response relationship.

Additional epidemiological evidence supporting a lack of effect of caffeine was supplied by Morgan et al. (1974). In a matched patient-control study of bladder cancer they examined the relationship of the disease to a number of factors, including caffeine intake, and found that consumption of tea and coffee did not increase the risk of disease.

On the other hand, Wynder and Goldsmith (1977) found a positive association between coffee drinking and bladder cancer in both men and women; the relative risk appeared slightly higher for men.

Mettlin and Graham (1979), in a retrospective study on dietary risk factors in human bladder cancer, reported some elevation of risk for heavy coffee drinking. There was an apparent protective effect of milk consumption that was not found to be a spurious result of lower caffeine intake. The authors point out the obvious difficulties of precise measurement of nutrition retrospectively and indicate the need for caution in evaluating these results. They relate their observations to those of Cole (1971), saying that while Cole found greater effects among females, they found significant smoking-adjusted risk for males with no elevation of risk evident among females. The Cole reference cited by these authors was the initial study, the findings of which were disputed by Cole and associates in the later studies. It is apparent, therefore, that Mettlin and Graham have indeed confirmed Cole's subsequent findings indicating no elevation of risk among females, although they failed to reference these later studies.

Morrison (1978) related bladder cancer incidence rates to per capita coffee imports for ten countries and analyzed time trends in these variables for the United

212

States and Denmark. Among the ten countries, there was a weak positive association between coffee and bladder cancer for both men and women. There was weak positive correlation of the time trends of coffee imports and bladder cancer incidence for men, but not women, in the United States. The trend of coffee imports for Denmark was dissimilar to both male and female trends in bladder cancer incidence. Because the relationships observed are neither strong nor consistent in direction, these results do not provide support for an association of coffee drinking with the development of bladder cancer.

Howe et al. (1980) examined the association between tobacco use, occupation, coffee, various nutrients and bladder cancer, and suggested that their data supported an association between coffee consumption and bladder cancer. However, they pointed out that the causality of the association must remain in doubt in view of a lack of dose-response relationship in their studies.

A perceived correlation between coffee consumption and national mortality from carcinoma of the kidney was reported by Shennan (1973). Subsequent to this report, a retrospective study of renal cancer with special reference to coffee consumption was carried out by Armstrong et al. (1976). Comparison of cancer patients with control patients showed no evidence of a positive association between type of renal cancer and coffee consumption.

Najem et al. (1982) conducted a case-control study on 75 bladder cancer patients and 142 controls matched for race, sex, age, birthplace and place of residence. Data were obtained on demographic and socioeconomic factors, lifetime occupational history, residency, family and medical history, history of smoking, history of drinking of coffee, cola beverages and alcohol, saccharin consumption and hair dye use.

The authors reported statistically significant associations with bladder cancer risk ratios of greater than 2.0 for cigarette smoking and for working in the dye, petroleum (fuel) and plastics industries. However, no statistically significant associations were found for cigar and pipe smoking, caffeine, saccharin and alcohol consumption, or lifetime occupational history other than working in the dye, petroleum and plastics industries. It is interesting to note there were no statistically significant differences between cases and controls in their consumption of coffee, cola, diet beverages and alcohol.

Morrison et al. (1982) evaluated the relation of coffee drinking to the incidence rate of cancer of the lower urinary tract ("bladder cancer"). Broadly based series of cases and series of controls drawn from the general population of each area were assembled and interviewed in Boston, Massachusetts (587 cases, 528 controls), Manchester, England (541 cases, 725 controls), and Nagoya, Japan (289 cases, 586 controls). Compared to drinkers of an average of less than one cup of coffee per day, those who drank more had a relative risk of bladder cancer estimated as 1.0 (95% confidence interval 0.8–1.2). With adjustment for cigarette smoking, only small and irregular changes in risk were seen with increasing coffee consumption. Duration of coffee drinking showed little relation to risk of bladder cancer. Apparent associations of coffee drinking and bladder cancer may be due to incomplete control of the effect of cigarette smoking. If there is a true association it is likely to be weak.

Marrett et al. (1983) carried out a case-control study designed to assess the relationship between use of coffee and tumors of the bladder. The study included all histologically confirmed bladder tumors identified through the Connecticut Tumor Registry between January 1978 and January 1979. Controls were selected from among the Connecticut population after age-sex stratification to give a distribution similar to that in the cases. Information on occupational exposures to known risk factors for bladder cancer, as well as tobacco, coffee, artificial sweetener and hair dye usage, was obtained through personal interviews with 412 patients and 493 controls. The unadjusted odds ratios for having ever consumed more than 100 cups of coffee as compared to 100 or fewer cups were found to be 4.0 (1.2–20.8) in males and 1.5 (0.5–5.4) in females (95% confidence intervals in parentheses). Similar results were obtained for current drinkers. Odds ratios for consuming more than seven cups per week relative to seven or fewer cups were slightly elevated in all but one of the 12 age-sex-smoking subgroups considered, although the confidence limits in these cases all included unity. Using logistic regression to adjust for the effects of age and smoking, bladder tumors were associated with total weekly consumption and with lifetime consumption ($P < 0.05$) in males, although no such effects were noted in females. A logistic regression analysis for different types of coffee yielded similar effects for ground and regular coffee, but not for instant and decaffeinated.

In summary, the above epidemiological studies do not indicate a direct relationship between coffee consumption and cancer of the urinary tract in man. This view is strengthened by the fact that the results of long-term coffee or caffeine feeding studies do not reveal any carcinogenic potential in the urinary tract in animals.

3.2 Cancer of the Pancreas

A recent epidemiological study dealing with coffee and cancer of the pancreas is that by MacMahon et al. (1981) in which 369 patients with histologically proved cancer of the exocrine pancreas and 644 control patients were questioned about their use of tobacco, alcohol, tea and coffee. A strong association between coffee consumption and pancreatic cancer was evident in both sexes. However, with tea consumption, slight inverse association appeared in both sexes but was not significant in either. It is important to note that the inverse association was observed with tea consumption greater than three cups per day, whereas there was an increased relative risk with one to two cups of coffee per day. This indicates that caffeine per se is not associated with an increased risk for pancreatic cancer. In discussing the results, MacMahon et al. (1981) noted that the positive association with coffee consumption must be evaluated with other data before serious consideration is given to the possibility of a causal relationship.

In a letter to the editor of the *New England Journal of Medicine,* Goldstein (1982) outlined a survey of patients at the Scripps Clinic that was undertaken to look for an association between coffee and cancer of the pancreas. He and his colleagues reviewed the records of 91 consecutive patients with histologically confirmed pancreatic carcinoma seen between 1973 and 1980. Forty-five consecutive patients with prostatic carcinoma and 48 consecutive patients with breast cancer seen between 1975 and 1980 were reviewed as a control group. The results are shown in Table 2.

Among patients with pancreatic carcinoma, 75 (82%) were coffee drinkers, as compared with 71 (76%) in the control group ($0.50 > P > 0.10$). The results failed to

Table 2. Coffee drinking by patients with pancreatic cancer and controls with breast or prostatic cancer

Group	Daily Consumption			
	0 cups	1–2 cups	3–4 cups	>5 cups
Pancreatic cancer (*n*=91)	16	48	19	8
Controls (*n*=93)	22	37	27	7

No significant difference between the groups $(0.50 > P > 0.10)$

demonstrate an association between coffee consumption and pancreatic carcinoma. Goldstein and colleagues note that they were unable to distinguish patients who drank coffee containing caffeine from those who drank decaffeinated coffee.

Feinstein et al. (1981) were harshly critical of the study by MacMahon et al. (1981) when they outlined problems encountered in etiological science and epidemiological case-control research. They identified a number of pertinent principles of case-control methodology and pointed out instances where these principles had not been followed, casting doubt on the validity of the findings of MacMahon et al.

Benarde and Weiss (1982) examined the temporal and spatial correlation between coffee consumption and pancreatic cancer. They found that data on per caput consumption of coffee and pancreatic cancer mortality in the United States since 1950 shows a temporal association. A rise and fall in coffee consumption was followed by a rise and fall in the incidence of pancreatic cancer, with roughly a 10-year lag. Nevertheless, there were inconsistencies in this relationship by sex and race. An unimpressive spatial relationship was also found between the consumption of coffee and pancreatic cancer mortality in 13 countries. While this suggests an association, major inconsistencies cast doubt on the possibility that the relationship is one of cause and effect. This may be due to confounding, particularly by cigarette smoking. The association between cigarette smoking and cancer of the pancreas is much more consistent with a causal relationship.

Benarde and Weiss (1982) point out several inconsistencies that cast doubt on a cause-and-effect relationship. Their cohort analysis (Benarde and Weiss 1977) showed a difference between white men and white women such that an increasing cohort effect in later birth cohorts was seen only in men. This would argue for a factor that differs in its impact on the sexes in whites. Such a factor is not likely to be an item like coffee, which is consumed equally by both sexes, unless one postulates a difference in susceptibility.

Benarde and Weiss point out that the higher incidence of pancreatic cancer in non-whites is not consistent with what is known of their coffee consumption relative to that of whites. They note that the spatial correlation found by Stock (1970) was limited to men and that the case-control study by Lin and Kessler (1981) found only an association between cancer and decaffeinated coffee which was limited to women. However, whereas the case-control study by MacMahon et al. (1981) indicated a fairly strong association in both sexes, there was no dose-response relationship in men and an irregular one in women.

In view of these inconsistencies, Benarde and Weiss (1982) conclude that a cause-and-effect relationship between coffee and pancreatic cancer has not been established.

Whittemore et al. (1983) examined precursors of pancreatic cancer in 50 000 men who had attended university between 1916 and 1950 or between 1931 and 1940. The subjects were studied for mortality through 1978. A small, non-significant positive association between pancreatic cancer and college coffee consumption was found. The authors conclude that the data from this study fail to show the strong positive association between coffee consumption and pancreatic cancer in men reported by MacMahon et al. (1981). A reduced risk, although the association was weak, was noted among those who drank tea during college.

3.3 Cancer of the Ovary

Trichopoulos et al. (1981) reported on an epidemiological study comparing 92 women with common epithelial tumors of the ovary to 105 women admitted for various orthopedic conditions. Questions asked of the women included their use of coffee and tobacco. While the authors found no association between smoking and ovarian cancer, they noted a statistically significant association between coffee drinking and ovarian cancer. The relative risk for women drinking two or more cups of coffee per day was 2.2 (95% confidence interval 1.0–4.8). All but 11 of the coffee drinkers prepared their coffee in the traditional way common to Greece, Turkey and the Middle East. The women were not questioned about methylxanthine consumption from sources other than coffee, so it is not possible to draw any conclusions about possible associations between ovarian cancer and caffeine or other methylxanthine consumption.

Hartge et al. (1982) examined data on coffee consumption as part of a case-control study on ovarian cancer. They compared 187 controls to 158 patients and found that altogether, women who drank coffee were apparently at greater risk than non-drinkers (estimated relative risk 1.3; 95% confidence interval 0.8–2.2), but those who drank most heavily were not at greatest risk. The relative risks among the 114 women who smoked were estimated as 0.8, 1.7 and 1.1 respectively for less than two cupfuls, two to three cupfuls, and four cupfuls or more per day. The corresponding relative risks among the non-smokers were estimated at 1.0, 1.9 and 1.5. These data indicate an apparently greater risk of ovarian cancer among women who drink coffee than among those who do not, but they do not indicate a relationship between dose and risk. The authors indicate that data from other studies would help to reveal whether there is an association between coffee drinking and ovarian cancer and, if so whether it is causal.

3.4 Conclusions

It is apparent that epidemiological studies in humans do not establish a causal relationship between caffeine consumption and cancer. When the results of animal studies and the epidemiological studies are evaluated together, they fail to provide substantive evidence of a link between caffeine consumption and cancer in man or other species. It is apparent that there is no evidence in the available epidemiological information that caffeine poses a hazard to the public when it is used at levels that are now current and in the manner now practiced.

4 Summary of Evidence on Mutagenicity

A chemical's mutagenic potential can be assessed in animals, in cell cultures from man and animals and in a variety of micro-organisms. The information derived from mutagenicity tests conducted with bacteria, yeast, mammalian cells and insects is also used in conjunction with other information to assess a chemical's carcinogenic potential. The mutagenic effects of caffeine are reviewed in detail by Haynes and Collins in Chap. 15 in this volume. A summary of two major reviews is included here for completeness.

The SCOGS (1978) summarized caffeine's mutagenic potential as follows:

"Caffeine causes chromosomal damage in certain microbial and other non mammalian test systems, and caffeine has similar effects at high concentrations on mammalian cells in culture in several in vitro tests. However, in vivo tests utilizing mice and rats have failed to demonstrate mutagenic effects of caffeine".

Previously, Kihlman (1977) concluded that available experimental evidence indicates that caffeine by itself has no mutagenic, chromosome-damaging, carcinogenic or teratogenic effects at the concentrations occurring in man as a result of normal levels of caffeine consumption. Kihlman believes that most of the available evidence suggests that caffeine may have anticarcinogenic effects rather than being a carcinogen or cocarcinogen.

Timson (1977) summarized caffeine's effects on genetic material as follows: "... the available evidence suggests that it is neither mutagenic in mammals nor synergistic with other mutagens".

It is noteworthy that caffeine has not shown mutagenicity in the widely used Ames screening test (McCann et al. 1975). Aeschbacher and Chappuis (1981) reported on the non-mutagenicity of urine from coffee drinkers. In these studies the urine of human coffee drinkers who ingested 12 g instant coffee per day for 4 days in a first experiment or 12 g within 2 h in a second experiment was fractionated by XAD-2 column chromatography. The non-polar urine fractions so obtained were not mutagenic in the Ames *Salmonella* tester strains TA98 or TA100 in either experiment with or without β-glucuronidase treatment of the urine. This study provides an additional piece of evidence supporting view that neither caffeine nor its metabolites possess carcinogenic potential. In contrast, the non-polar urine fraction of subjects who smoked 20–30 cigarettes per day for 4 days in the first experiment or 7–18 cigarettes within 7 h in the second experiment was mutagenic when metabolically activated.

In conclusion, the evidence available from animal studies, human epidemiological studies, studies on chemical characteristics, metabolism, physiology and toxicology, and mutagenicity, other short-term studies, and the long history of use in man provides reassurance that caffeine is without carcinogenic potential.

References

Aeschbacher HU, Chappuis C (1981) Non-mutagenicity of urine from coffee drinkers compared with that from cigarette smokers. Mutat Res 89: 161–177

Andrews AW, Fornwald JA, Lijinsky W (1980) Nitrosation and mutagenicity of some amine drugs. Toxicol Appl Pharmacol 52: 237–244

Archer MC, Eng VWS (1981) Quantitative determination of carcinogens and mutagens as alkylating agents following chemical activation. Chem Biol Interact 33: 207–214

Armstrong B, Garrod A, Doll R (1976) A retrospective study of renal cancer with special reference to coffee and animal protein consumption. Br J Cancer 33: 127–136

Armuth V, Berenblum I (1981) The effect of caffeine on two stage carcinogenesis and on complete systemic carcinogenesis. Carcinogenesis 2: 977–979

Arnaud MJ (1976) Identification, kinetic and quantitative study of [2–^{14}C] and [1-Me-^{14}C] caffeine metabolites in rat's urine by chromatographic separations. Biochem Med 16: 67–76

Bauer AR Jr, Rank RK, Kerr R, Straley RL, Mason JD (1977) The effects of prolonged coffee intake on genetically identical mice. Life Sci 21: 63–70

Benarde MA, Weiss W (1977) A cohort analysis of pancreatic cancer, 1939–1969. Cancer 39: 1260–1263

Benarde MA, Weiss W (1982) Coffee consumption and pancreatic cancer: temporal and spatial correlation. Br Med J 284: 400–402

Booth J, Boyland E (1953) The reaction of the carcinogenic dibenzcarbazoles and dibenzacridines with purines and nucleic acid. Biochim Biophys Acta 12: 75–87

Bross DJ, Tidings J (1973) Another look at coffee drinking and cancer of the urinary bladder. Prev Med 2: 455–461

Brune H, Deutsch-Wenzel R, Habs M, Ivankovic S, Schmahl D (1981) Investigation of the tumorigenic response to benzo(a)pyrene in aqueous coffee solution applied orally to Sprague-Dawley rats. J Cancer Res Clin Oncol 102: 153–157

Caldwell J, O'Gorman J, Adamson RH (1981) The fate of caffeine in three non-human primates. Biochem Soc Abstr (Southampton Meeting), 8 January, p 24

Challis BC (1973) Rapid nitrosation of phenols and its implications for health hazards from dietary nitrites. Nature 244: 466

Challis BC, Bartlett CD (1975) Possible cocarcinogenic effects of coffee constituents. Nature 254: 532–533

Clayson DB, Garner RC (1976) Carcinogenic aromatic amines. In: Searle CE (ed) Chemical carcinogens. American Chemical Society, Washington (ACS monograph 173, pp 435–437)

Cohen MH (1973) Enhancement of the anti-tumor effect of 1,3-bis-(2-chloroethyl)-1-nitrosourea by cholopromazine and caffeine. J Natl Cancer Inst 51: 1323

Cole P (1971) Coffee drinking and cancer of the lower urinary tract. Lancet 1: 1335–1337

Denda A, Inui S, Takahashi S, Yoshimura H, Miuagi N, Konishi Y (1979) Inhibitory effect of caffeine on pancreatic tumors induced by 4-hydroxyaminoquinoline 1-oxide after partial pancreatectomy in rats. Igaku No Ayumi 108: 224

Federal Register (1980) 45: 69825

Feinstein A, Horwitz R, Spitzer W, Battista R (1981) Coffee and pancreatic cancer: the problems of etiologic science and epidemiologic case-control research. JAMA 246: 957–961

Fraumeni JF, Scotto J, Dunham LJ (1971) Coffee-drinking and bladder cancer. Lancet 2: 1204

Goldstein A, Aronow L, Kalman SM (1974) Principles of drug action: the basis of pharmacology. Wiley, New York

Goldstein HR (1982) No association found between coffee and cancer of the pancreas. N Engl J Med 306: 997

Goth R, Cleaver JE (1976) Metabolism of caffeine to nucleic acid precursors in mammalian cells. Mutat Res 36: 105–114

Grasso P, Goldberg L (1966) Subcutaneous sarcoma as an index of carcinogenic potency. Food Cosmet Toxicol 4: 297–320

Hartge P, Lesher LP, McGowan L, Hoover R (1982) Coffee and ovarian cancer. Int J Cancer 30/4: 531–532

Howe GR, Burch JD, Miller AB, Cook GM, Esteve J, Morrison B, Gordon P, Chambers LW,

Foder G, Winsor GM (1980) Tobacco use, occupation, coffee, various nutrients, and bladder cancer. J Natl Cancer Inst 64/4: 701–713

Ito N (1978) In vivo short-term and long-term tests on caffeine. First International Caffeine Committee Workshop, Keauhou-Kona, Hawaii, 8–10 November

Johansson SL (1981) Carcinogenicity of analgesics: long term treatment of Sprague-Dawley rats with phenacetin, phenazone, caffeine and paracetamol (acetamidophen). Int J Cancer 27: 521–529

Kakunaga T (1975) Caffeine inhibits cell transformation by 4-nitro-quinoline-1-oxide. Nature 258: 248–250

Kihlman BA (1977) Caffeine: a chemical hazard in the environment of man? Caffeine and chromosomes. Elsevier, Amsterdam, pp 407–415

Leitner J, Shear MJ (1943) Quantitative experiment on the production of subcutaneous tumors in strain. A mice with marginal doses of 3,4-benzpyrene. J Natl Cancer Inst 3: 455

Lin RS, Kessler II (1981) A multifactorial model for pancreatic cancer in man – epidemiological evidence. JAMA 245: 147–152

Macklin AW, Szot RJ (1980) Eighteen month oral study of aspirin, phenacetin and caffeine in C57BL/6 mice. Drug Chem Toxicol 3/2: 135–163

MacMahon B, Yen S, Trichopoulos D, Warren K, Nardi G (1981) Coffee and cancer of the pancreas. N Engl J Med 304: 630–633

Marrett LD, Walter SD, Meigs JW (1983) Coffee drinking and bladder cancer in Connecticut. Am J Epidemiol 117: 113–127

McCann J, Choi E, Yamasaki E, Ames B (1975) Detection of carcinogens as mutagens in the *Salmonella*/microsome test: assay of 300 chemicals. Proc Natl Acad Sci USA 72 (12): 5135–5139

Meier-Bratschi A (1980) Second report: alkylation of DNA by caffeine. Interim report

Mettlin C, Graham S (1979) Dietary risk factors in human bladder cancer. Am J Epidemiol 110/3: 255–263

Miller EC, Miller JA (1971) Chemical carcinogenesis: mechanisms and approaches to its control. J Natl Cancer Inst 47: v–xiv

Miyata Y, Hagiwara A, Nakatsuka T (1980) Effects of caffeine and saccharin on DNA in the bladder epithelium of rats treated with N-butyl-N-(3-carboxy-propyl)-nitrosamine. Chem Biol Interact 29: 291–302

Mohr U, Althoff J, Morgareidge K (1982) The influence of caffeine on the incidence of "spontaneous" tumors in Wistar derived rats. Fourth International Caffeine Committee Workshop, Athens, Greece, 18–21 October

Morgan RW, Jain MG (1974) Bladder cancer: smoking, beverages and artificial sweeteners. Can Med Assoc J 111: 1067–1070

Morrison AS (1978) Geographic and time trends of coffee imports and bladder cancer. Eur J Cancer 14/1: 51–54

Morrison AS, Buring JE, Verhoek WG, Aoki K, Leck I, Ohno Y, Obata K (1982) Coffee drinking and cancer of the lower urinary tract. J Natl Cancer Inst 68: 91–94

Najem R, Louria D, Seebode J, Thind I, Prusakowski J, Ambrose R, Fernicola A (1982) Lifetime occupation, smoking, caffeine, saccharine, hair dyes and bladder carcinogenesis. Int J Epidemiol 11: 212–217

Nakanishi K, Fukushima S, Shibata M, Shirai T, Ogiso T, Ito N (1978) Effects of phenacetin and caffeine on the urinary bladder of rats treated with N-butyl-N-(4-hydroxybutyl)-nitrosamine. Gan 69: 395–400

Nakanishi K, Hirose M, Ogiso T, Hasegawa P, Arie M, Ito N (1980) Effects of sodium saccharin and caffeine on the urinary bladder of rats treated with N-butyl-N-(4-hydroxybutyl)-nitrosamine. Gan 71: 490–500

National Cancer Institute (1978) Bioassay of mixture of aspirin, phenacetin, and caffeine for possible carcinogenicity. NCI-CG-TR-67

Nomura T (1976) Diminution of tumorigenesis initiated by 4-nitroquinoline 1-oxide post-treatment with caffeine in mice. Nature 260: 547–549

Nomura T (1980) Timing of chemically induced neoplasia in mice revealed by the antineoplastic action of caffeine. Cancer Res 40: 1332–1334

Palm EP (1978) Two-year toxicity study of fresh-brewed coffee in rats initially exposed in utero. First International Caffeine Committee Workshop Keauhou-Kona, Hawaii, 8–10 November

Palm PE, Rohovsky MW, Arnold EP, Rachwall PC, Nick MS, Valentine JR, Doerfler TE (1983) Two year toxicity carcinogenicity study of fresh-brewed coffee in rats initially exposed in utero. Toxicol Appl Pharmacol (in press)

Pohle W, Fritzsche H (1981) DNA-caffeine interactions. Evidence of different binding modes by infrared spectroscopy. Stud Biophys 82: 81–96

Reddi PK, Constantinides SM (1972) Partial suppression of tumor production by di-butyryl-cyclic AMP and theophylline. Nature 238: 286

Report of the Interagency Regulatory Liaison Group (1979) Work Group on risk assessment: scientific bases for identification of potential carcinogens and estimation of risks. J Natl Cancer Inst 63: 245–268

Richardson CL, Grant AD, Schulman GE (1981) The interaction of caffeine and other xanthine analogs with DNA is measured by competitive fluorescence polarization. Environmental Mutagen Society, Abstract Ac-5, p 101

Rothwell K (1974) Dose related inhibition of chemical carcinogenesis in mouse skin by caffeine. Nature 252: 69–70

Schlatter C (1979) Research proposal "Alkylation of DNA by caffeine". Interim report

Schmauz R, Cole P (1974) Epidemiology of cancer of the renal pelvis and ureter. J Natl Cancer Inst 52: 1431–1434

SCOGS (1978) Evaluation of health aspects of caffeine as a food ingredient, SCOGS-89. Federation of American Societies for Experimental Biology, Bethesda/Md

Shennan DH (1973) Renal carcinoma and coffee consumption in 16 countries. Br J Cancer 28: 473–474

Simon D, Yen S, Cole P (1975) Coffee-drinking and cancer of the lower urinary tract. J Natl Cancer Inst 54: 587

Stock P (1970) Cancer mortality in relation to national consumption of cigarettes, solid fuel, tea, and coffee. Br J Cancer 24: 215–225

Szczawinska K, Ginelli E, Bartosek I, Gambazza C, Pantarotto C (1981) Caffeine does not bind covalently to liver microsomes from different animal species and to proteins and DNA from perfused rat liver. Chem Biol Interact 34: 345–354

Takayama S, Kuwabara N (1982) Long-term study on the effect of caffeine in Wistar rats. Gan 73: 365–371

Takayama S, Kuwabara N, Sugimura T (1978) Induction by caffeine of various tumors in Wistar rats. First International Caffeine Committee Workshop, Keauhow-Kona, Hawaii, 8–10 November

Takeda Y, Kanaya H (1981) Formation of nitroso compounds and mutagens by drug/nitrite interaction. Cancer Lett 12: 81–86

Thayer PS, Palm PE (1975) A current assessment of the mutagenic and teratogenic effects of caffeine. Crit Rev Toxicol 3: 345–369

Timson J (1977) Caffeine. Mutat Res 47: 1–52

Trichopoulos D, Rapapostolou M, Polychronpoulou A (1981) Coffee and ovarian cancer. J Cancer 28: 691–693

Weil-Malherbe H (1946) The solubilization of polycyclic aromatic hydrocarbons by purines. Biochem J 40: 351–363

Weinberger MS, Friedman L, Farber TM, Moreland FM, Peters EL, Gilmore CE, Khan MA (1978) Testicular atrophy and impaired spermatogenesis in rats fed high levels of the methylxanthines caffeine, theobromine, or theophylline. J Environ Pathol Toxicol 1: 669–688

Whittemore AS, Paffendarger RS Jr, Anderson K, Halpern J (1983) Early precursors of pancreatic cancer in college men. J Chronic Dis 36: 251–256

WHO International Agency for Research on Cancer (1979) IARC monographs on the evaluation of the carcinogenic risk of chemicals to humans, vol 21, p 14

Wurzner HP, Lindstron E, Vuataz L (1977) A 2-year feeding study of instant coffees in rats. I. Body weight, food consumption, haematological parameters and plasma chemistry. Food Cosmet Toxicol 15: 7–16

Wynder EL, Goldsmith R (1977) The epidemiology of bladder cancer. A second look. Cancer 40: 1246–1268

Zeitlin BR (1972) Coffee and bladder cancer. Lancet 1: 1066

XV The Mutagenic Potential of Caffeine

R. H. Haynes and J. D. B. Collins

1 Introduction

In this paper we evaluate the available data on the mutagenic potential of caffeine and discuss its possible risk to man. A primary consideration in risk assessment is to compare the doses to which average human subjects may be exposed with those required to produce measurable genetic effects in various test systems.

Caffeine is able to enter gonadal and fetal tissue and attain the same concentrations there as in circulating plasma. It has been estimated that the germ cells of a person who drinks tea or coffee several times daily are exposed for considerable periods of the day to about 1 mg caffeine/liter tissue water ($5.2 \times 10^{-6} M$); maximum exposures for the heaviest caffeine users are unlikely ever to exceed 10 mg/liter tissue water, equivalent to a 0.001% (w/v) solution of caffeine. In most of the genetic studies reviewed, the caffeine concentrations employed ranged from 0.002% to 2%, with the commonest exposure being 0.2%, a level some 200-fold greater than estimated exposures for the heaviest caffeine consumers. It should also be noted that the estimated level for human lethality is about 0.01% (Neims 1981); thus, the exposures generally required to produce genetic activity by caffeine have been about 20 times greater than the lethal dose for man. These dose ranges must be borne in mind when considering the practical significance of any data from short-term mutagenicity tests. This is especially true in view of the reported existence of an *apparent* threshold for mutation induction by caffeine at doses which extend up to 400 times the maximum exposure expected for the heaviest consumers of caffeine (Amacher et al. 1980).

Caffeine, alone or in combination with other agents, has been reported to have cytotoxic, DNA replicative, genetic, carcinogenic, and teratogenic effects, but contradictory results have been obtained and the overall picture is confused. Caffeine appears to induce gene mutations in bacteria and fungi, but its ability to cause point mutations in higher organisms is not well documented. It produces chromosomal aberrations in both plant and animal cells, although high concentrations are needed (around $10^{-2} M$) to provoke these effects. Overall, the available data indicates no significant risk of gene mutations or chromosomal aberrations at dose levels of caffeine comparable to normal human exposures. Caffeine also can potentiate the genetic effects of other agents, including radiation and chemicals. At least some of these effects can be attributed to its action in modifying DNA repair processes: effects on photoreactivation, excision repair, and postreplication repair have been reported in various organisms. Also there is evidence that caffeine may affect normal

DNA nucleotide precursor pool balances, which, when altered, can induce genetic alterations in cells.

On the basis of our review of current literature, we conclude that no significant genetic risk to man can be associated with current levels of caffeine consumption.

2 Exposure

It has been estimated that if a person drinks coffee or tea several times daily, the germ cells are bathed for considerable periods in a caffeine solution estimated to be about 1 µg/ml (Goldstein and Warren 1962) or 1 mg/liter (kg) tissue water $(5.2 \times 10^{-6}\ M)$. The tissues of heavy coffee or tea drinkers may contain at times as much as 5 mg/liter or $2.5 \times 10^{-5}\ M$, but the concentration is unlikely to ever exceed 10 mg/liter or $5 \times 10^{-5}\ M$ (Kihlman 1974).

3 Results of Mutagenicity Tests

3.1 Gene Mutations

There is considerable evidence that caffeine is mutagenic in bacteria and fungi (Fishbein et al. 1970; Kihlman 1977; Timson 1977). Furthermore, the mutagenic effects in *Escherichia coli* of commercial instant coffee products have been correlated with their caffeine content (Clarke and Shankel 1977). However, the ability of caffeine to cause point mutations in higher organisms is not as well documented. Table 1 lists the principal systems in which caffeine has been tested for mutagenicity, and we discuss some of the highlights from this table.

There is evidence in *E. coli* K-12 (Clarke and Wade 1975) that caffeine acts as a frameshift mutagen, and this has been attributed to its ability to intercalate between base pairs in DNA (Kihlman 1977). On the other hand, caffeine appears not to be a mutagen in *Salmonella*, with or without metabolic activation (King et al. 1979; McCann et al. 1975), and it has been reported even to have *antimutagenic* activity in reducing the his^- to his^+ mutation rate in the stationary phase of *E. coli* 15 (Grigg and Stuckey 1966). Also, caffeine was not found to be mutagenic in host-mediated assays when three histidine mutants (Gabridge and Legator 1969) or the G-46 mutant (Legator 1970) of *Salmonella typhimurium* were used in mice. This result has been confirmed recently by King et al. (1979). Despite these conflicting results, a majority of the available reports, of which only a few are listed in Table 1, confirm the mutagenic potential of caffeine in micro-organisms. Unfortunately, the negative findings remain for the most part unexplained.

The question of caffeine mutagenicity in *Drosophila melanogaster* is still unresolved (Kihlman 1974; Timson 1977). Andrew (1959) first detected a weak but definite positive effect in the sex-linked recessive lethal test, but the results were not confirmed by Yanders and Seaton (1962), who repeated the experiments at the same doses. Negative results were also obtained by Alderson and Khan (1967), Clark and Clark (1968), and Forbes (1971). However, positive results have been obtained by others (Ostertag and Haake 1966; Shakarnis 1970). With the exception of a study in

Table 1. Gene mutations

System	Description	Result	Reference	Comments
1. Bacteria				
E. coli	Back-mutation to phage resistance	Mutagenic	Gezelius and Fries (1952) Glass and Novick (1959)	Concentrations of 0.015% $(7.7 \times 10^{-4}\ M)$ and 0.6% $(3.12 \times 10^{-2}\ M)$
	Mutation to streptomycin nondependence	Mutagenic	Demerec et al. (1948) Demerec et al. (1951) Novick (1956)	Concentrations of 2.1% $(1.1 \times 10^{-1}\ M)$
E. coli K-12 strain ND160	Back-mutation *lac⁻* to *lac⁺*	Mutagenic	Clarke and Wade (1975)	Evidence it acts as a frameshift mutagen
S. typhimurium (Ames test)	Back-mutation *his⁻* to *his⁺* with and without metabolic activation	Non-mutagenic	McCann et al. (1975) King et al. (1979)	Concentration 6 mg/plate
E. coli 15	Back-mutation *his⁻* to *his⁺* in stationary phase cultures of *E. coli* 15	Anti-mutagenic	Grigg and Stuckey (1966)	Concentration $(8 \times 10^{-3}\ M)$ reduced *his⁻* to *his⁺* mutation rate by more than 90%
2. Fungi				
Ophiostoma multiannulatum	Forward mutations for physiological and morphological endpoints	Mutagenic	Fries and Kihlman (1948)	Concentration 0.2% $(10^{-2}\ M)$
3. Host-mediated assay	*S. typhimurium* in mice	Non-mutagenic	Gabridge and Legator (1969) Legator (1970) King et al. (1979)	$10^{-3}\ M$/kg
4. Insects				
D. melanogaster	Sex-linked, recessive, lethals	Mildly mutagenic	Andrew (1959)	Concentration 0.25% $(1.3 \times 10^{-2}\ M)$ in agar of larvae and 0.5% $(2.6 \times 10^{-2}\ M)$ injected adults
		Non-mutagenic	Yanders and Seaton (1962)	Same doses as above plus 0.5% $(1.3 \times 10^{-2}\ M)$ in agar of larvae
		Non-mutagenic	Alderson and Khan (1967)	
		Non-mutagenic	Clark and Clark (1968)	Experiments done in same laboratory as Andrew (1959)

Table 1. (continued)

System	Description	Result	Reference	Comments
		Non-mutagenic	Forbes (1971)	
		Mutagenic	Ostertag and Haake (1966)	Larvae exposed for 1 h to 1% $(5.2 \times 10^{-2}\ M)$ caffeine
		Mutagenic	Shakarnis (1970)	Females exposed to 0.115% $(5.9 \times 10^{-3}\ M)$ caffeine
Bombyx	Dominant, lethals	Non-mutagenic	Murota and Murakami (1976)	
5. Mammalian cells in culture				
Chinese hamster cells	Mutation to auxotrophy	Non-mutagenic	Kao and Puck (1969)	
XP variants (human cells)	Mutation to 8-aza-quanine resistance	Non-mutagenic	Maher et al. (1976)	
6. Mammals				
Mice	Specific locus	Non-mutagenic	Lyon et al. (1962)	Concentration 0.1% $(5.2 \times 10^{-3}\ M)$ in drinking water

the silkworm, in which caffeine failed to induce dominant lethal mutations (Murota and Murakami 1976), there is no data on mutagenic effects of caffeine in other insects (Timson 1977). It is worth noting that even those investigators who reported positive results have commented on the lack of reproducibility in replicate experiments (Fishbein et al. 1970). Clark and Clark (1968) summarized the problem best when they wrote "If it were not for the significance of caffeine as a potential mutagen in man, further efforts to study its genetic effects in higher organisms would scarcely be justified."

Although it has been suggested that caffeine may be mutagenic in mammalian cells (Ostertag and Greif 1967), direct evidence for this is almost nil (Timson 1977). A study with several lines of cultured Chinese hamster cells failed to provide evidence that caffeine induces point mutations (Kao and Puck 1969). Data obtained with cultured human cells (XP variants) also failed on indicate any mutagenic effect (Maher et al. 1976). Only one assay for gene mutations in intact mammals has been reported for caffeine; Lyon et al. (1962) obtained negative results in the specific locus test.

Thus, although caffeine is considered to be mutagenic in micro-organisms, the same conclusion cannot be made for mammals or even for cultured mammalian cells. It appears that metabolic responses to caffeine in micro-organisms are diverse and different from those in mammals; this may be one reason for these differences in response (Timson 1977).

There is no doubt that caffeine and several other methylated oxypurines cause chromosomal aberrations in both plant and animal cells, although quite high concentrations are needed (about $10^{-2} M$) (Kihlman 1974). The number of chromosome breaks induced appears generally to be proportional to dose (Fishbein et al. 1970). Evidence of caffeine-induced chromosomal aberrations was first presented by Kihlman and Levan (1949), who worked with *Allium cepa* (onion) root tips; since that time similar phenomena have been observed in other plants as well. Table 2 lists some of the systems in which caffeine has been tested for induction of chromosomal aberrations.

The fact that caffeine is capable of producing chromosomal aberrations in cultured mammalian cells was first reported by Ostertag et al. (1965) in HeLa cells. Since that time other data have been accumulated on caffeine-induced chromosomal aberrations (Table 2). Chinese hamsters given caffeine directly by incubation were found to have about a 50% increase in sister chromatid exchanges (SCEs) in their bone marrow cells at the highest doses (Basler et al. 1979). Negative results have been reported for SCE induction by others such as Shiraishi and Sandberg (1976) who exposed human lymphocytes in vitro to millimolar concentrations of caffeine. While these conflicting results are unexplained, support for induction of SCEs by caffeine was recently provided by Guglielmi et al. (1982), who found a non-linear dose-dependent increase in SCEs from chronic exposure of human peripheral lymphocytes in vitro to millimolar concentrations of caffeine. Matter and Grauwiler (1974), however, found that intraperitoneal injections of caffeine did not induce micronucleus formation in bone marrow cells of mice. Overall, the studies show that chromosomal aberrations can be induced by caffeine but not at levels comparable to normal consumption of caffeine-containing beverages (Fishbein et al. 1970; Timson 1977).

Caffeine also has been reported to cause both X-chromosome loss and non-disjunction in *D. melanogaster*. As is the case with point mutations in this organism, there are conflicting reports regarding the action of caffeine. The former effect is well supported by experimental evidence (Clark and Clark 1968; Mittler et al. 1967a; Ostertag and Haake 1966) showing that caffeine can induce the loss of sex chromosomes in both sexes, but the maximum effect was only to double the spontaneous mutation rate, an increase which is far from impressive (Timson 1977). The data on non-disjunction were too variable to permit any conclusion (Kihlman 1977).

In mice, several studies have failed to provide any evidence for genetic effects, although near-lethal concentrations were used (Kihlman 1977). The only study in which caffeine was found to produce an increase in the frequency of dominant lethals is that of Kuhlmann et al. (1968). However, this study has been severely criticized by others (Adler 1970; Röhrborn 1972) as being founded on invalid or inferential data.

Table 2. Effects on chromosomes

System	Result	Reference	Comments
1. Plants			
Allium cepa root tips	Induced chromosomal aberrations including fragmentation, sister chromatid reunion, and reciprocal translocations	Kihlman and Levan (1949)	Concentration 0.02%–0.4% caffeine
Pisum sativum	Chromosome damage	Kihlman (1952)	
Allium satium root tips	Induced formation of chromosome bridges, fragments, chromatid exchanges, ring chromosomes and micronuclei	Koertung-Keiffer and Mickey (1969)	Concentration 0.1%–0.5% caffeine
Nordeum vulgare barley	Chromosome damage	Yamamoto and Yamaguchi (1969)	Concentration 0.06%–0.1%
Allium proliferum root tips	Chromosomal aberrations	Kihlman et al. (1971)	Concentration $10^{-2}-2 \times 10^{-2}\ M$
Callisia fragrans	Chromosome damage	Roy (1973)	
Vicia faba	Chromatid aberrations but no increase in number of SCEs	Kihlman and Sturelid (1975)	
Coreopis tinctoria	Chromosome damage	Batkyan and Pogosyan (1976)	
2. Insects			
D. melanogaster	X-chromosome loss, slightly reduced non-disjunction rate	Ostertag and Haake (1966)	Exposure of larvae to 1% caffeine for 1 h, increase of XO males but no increase of XXY females, which would be expected if due to non-disjunction
	X-chromosome loss, no increase in number of translocations	Mittler et al. (1967a)	Concentration of 0.123% ($6.3 \times 10^{-3}\ M$) caffeine, significant increase in number of XO males
	and		and
	increased non-disjunction	Mittler et al. (1967b)	large increase in number of non-disjunction females (XXY), i.e., chromosome loss was due to non-disjunction
	Very low incidence of chromosome loss	Clark and Clark (1968)	Increase in XO males but no clear effect on XXY females
3. Cultured mammalian cells HeLa cells (human)	Chromatid breaks	Ostertag et al. (1965)	Exposed for 1 h to caffeine concentrations of 0.05%–1.0% ($2.6 \times 10^{-3}-5.2 \times 10^{-2}\ M$)

226

Table 2. (continued)

System	Result	Reference	Comments
Chinese hamster cells	Induced chromosome rearrangements	Kao and Puck (1969)	Dose of 0.6% (3.1×10^{-2} M) caffeine
Human lymphocytes and human embryonic tissue	Induced high frequency of aberrations, mainly gaps and breaks	Lee (1971)	Induced at relatively high caffeine concentrations
HeLa cells	No chromosomal aberrations	Thayer et al. (1971)	Continuous normal consumption doses 20 mg/ml caffeine
Human lymphocytes in vivo and in vitro	No chromosomal aberrations at normal consumption levels, but aberrations at very high doses	Weinstein et al. (1972)	Chromosome aberrations induced at high doses (800 mg/day). Patients had plasma levels of 30 mg/l or 1.5×10^{-4} M, which corresponds to 8 cups of coffee per day, but when 250–750 mg/l was added as well in culture, aberrations were produced
HeLa cells	No chromosomal aberrations	Bishun et al. (1973b)	Continuous normal consumption doses
	Induced chromosome breaks and rearrangements	Bishun et al. (1973a)	Dose of 160 mg/ml (16%) caffeine (i.e., 8–32 times the transitory level normally experienced in man)
Human lymphocytes	No induction of SCEs	Shiraishi and Sandberg (1976)	In vitro exposure to millimolar concentrations of caffeine
Human peripheral lymphocytes	Non-linear dose-dependent increase in SCEs	Guglielmi et al. (1982)	Chronic in vitro exposure to millimolar concentrations of caffeine
4. Mammals Mice	Increase in SCEs of bone marrow cells	Basler et al. (1979)	Caffeine administered directly by incubation
	No increase in micronucleus of bone marrow cells	Matter and Grauwiler (1974)	Intraperitoneal injections of caffeine into mice
Mice dominant lethal	Mutagenic	Kuhlmann et al. (1968)	Administration of caffeine 0.02%–0.5% in drinking water for 100–140 days
	Non-mutagenic	Adler (1969)	Dose 250 mg/kg body weight
	Non-mutagenic	Epstein et al. (1970)	Caffeine injected intraperitoneally into male mice at doses from 168 to 240 mg/kg body weight

Table 2. (continued)

System	Result	Reference	Comments
	Non-mutagenic	Röhrborn (1972)	Caffeine in drinking water corresponded to daily intake of 3.39–514.3 mg/kg body weight
	Non-mutagenic	Thayer and Kensler (1973)	Caffeine in drinking water corresponded to daily intake of 3.6–122 mg/kg body weight

3.3 Caffeine in Combination with Other Agents

Caffeine has been found to be both synergistic and antagonistic towards the effects of other mutagens (Kihlman 1974, 1977; Legator and Zimmering 1979). In this section we discuss examples for these combined effects in micro-organisms, *Drosophila melanogaster*, plants, and mammalian cells in culture.

3.3.1 Micro-organisms

In bacteria capable of excising ultraviolet (UV) light-induced pyrimidine dimers from their DNA, UV-induced mutation frequencies are greatly enhanced by postirradiation incubation in the presence of caffeine. Lieb (1961) reported that addition of caffeine to the growth medium of UV-irradiated *E. coli* B/r *try⁻* immediately after irradiation caused about ten times as many *try⁺* mutants as UV alone. The effect of caffeine can be largely reversed by treating the cells with photoreactivating light after UV irradiation but prior to plating (Shankel and Kleinberg 1967). It was suggested that the caffeine-induced increase in mutation frequency was caused by an inhibition of dimer excision by caffeine (Timson 1977). In excision-deficient bacteria, caffeine does not enhance, but rather reduces, UV-induced mutation frequencies (Lieb 1961; Shankel and Kleinberg 1967; Witkin and Farquharson 1969). Also, Clarke (1970) found that the yield of *try⁺* mutants in an *hcr⁺* strain of *E. coli* B/r treated with nitrous acid was enhanced, but when *hcr⁻* strain was used, caffeine had an antimutagenic effect. The antagonistic effects on UV- and nitrous acid-induced mutations in these two cases has been interpreted as caffeine inhibition of an error-prone, postreplicative, recombinational repair process. This repair mechanism is believed to err in filling postreplicative gaps (opposite pyrimidine dimers) in the DNA of UV-irradiated bacteria.

Investigations carried out in yeast suggest that the effect of caffeine on UV-induced mutations is restricted to recombinational repair systems (Legator and Zimmering 1979). Sarachek et al. (1970) have shown that caffeine-sensitive excision repair does not occur in *Candida albicans*. In *Schizosaccharomyces pombe*, Clarke (1968) reported that the effect of caffeine on mutation frequency is dependent on the UV dose. At high doses he observed a synergistic effect of caffeine on the pro-

228

duction of prototrophic revertants, at low doses an antimutagenic effect. It has been proposed both by Loprieno and by Clarke that this antimutagenic effect reflects caffeine modification of a recombinational repair system (Legator and Zimmering 1979).

In the slime mold *Physarum polycephalum,* Haugli and Dove (1972) found that caffeine acts synergistically with UV to increase the mutation frequency. In this situation, caffeine is believed to act by inhibition of excision repair (Kihlman 1977). Thus, there is evidence in bacterial, yeast, and slime mold systems that caffeine can act either synergistically or antagonistically with other mutagens. Caffeine appears to exert these effects through interaction with various DNA repair mechanisms.

3.3.2 Drosophila melanogaster

While caffeine alone does not appear mutagenic in Oregon-R stocks, Yeomans et al. (1972) found it to be synergistic with gamma radiation in the production of sex-linked lethals. Mendelson (1974) observed increased X-ray-induced dominant lethals in some but not all strains of *D. melanogaster* after caffeine treatment. No such enhancing effect of caffeine occurred on the yield of dominant lethals when *D. melanogaster* was treated with ethyl methanesulfonate (EMS) or 1,2:3,4-diepoxybutane (DEB), but an enhancement after X-irradiation was reported by Watson (1975). Caffeine has been shown to act synergistically with UV light in the production of non-disjunction and crossing-over (Venkatasetty 1972).

Thus, the effects in *Drosophila* of caffeine in combination with other agents appears similar to results discussed for caffeine alone. Overall, it seems safe to conclude that caffeine does not strongly enhance mutagenic responses to other agents in *D. melanogaster,* but it may be weakly mutagenic in certain circumstances, depending on the stock used, means of administration, sex treated, and medium used (Timson 1977).

3.3.3 Plants

Reports regarding potentiation by caffeine of chromosome damage induced by ionizing radiation are also mixed. Enhancement effects have been found in barley (Ahnström and Natarajan 1971), *Crepes* (Ehliseyenko 1970), and rye seed, but negative results have been reported in *Vicia faba* (Swietlinska and Zuk 1974). However, experiments on the effects of caffeine on chemically-induced aberrations in *Vicia* root tips indicate potentiation (Legator and Zimmering 1979). The chemicals with which caffeine has shown potentiation include mono-, bi-, and polyfunctional alkylating agents, 4-nitroquinilone-1-oxide (4NQO), maleic hydrazide, and ethanol (Kihlman et al. 1973; Schöneich et al. 1970).

3.3.4 Mammalian Cells in Culture

The ability of caffeine in combination with other chemical mutagens to induce chromosomal aberrations and gene mutations has been studied in Chinese hamster and human cells. The frequency of mutation to ouabain resistance after EMS treatment was enhanced by caffeine in Chinese hamster cells (Turnbull 1975). Similarly, Maher et al. (1976) found caffeine synergistic with UV-induced mutations in human xeroderma pigmentosum variant cells. Experiments on the effects of caffeine on UV-induced mutants resistant to 8-azaguanine in Chinese hamster cells have produced apparently conflicting results. Roberts and Sturrock (1973) found an increase in 8-azaguanine resistant mutants with 0.75 mM caffeine following treatment with N-methyl-N-nitrosourea (MNU). On the other hand, Trosko and Chu (1971) reported that caffeine acts as an antimutagen to reduce the frequency of both spontaneous and UV-induced mutations in Chinese hamster cells. Fox (1974), however, concluded that this apparent reduction in mutation frequency after caffeine treatment was attributable to a delay in expression of UV-induced mutation rather than a *bona fide* antimutagenic effect, since it was found that if the expression period was extended, the mutation frequency in the caffeine-treated series surpassed that of the controls. The delay was dependent on the dose of caffeine used. Also, it has been suggested that caffeine does not increase mutation frequency but instead converts sublethal to lethal damage in alkylated and UV-irradiated Chinese hamster cell strain V79 (Fox 1977). Experiments with EMS treatment of V79 cells (Simons et al. 1977) support this idea and indicate that caffeine blocks a repair process which results in enhanced killing but has no effect on the error frequency of repair lesions. Thus, caffeine does not appear to be an efficient producer of gene mutations in Chinese hamster cells.

The evidence for possible genotoxicity is more conclusive in assays for chromosomal aberrations. Significant increases in chromosomal rearrangements after caffeine treatment were observed in an MNU-exposed pseudodiploid Chinese hamster cell line (Fujiwara 1975a) and a UV-exposed endoreduplicated Chinese hamster cell line (Fujiwara 1975b). Similar results were found by others for diploid Chinese hamster cells and plant cells (Legator and Zimmering 1979). In a cultured human lymphocytes study, Brøgger (1973) observed that 10^{-3} M caffeine enhanced the number of chromosome breaks and exchanges induced by X-irradiation at 50, 100, and 200 rads. In the same system, others (Timson 1977) noticed caffeine enhancement of all types of damage induced by mitomycin C (at 0.1 and 0.5 mg/ml) and methyl methanesulphonate (at 2×10^{-5} M and 2×10^{-4} M).

3.4 Summary and Risk Evaluation for Genetic Effects

Although it has been suggested that caffeine may be mutagenic in mammals and man, no unequivocal or conclusive evidence exists to support this contention, which is based on extrapolation from early observations in lower organisms. These latter studies were generally performed at caffeine concentrations far exceeding normal levels of exposure in man. Most of the experiments summarized in Table 1 were done with concentrations of 0.02%–2.0% caffeine, about 40–4000 times the gonadal dose expected for heavy coffee drinkers (5 mg/liter or 0.0005% caffeine). Data on induction of chromosome damage was obtained at similar dose levels. These levels of exposure also greatly exceed the presumed lethal dose for caffeine in man (estimated to be amounts in excess of 100 mg/liter plasma or 0.01% w/v) (Neims 1981). On the other hand, the concentrations needed to enhance chromosome damage caused by other agents are lower than those which could be associated with any genetic effects of caffeine alone. Kihlman reports the "threshold" for potentiating effects to be 60 mg/liter, a level that is still 6–12 times higher than the concentration one is ever likely to encounter in human tissue (Kihlman 1974). Thus, we believe that the mutagenic risk to man from caffeine is insignificant primarily because genotoxic effects, when found, seem to occur only at caffeine levels far exceeding normal human exposures and at levels far above the estimated human lethal dose.

The dose level required to induce mutagenic responses is an important consideration when evaluating the mutagenic potential of any agent. It is possible that there may exist an "apparent" threshold within which any genetic effects are not detectable because they lie beyond the limit of resolution of the assay systems employed. Such threshold dose levels are thought to exist for a variety of chemical mutagens (Brusick 1980; Tazima 1981; Amacher et al. 1980). Unfortunately, the possible existence of a mutagenic threshold for caffeine has not been resolved. Amacher et al. (1980) recently reported data which may indicate the presence of a "no-effect dose" range up to concentrations of 1.52×10^{-2} M to 2.64×10^{-2} M; furthermore, the reported increase in mutation *frequency* for doses above 3×10^{-2} M could be attributed to the toxic effects of caffeine rather than to any enhanced mutagenic response.

Timson (1972) has suggested that the mutagenic threshold of caffeine in man may be the same as the antimitotic threshold and that therefore the actual yield of viable mutants produced by caffeine would be extremely low. Timson (1977) also suggested that the clastogenic effects of caffeine, even at low doses, might prevent the multiplication of any putative caffeine-induced mutants. These considerations, together with the relatively short half-life of caffeine in the body, support the concept that the mutagenic risk to man of caffeine is negligible or non-existent.

4 Related Effects of Caffeine

4.1 Crossing-over

Caffeine has been found to have primarily an inhibiting effect on recombination, although a stimulating effect also has been observed in plant systems. The frequency of mitotic crossing-over in seeds of *Glycine max* and in cell cultures of *Nicotiana tabaccum* was greatly increased by caffeine exposure (Carlson 1974; Vig 1972). However, studies in the yeast *S. pombe* revealed a significant decrease in meiotic recombination and an increase in mitotic gene conversion between closely linked heteroallelic markers (Loprieno et al. 1974). Based on the assumption that meiotic recombination requires DNA strand breakage and degradation, whereas mitotic gene conversion may depend primarily on repair to correct mismatched bases at heterozygous sites, it has been suggested that the reduction of meiotic crossing-over may be caused by a caffeine-DNA interaction which inhibits DNA degradation (Anmad and Leopold 1973; Loprieno et al. 1974). As a result of this interaction more stable pairing might occur at the level of mismatched bases, thereby generating an increase in mitotic gene conversion.

Witkin and Farquharson (1969) reported that 0.2% (10^{-2} M) caffeine in the plating medium of *E. coli* reduces recombination frequency by 50%. Similarly, Yefremova and Filippova (1974) found a 50% decrease in frequency of crossing-over in *Drosophila*. Thus, most available evidence indicates that caffeine acts primarily to reduce recombination frequencies.

4.2 DNA Repair

It is likely that at least some of the effects of caffeine are attributable to its ability to modify DNA repair processes. The data reviewed here indicate that caffeine affects photoreactivation, excision repair, and postreplication repair. A more extensive discussion of this topic can be found in Chap. 16 in this volume.

Harm (1970) reported caffeine to be a competitive inhibitor of photoreactivation in *E. coli*. This inhibition is thought to result from competition between caffeine and the photoreactivating enzyme for pyrimidine dimer sites in DNA (Legator and Zimmering 1979), and is consistent with the finding that caffeine interacts with partially denatured DNA (T'so and Lu 1964).

Caffeine also affects DNA excision repair (Lumb et al. 1968; Witkin 1959). Enhancement of cell killing and mutation frequency is believed to reflect caffeine inhibition of the removal of UV photoproducts prior to replication, rather than caffeine-mediated errors in excision repair. This surmise is based on the fact that the inhibitory effect of caffeine is reversible prior to the first post-treatment division, either by diluting out the caffeine directly or by giving the cells an increased opportunity to dilute out the caffeine themselves by prolonging the period between caffeine treatment and division (Witkin 1959).

There is also evidence that caffeine can affect postreplication recombinational repair. Witkin and Farquharson (1969) first observed that the frequency of UV-induced mutation in excision-deficient strains (*hcr* strains) was modified in a singular manner by caffeine. Although the addition of caffeine in the *hcr* strain enhanced UV cell killing, it dramatically *reduced* the frequency of induced mutations. The antagonistic effect of caffeine on UV-induced mutations has been explained on the basis of caffeine inhibition of an error-prone, postreplicative, recombinational repair process. This repair mechanism is believed to err in filling postreplicative gaps (opposite pyrimidine dimers) in the DNA of UV-irradiated bacteria.

Thus, the available evidence indicates that caffeine can affect various DNA repair processes in bacteria. Similar results have been found in some but not all cultured mammalian cells. The data for mammalian cells has recently been reviewed by Timson (1977).

It has been established recently that genetic effects can be produced not only by radiation and chemical attack upon DNA, but also by disturbances in deoxyribonucleotide precursor pools (Kunz 1982). For example, thymidylate starvation has been found to be mutagenic in a variety of prokaryotes such as *E. coli* (Coughlin and Adelberg 1956) and *S. typhimurium* (Bresler et al. 1970). In yeast, thymidylate starvation, induced directly or by antifolate drugs, is recombinagenic but not mutagenic (Kunz et al. 1980). However, excess thymidylate is mutagenic in yeast. In these ways diverse genetic effects can be produced whose nature and magnitude seems to depend, rather surprisingly, on the precise status of the pools during cell growth.

Recent work indicates that caffeine, a purine analog, may affect DNA precursor metabolism. Waldren and Patterson (1979) observed that at doses which enhance the killing action of UV light, caffeine inhibits both de novo synthesis and also the utilization of exogenous purines in cultured Chinese hamster ovary cells. Furthermore, other workers have found that caffeine inhibits incorporation of thymidine into DNA both in prokaryotic and eukaryotic cells (Grigg 1968; Lehman and Kirk-Bell 1974). In *E. coli* it has been suggested that this inhibition could be caused by a caffeine-induced inhibition of thymidine kinase or, more likely, an effect of caffeine on the DNA synthesis process itself (Sandlie et al. 1980).

Recently, Sandlie and Kleppe (1982) have shown that although thymidine kinase is inhibited by caffeine in vivo, intracellular concentrations of dTTP, which one would consequently expect to decrease, actually *increase* significantly. Thus, the major effect of caffeine appears to be caused by inhibition of processes that involve dTTP. In these experiments intracellular concentrations of the other nucleoside triphosphate pools were only slightly increased by caffeine.

Guglielmi et al. (1982) recently showed that chronic exposure to caffeine leads to a dose-dependent increase in frequency of SCEs in human peripheral blood lymphocytes. They concluded that this arose as a result of inhibition of DNA synthesis and proposed that this was brought about by the inhibition of de novo synthesis of endogenous purines and also the transport and utilization of exogenous purines. Thus, the genetic effects of caffeine may be mediated not only by effects on DNA repair, but also by effects on DNA precursor utilization or biosynthesis.

Clearly, more work should be done along these lines. It is possible that the confused or contradictory reports on the various putative genetic effects of caffeine may be attributed in part to unknown nucleotide pool fluctuations which can either increase or decrease mutational responses, depending on the status of the pools in the particular systems employed.

5 Conclusions

Caffeine is a purine analog and an inhibitor of DNA repair. There is widespread consumption of caffeine in the human diet at levels which can cause both physiological and behavioral effects. Consequently, a great deal of work of a genetic nature has been done on caffeine.

A variety of positive and negative mutagenic test results have been observed for caffeine. In sum, the rather large body of available data contains results which, all too frequently, seem inconsistent with one another. Thus, it is difficult to come to any clear or straightforward conclusions regarding the genotoxic potential of caffeine. This is a good illustration of the fact that when the biochemical responses to a compound such as caffeine are not fully understood, a proliferation of data from short-term tests in diverse organisms can confuse rather than clarify mutagenic risk assessment. Where mutagenic effects have been observed for caffeine, they have been relatively small and have occurred at doses often orders of magnitude greater than the estimated lethal dose for humans. In such cases, some people will take the most cautious approach and conclude that caffeine should be "banned" because some mutagenicity tests have shown positive results. Others, however, may argue the opposite and say that there is no proven genotoxic risk from caffeine since the agent did not show consistently significant, positive results in all assays.

For our part, we feel that the common-sense conclusion must be that normal levels of caffeine consumption, at least in the form of beverages, poses no mutagenic hazard. However, this conclusion is based mainly on the fact that human exposure to caffeine occurs at levels far below those used in the genetic tests, rather than the outcome of the tests themselves.

From past experience with radiation it is known that an important consideration is the question of a threshold dose level. If there is no mutagenic threshold for caffeine, then in a large population even very small doses may be expected to affect a small number of individuals and therefore some population risk would be associated with caffeine consumption. How small this risk is will probably determine how "acceptable" regulatory agencies judge it to be. An essential need, therefore, is to determine whether or not a threshold exists for caffeine's mutagenic effects in those assays where such effects have been observed. One study is available which seems to indicate that a threshold level may exist. Under these circumstances the old toxicologist's dictum, "it is not the drug, but rather the dose which is the poison" should prevail. In either event we are forced to conclude that caffeine poses no significant genetic hazard to humans at normal levels of consumption.

Acknowledgement. We thank Mr. John Wassom of the Environmental Mutagen Information Center for his valuable assistance in a computer search of the literature.

References

Adler ID (1969) Does caffeine induce dominant lethal mutations in mice? Humangenetik 7: 137–148

Adler ID (1970) The problem of caffeine mutagenicity. In: Vogel F, Röhrborn G (eds) Chemical mutagenesis in mammals and man. Springer, Berlin Heidelberg New York, pp 383–403

Ahnström G, Natarajan AT (1971) Repair of gamma-ray and neutron-induced lesions in germinating barley seeds. Int J Radiat Biol 19: 433–443

Alderson T, Khan AH (1967) Caffeine-induced mutagenesis in *Drosophila*. Nature 215: 1080

Amacher DE, Paillet SC, Turner GN, Ray VE, Salsburg DS (1980) Point mutations at the thymidine kinase locus in L5178Y mouse lymphoma cells. II. Test validation and interpretation. Mutat Res 72: 447–474

Andrew LE (1959) The mutagenic activity of caffeine in *Drosophila*. Am Nat 93: 135–138

Anmad A, Leopold U (1973) On a possible correlation between fine structure and map expansion and reciprocal recombination based on crossing over. Mol Gen Genet 123: 143–158

Axelrod J, Reichenthal J (1953) The fate of caffeine in man and a method for its estimation in biological material. J Pharmacol Exp Ther 107: 519

Basler A, Bachmann U, Roszinsky-Köcher G, Röhrborn G (1979) Effects of caffeine on sister chromatid exchanges in vivo. Mutat Res 59: 209–214

Batkyan GG, Pogosyan VS (1976) Investigation of caffeine action in different tissues of Coreopsis (*Coreopsis tinctoria* Nutt.). Tsitol Genet 10: 240–243

Bertrand M, Schwam E, Frandon A, Vagne A, Alary J (1965) Sur un effet teratogène systématique et spécifique de la caféine chez les rongeurs. CR Soc Biol (Paris) 159: 2199–2101

Bishun N, Williams D, Mills J (1973a) The cytogenetic effects of caffeine on two tumour cell lines. Mutat Res 21: 186–187

Bishun NP, Williams DC, Raven RW (1973b) Chromosome damage to HeLa cells grown continuously in caffeine. Mutat Res 17: 145–146

Bresler S, Mosevitsky M, Vyacheslavov L (1970) Complete mutagenesis in a bacterial population induced by thymine starvation on solid media. Nature 225: 764–766

Brøgger A (1973) Caffeine-induced enhancement of chromosome damage. Genetics 74: S31

Brusick D (ed) (1980) Principles of genetic toxicology. Plenum, New York London

Carlson PS (1974) Mitotic crossing-over in a higher plant. Genet Res 24: 109–112

Clark AM, Clark EG (1968) The genetic effects of caffeine on *Drosophila melanogaster*. Mutat Res 6: 227–234

Clarke CH (1968) Differential effects of caffeine in mutagen-treated *Schizosaccharomyces pombe*. Mutat Res 5: 33–40

Clarke CH (1970) Repair systems and nitrous acid mutagenesis in *E. coli* B/r. Mutat Res 9: 359–368

Clarke CH, Shankel DM (1977) Reversion induction in lac Z frameshift mutants of *E. coli* K12. Mutat Res 46: 243

Clarke CH, Wade MJ (1975) Evidence that caffeine, 8-methoxysporalen, and steroid diamines are frameshift mutagens for *E. coli* K-12. Mutat Res 28: 123–126

Cole P (1971) Coffee-drinking and cancer of the lower urinary tract. Lancet 1: 1335–1337

Cornish H, Christman AA (1957) A study of the metabolism of theobromine, theophylline, and caffeine in man. J Biol Chem 228: 315–323

Coughlin CA, Adelberg EA (1956) Bacterial mutation induced by thymine starvation. Nature 178: 531–532

Demerec M, Wallace B, Witkin EM (1948) The gene. Carnegie Inst Washington Yearb 47: 169–176

Demerec M, Bertani G, Flint J (1951) A survey of chemicals for mutagenic action on *E. coli*. Am Nat 85: 119

Donovan PJ, DiPaolo JA (1974) Caffeine enhancement of chemical carcinogen-induced transformation of cultured Syrian hamster cells. Cancer Res 34: 2720–2727

Ehliseyenko NN (1970) Modification of chromosome radiation lesion in roots of *Crepis capillaris*. Radiobiologiia 10: 449–503

Epstein SS, Bass W, Arnold E, Bishop Y (1970) The failure of caffeine to induce mutagenic effects or to synergize the effects of known mutagens in mice. Food Cosmet Toxicol 8: 381–401

Federal Register (1980) 45/205: 69616–69638

Fishbein L, Flamm WG, Falk HL (eds) (1970) Chemical mutagens. Academic, New York, pp 39–53, 246–291

Forbes C (1971) The influence of caffeine on the sex-linked lethal frequency in *D. melanogaster*. Genetics 68: S20

Fox M (1974) The effect of post-treatment with caffeine on survival and UV-induced mutation frequencies in Chinese hamster cells and mouse lymphoma cells in vitro. Mutat Res 24: 187–204

Fox M (1977) A caffeine insensitive error-prone repair process in V79 Chinese hamster cells? Mutat Res 46: 118

Fries N, Kihlman B (1948) Fungal mutations obtained with methyl xanthines. Nature 162: 573–575

Fujiwara Y (1975a) Caffeine-sensitive post-replication repair of N-methyl-N-nitrosourea damage in mouse L cells. Mutat Res 31: 260–261

Fujiwara Y (1975b) Postreplication repair of UV damage to DNA, DNA-chain elongation and effects of metabolic inhibitors in mouse L cells. Biophys J 15: 403–415

Gabridge MG, Legator MS (1969) A host-mediated microbial assay for the detection of mutagenic compounds. Proc Soc Exp Biol Med 130: 831–834

Gezelius K, Fries N (1952) Phage resistant mutants induced in *E. coli* by caffeine. Hereditas 38: 112–114

Gilbert EF, Pistey WR (1973) Effect on the offspring of repeated caffeine administration to pregnant rats. J Reprod Fertil 34: 495–499

Glass EA, Novick A (1959) Induction of mutation in chloramphenicol-inhibited bacteria. J Bacteriol 77: 10–16

Goldstein A, Warren R (1962) Passage of caffeine into human gonadal and fetal tissue. Biochem Pharmacol 11: 166–168

Goodman LS, Gilman A (eds) (1967) The pharmacological basis of therapeutics, 3rd edn. Macmillan, New York, p 354

Grigg GW (1968) Caffeine-death in *Escherichia coli*. Mol Gen Genet 102: 316

Grigg GW, Stuckey J (1966) The reversible suppression of stationary phase mutations in *E. coli* by caffeine. Genetics 53: 823–834

Guglielmi GE, Vogt TF, Tice RR (1982) Induction of sister chromatid exchanges and inhibition of cellular proliferation in vitro. I. Caffeine. Environ Mutagen 4: 191–200

Harm W (1970) Analysis of photoenzymatic repair of UV lesions in DNA by single light flashes. VIII. Inhibition of photoenzymatic repair of UV lesions in *E. coli* DNA by caffeine. Mutat Res 10: 319–333

Haugli FB, Dove WF (1972) Mutagenesis and mutant selection in *Physarum polycephalum*. Mol Gen Genet 118: 109–124

Kakunaga T (1975) Caffeine inhibits cell transformation by 4-nitroquinoline-1-oxide. Nature 258: 248–250

Kao FT, Puck TT (1969) Genetics of somatic mammalian cells. IX. Quantitation of mutagenesis by physical and chemical agents. J Cell Physiol 74: 245–258

Kihlman BA (1952) A survey of purine derivatives as inducers of chromosome changes. Hereditas 38: 115–127

Kihlman BA (1964) The production of chromosome aberrations by streptonigrin in *Vicia faba*. Mutat Res 1: 54–62

Kihlman BA (1974) Effects of caffeine on the genetic material. Mutat Res 26: 53–71

Kihlman BA (ed) (1977) Caffeine and chromosomes. Elsevier/North-Holland, New York

Kihlman BA, Levan A (1949) The cytological effect of caffeine. Hereditas 35: 109–111

Kihlman BA, Odmark G (1965) Deoxyribonucleic acid synthesis and the production of chromosomal aberrations by streptonigrin, 8-ethoxycaffeine, and 1, 3, 7, 9-tetramethyluric acid. Mutat Res 2: 494–505

Kihlman BA, Sturelid S (1975) Enhancement by methylated oxypurines of the frequency of induced chromosomal aberrations. III. The effect in combination with X-rays in root tips of *Vicia faba*. Hereditas 80: 247–254

Kihlman BA, Sturelid S, Norlen K, Tidriks D (1971) Caffeine, caffeine derivitives and chromosomal aberrations. II. Different responses of *Allium* root tips and Chinese hamster cells to treatments with caffeine, 8-ethoxycaffeine, and 6-methylcoumarin. Hereditas 69: 35–50

Kihlman BA, Sturelid S, Hartley-Asp B, Nilsson K (1973) Caffeine potentiation of the chromosome damage produced in bean root tips and in Chinese hamster cells by various chemical and physical agents. Mutat Res 17: 271–275

King MT, Beikirch H, Eckhardt K, Gocke E, Wild D (1979) Mutagenicity studies with X-ray contrast media, analgesics, antipyretics, antirheumatics, and some other pharmaceutical drugs in bacterial, drosophila, and mammalian test systems. Mutat Res 66: 33–43

Koerting-Keiffer LE, Mickey GH (1969) Einwirkung von Koffein auf Chromosomen. Z Pflanzenzucht 61: 244–251

Kuhlmann W, Fromme HG, Heege EM, Ostertag W (1968) The mutagenic action of caffeine in higher organisms. Cancer Res 28: 2375–2389

Kunz BA (1982) Genetic effects of deoxyribonucleotide pool imbalances. Environ Mutagen 4: 695–725

Kunz BA, Barclay BJ, Game JC, Little JG, Haynes RH (1980) Induction of mitotic recombination in yeast by starvation for thymine nucleotides. Proc Natl Acad Sci USA 77: 6057–6061

Lee S (1971) Chromosome aberrations induced in cultured human cells by caffeine. Jpn J Genet 46: 337–344

Legator MS (1970) The host-mediated assay, a practical procedure for evaluating potential muta-

236

genic agents. In: Vogel F, Röhrborn G (eds) Chemical mutagenesis in mammals and man. Springer, Berlin Heidelberg New York, pp 260–270

Legator MS, Zimmering S (1979) Review of the genetic effects of caffeine. J Environ Sci Health [C] 13/12: 135–188

Lehmann AR, Kirk-Bell S (1974) Effects of caffeine and theophylline on DNA synthesis in unirradiated and UV-irradiated mammalian cells. Mutat Res 26: 73

Lieb M (1961) Enhancement of ultraviolet-induced mutations in bacteria by caffeine. Z Vererbungsl 92: 416–429

Linn S, Schoenbaum SC, Monson RR, Rosner B, Stubblefield PG, Ryan KJ (1982) No association between coffee consumption and adverse outcomes of pregnancy. N Engl J Med 306/3: 141–145

Loprieno N, Barale R, Baroncelli S (1974) Genetic effects of caffeine. Mutat Res 26: 83–87

Lumb J, Sideropoulos A, Shankel D (1968) Inhibition of dark repair of ultraviolet damage in DNA by caffeine and 8-chlorocaffeine. Kinetics of inhibition. Mol Gen Genet 102: 108–111

Lyon MF, Philips RJS, Searle AG (1962) A test for mutagenicity of caffeine in mice. Z Vererbungsl 93: 7–13

Maher VM, Ouellette LM, Curren RD, McCormick JJ (1976) Caffeine enhancement of the cytotoxic and mutagenic effect of ultraviolet irradiation in a xeroderma pigmentosum variant strain of human cells. Biochem Biophys Res Commun 71: 228–234

Matter BE, Grauwiler J (1974) Micronuclei in mouse bone-marrow cells. A simple in vivo model for the evaluation of drug-induced chromosomal aberrations. Mutat Res 23: 239–249

McCann J, Choi E, Yamasaki E, Ames BN (1975) Detection of carcinogens as mutagens in the Salmonella/microsome test: a assay of 300 chemicals. Proc Natl Acad Sci USA 72/12: 5135–5139

Mendelson D (1974) The effect of caffeine on repair systems in oocytes of D. melanogaster I. Mutat Res 22: 145–156

Mirvish SS, Cardesa A, Wallcave L, Shubik P (1975) Induction of mouse lung adenomas by amines or ureas plus nitrite and by N-nitroso compounds: Effect of ascorbate, gallic acid, thiocynate and caffeine. J Natl Cancer Inst 55: 633–636

Mittler S, Mittler JE, Tonetti AM, Szymczak ME (1967a) The effect of caffeine on chromosome loss and nondisjunction in Drosophila. Mutat Res 4: 708–710

Mittler S, Mittler JE, Owens SL (1967b) Loss of chromosomes and nondisjunction induced by caffeine in Drosophila. Nature 214: 424

Mulvihill JJ (1973) Caffeine as teratogen and mutagen. Teratology 8: 69–72

Murota T, Murakami A (1976) Induction of dominant lethal mutations by alkylating agents in germ cells of the silkworm Bombyx mori. Mutat Res 38: 343–344

Neims A (1981) Third international caffeine workshop Nutr Rev 39/4: 184

Novick A (1956) Mutagens and antimutagens. Brookhaven Symp Biol 8: 201–214

Ostertag W, Greif BJ (1967) Die Erzeugung von Chromatidenbrüchen durch Coffein in Leukocytenkulturen des Menschen. Humangenetik 3: 282–294

Ostertag W, Haake J (1966) The mutagenicity in D. melanogaster of caffeine and other compounds which produce chromosome breakage in human cells in culture. Z Vererbungsl 98: 299–308

Ostertag W, Duisberg E, Stürmann M (1965) The mutagenic activity of caffeine in man. Mutat Res 2: 293–296

Roberts JJ, Sturrock JE (1973) Enhancement by caffeine of N-methyl-N-nitrosourea-induced mutations and chromosome aberrations in Chinese hamster cells. Mutat Res 20: 243–255

Röhrborn G (1972) Mutagenitätsuntersuchungen an Mäusen nach chronischer Behandlung mit Coffein. Z Ernährungswiss [Suppl] 14: 54–67

Roy SC (1973) Comparative effects of colchicine, caffeine and hydroquionone on nodal roots of Callisia fragrans. Biol Plant 15: 383–390

Sandlie I, Kleepe K (1982) Effect of caffeine on nucleotide pools in Escherichia Coli. Chem Biol Interact 40: 141–148

Sandlie I, Solberg K, Kleepe K (1980) The effect of caffeine on cell growth and metabolism of thymidine in Escherichia coli. Mutat Res 73: 29

Sarachek A, Bish JT, Ireland R (1970) Relative susceptibilities of caffeine-sensitive and caffeine-resistant strains of Candida albicans to inactivation and mutation by ultraviolet radiation. Arch Mikrobiol 74: 244–257

Schöneich J, Michaelis A, Rieger R (1970) Coffein und die chemische Induktion von Chromatiden Aberrationen bei Vicia faba und Ascitestumoren der Maus. Biol Zentralbl 89: 49–63

Shakarnis VF (1970) Comparative study of the action of caffeine on X chromosome nondisjunction and recessive sex-linked lethal mutations in females of various *D. melanogaster* lines. Sov Genet 6: 921–924

Shankel DM, Kleinberg JA (1967) Comparison of mutational synergism elicited by caffeine and acriflavin with ultraviolet light. Genetics 56: 589

Shiraishi Y, Sandberg AA (1976) Caffeine and sister chromatid exchange. Proc Jpn Acad 52: 379–382

Simon D, Yen S, Cole P (1975) Coffee drinking and cancer of the lower urinary tract. J Natl Cancer Inst 54: 587–591

Simons JWIM, van Zeeland AA, Knaap AGAC (1977) Mutation induction and analysis of repair processes in mammalian cells in vitro. Mutat Res 46: 156

Swietlińska Z, Zuk J (1974) Effects of caffeine on chromosome damage induced by chemical mutagens and ionizing radiation in *Vicia faba* and *Secale cereale*. Mutat Res 26: 89–97

Tazima Y (1981) Apparent threshold and its significance in the assessment of risks due to chemical mutagens. In: Sugimura T, Kondo S, Takebe H (eds) Environmental mutagens and carcinogens. University of Tokyo Press, Tokyo

Terada M, Nishimura H (1975) Mitigation of caffeine-induced teratology in mice by prior chronic caffeine ingestion. Teratology 12: 79–82

Thayer PS, Kensler CJ (1973) Exposure of four generations of mice to caffeine in drinking water. Toxicol Appl Pharmacol 25: 169–179

Thayer PS, Himmelfarb P, Liss RH, Carlson BL (1971) Continuous exposure of HeLa cells to caffeine. Mutat Res 12: 197–203

Timson J (1972) Effect of theobromine, theophylline and caffeine on the mitosis of human lymphocytes. Mutat Res 15: 197–201

Timson J (1977) Caffeine. Mutat Res 47: 1–52

Trosko JE, Chu EHY (1971) Effects of caffeine on the induction of mutations in Chinese hamster cells by ultraviolet light. Mutat Res 12: 337–340

Ts'o PO, Lu P (1964) Interaction of nucleic acids. I. Physical binding of thymine, adenine, steroids, and aromatic hydrocarbons to nucleic acid. Proc Natl Acad Sci USA 51: 17–24

Turnbull D (1975) Factors affecting the response of Chinese hamster cells to mutagenic alkylating agents. PhD Thesis, Sussex University

Venkatasetty R (1972) Genetic variation induced by radiation and chemical agents in *Drosophila melanogaster*. Diss Abstr [B] 32: 5047–5048

Vig BK (1972) Effect of caffeine and other antimetabolites on the induction of somatic crossing-over in *Glycine max* (soybean). Genetics 71: S66

Waldren CA, Patterson D (1979) Effects of caffeine on purine metabolism and ultraviolet light-induced lethality in cultured mammalian cells. Cancer Res 39: 4975–4982

Warren RN (1969) Metabolism of xanthine alkaloids in man. J Chromatogr 40: 468–469

Watson WAF (1975) Lack of an effect of caffeine on repair systems in oocytes of *D. melanogaster* following treatment of mature sperm with alkylating agents. Mutat Res 33: 395–398

Weinstein D, Mauer I, Solomon HM (1972) The effect of caffeine on chromosomes of human lymphocytes in vivo and in vitro studies. Mutat Res 16: 391–399

Witkin E (1959) Post-irradiation metabolism and the timing of ultraviolet-induced mutations in bacteria. In: Proceedings of the Xth international Congress on Genetics, vol 1. University of Toronto Press, Toronto, pp 280–299

Witkin EM, Farquharson EL (1969) Enhancement and diminution of ultraviolet light initiated mutagenesis by post-treatment with caffeine in *E. coli*. In: Wolstenholme GEW, O'Connor M (eds) Ciba Foundation symposium on mutation as a cellular process. Churchill, London, pp 36–49

Yamamoto K, Yamaguchi H (1969) Inhibition by caffeine of the repair of X-ray-induced chromosome breaks in barley. Mutat Res 8: 428–430

Yanders AF, Seaton RK (1962) The lack of mutagenicity of caffeine in *Drosophila*. Am Nat 96: 277–280

Yefremova GI, Filippova LM (1974) Effect of caffeine on crossing-over in *Drosophila melanogaster*. Mutat Res 23: 347–352

Yeomans TC, Hilliker AJ, Holm DG (1972) Recessive lethals in Drosophila sperm: Synergism of caffeine and gamma radiation. Can J Genet Cytol 14: 741

Yielding LW, Riley TL, Yielding KL (1976) Preliminary study of caffeine and chloroquine enhancement of X-ray-induced birth defects. Biochem Biophys Res Commun 68: 1356–1361

XVI Mechanism of Potentiation by Caffeine of Genotoxic Damage Induced by Physical and Chemical Agents: Possible Relevance to Carcinogenesis

J. J. Roberts

1 Introduction

In a number of eukaryotic higher organisms, post-treatment with methylated xanthines, and caffeine in particular, has been found to potentiate the lethal and chromosome-damaging effects of a number of physical and chemical agents. Despite many years of intensive study, there is still discussion as to which of the various effects of caffeine that can be observed in treated or untreated cells are most directly responsible for the enhancement of what are thought to be manifestations of genotoxic damage resulting from modifications to cellular DNA or chromatin. Difficulties in the interpretation of many of these observations arise partly because of the lack of a uniform response by mammalian cells, not only to the initial damaging agents themselves, but also to their subsequent post-treatment incubation in the presence of caffeine. Many of the effects of caffeine on damaged cells have been described in detail previously, and the reader is referred to reviews by Kihlman (1977) and Roberts (1978) for references. It has generally been concluded that one of the major effects of caffeine in treated cells is its ability to change the normal mode of DNA replication in damaged cells. This chapter will therefore examine these particular effects of caffeine in UV- and X-irradiated and chemically modified cells and attempt to assess their significance with regard to potentiation of genotoxic damage. The relationship between such caffeine-induced perturbations of DNA synthesis and the ability of caffeine to modify the mutagenic and carcinogenic effects of genotoxic agents will then be discussed. Initially some of the features of the potentiation by caffeine of the lethal and chromosome-damaging effects of genotoxic compounds will be summarised.

2 Enhancement by Caffeine of Toxicity and Chromosomal Damage Induced by Chemical Agents

Numerous examples are available of the ability of caffeine to enhance the lethal effects of various DNA-damaging agents in a variety of biological systems, including yeast, barley, rodent and some, but not apparently all, human cells (see Roberts 1978 for references). Potentiation of sulphur mustard-induced toxicity was achieved in Chinese hamster cells by non-toxic concentrations of caffeine, and the effect increased markedly with increasing caffeine concentrations (Roberts and Ward 1973). Concentrations of at least $0.1 \, \text{m}M$, however, seem to be required to produce measurable enhancement of toxicity. The increase in toxicity induced by caffeine can result in both the elimination of the shoulder, and a decrease in the slope, of a semilogarithmic survival curve. The temporal aspects of such potentiation indicate that enhancement of toxicity can only be achieved for a limited time after the initial insult. It appears that for both UV irradiation and a number of chemical agents, in various eukaryotic and prokaryotic systems, that the maximum sensitisation is only achieved when cells have passed through at least one DNA-synthesising (S) phase of the cell cycle in the presence of caffeine. Thus using G_1-treated synchronous populations of hamster cells it could be shown that the potentiation of cell killing persisted only during the first S phase after treatment of cells with sulphur mustard but during at least two S phases (> 40 h) after treatment with N-methyl-N-nitroso-urea (MNU) (Roberts and Ward 1973). It thus appeared that some damage (presumably in DNA) persisted into the daughters of MNU-treated cells, and further that the repair of such damage could be influenced by caffeine. Clearly a knowledge of the time following treatment with chemical agents during which caffeine can potentiate genotoxic damage is essential for an understanding of the possible role that caffeine might play in modifying the carcinogenic response of an agent due to effects on DNA repair processes. It now seems that for some agents and cells, incubation with caffeine in the post-DNA-synthesising (G_2) phase of the cell cycle is additionally required for maximum sensitisation (see Lau and Pardee 1982).

It has become apparent during the past few years that there is a direct relationship between the amount of chromosomal damage present in cells and the reproductive cell death induced by a number of physical and chemical agents. Not surprisingly, therefore, it has been found that the potentiation of cell death by post-treatment incubation in the presence of caffeine should be accompanied by a corresponding potentiation of chromosomal damage. Thus in the case of Chinese hamster cells treated with either MNU or *cis*-platinum(II)diammine dichloride (cisplatin), there is a direct relationship between the number of cells exhibiting chromosomal aberrations and the number of cells which fail to divide to form colonies (see Roberts 1978 for references). Just as caffeine potentiation of cell death was shown to be dependent on its presence during the S phase following treatment with UV irradiation and a number of chemical substances, so for these same agents potentiation of chromosome damage is also greatest when caffeine is present during this same phase (Kihlman 1977); although, as with enhancement of toxicity, the presence of caffeine during the G_2 phase of the cell cycle can also increase chromosomal damage at the following mitosis. These various findings therefore suggest that caffeine induces its effect both by interfering with the normal mode of DNA replication in cells treated with DNA-damaging agents, and also possibly by interfering with a post-DNA-synthesis cellular repair process that repairs damage induced during DNA synthesis.

3 Effects of Caffeine Alone on Normal DNA Replication

Caffeine at relatively high concentrations has been reported to inhibit DNA synthesis in HeLa cells (Cleaver 1969) and in first-instar larvae of *Drosophila melanogaster* and in opossum lymphocytes (Boyd and Presley 1974). There is good evidence that an apparent depression of DNA synthesis can be due to an effect on the utilisation of labelled DNA precursors in a number of different biological systems. However, no effect of caffeine on pool sizes was demonstrated by Painter (1980) in a line of Chinese hamster V79 cells used for a detailed study of caffeine effects on replicon initiation (see below).

Pulse-labelled, nascent DNA synthesised in the presence of caffeine or theophylline (in the dose range $1-3 \times 10^{-3}$ M) was shown by Lehmann (1972) and Lehmann and Kirk-Bell (1974) to be smaller than that in similarly labelled mouse cells incubated in caffeine-free medium. The data suggested that this was the result of DNA being synthesised in smaller replicating units rather than due to gaps being formed in normal-sized replicons. The accumulation of DNA, bifilarly labelled with 5-bromodeoxyuridine (BUDR), in the first round of DNA synthesis in human lymphoblastoid cells was similarly attributed to the decreased chain elongation along with the initiation of replication at additional sites in cells treated with caffeine (Tatsumi and Strauss 1979).

Before describing the effects of caffeine on DNA synthesis in cells treated with genotoxic agents I will briefly describe some of the effects of the agents alone on DNA synthesis.

4 Effects of Genotoxic Agents on DNA Synthesis

The ability of genotoxic chemical and physical agents to inhibit, selectively, DNA replication in preference to exerting effects on RNA and protein synthesis has long been recognised. Frequently, cells exhibit a progressive depression in the rate of synthesis of nascent, pulse-labelled DNA following short treatments with various agents. In cells treated with minimally toxic doses, this early depression in rate of DNA synthesis is frequently partially reversed several hours later (Roberts et al. 1971). Subsequent later effects on the rate of DNA synthesis in asynchronous cell cultures probably reflect the agent-induced inhibition of mitosis and the delayed progression into the S phase of the following cell cycle, as observed in studies using synchronised cell cultures (Roberts et al. 1971; Plant and Roberts 1971 a, b; Fraval and Roberts 1978 a, b).

It has been shown that this early inhibition of DNA synthesis is frequently due to inhibition of replicon initiation, as indicated by a decrease in the number of counts in that region of a sucrose gradient of pulse-labelled DNA ($\sim 10^{-1}$), that corresponds to DNA molecules of around 2×10^7 daltons. An effect on replicon initiation has been demonstrated in both human and rodent cells treated with a variety of physical and chemical agents. In X-irradiated cells, the selective inhibition of replicon initiation, with little effect on DNA chain elongation (see below), gives rise to a population of labelled DNA molecules, the majority of which have molecular weights larger than that of those synthesised in the control cells. Painter and Young (1976) suggested that a single lesion within a DNA segment of about 10^9 daltons blocks the initiation of DNA synthesis in that entire segment, possibly following an alteration in the conformation of DNA.

In addition to the inhibition of replicon initiation, certain physical and chemical agents can also affect the rate at which nascent DNA can increase in size to high-molecular-weight, template-sized molecules that can be visualised in sucrose gradients with sedimentation values in excess of 120S. It has been found that while certain agents like X-rays and 4-nitroquinoline-1-oxide (4NQO) predominantly affect DNA initiation, for other agents, such as adriamycin, inhibition of initiation was not as important as the effect on chain elongation. With agents such as ethyleneimine, inhibition of DNA synthesis appears to be due to an equal combination of inhibition of initiation and chain elongation (Painter 1978). The relative contribution of these two effects to the overall inhibition of DNA synthesis induced by a particular agent is likely to depend on the nature of lesions introduced into DNA and on whether they are recognised by excision repair enzymes, as well as on the extent to which the agent induces, either directly or indirectly, X-ray-like breaks in DNA (see above). Dramatic effects on the rate of elongation of DNA in Chinese hamster cells treated with the reactive hydrocarbons 7-bromomethylbenz[a]anthracene (Roberts et al. 1977; Friedlos and Roberts 1978) or the diolepoxide of benzo[a]pyrene (Roberts et al. 1978; Hsu et al. 1979) can result in the transient formation of DNA molecules equal in size to the distance between lesions on one strand of DNA, and in a considerable prolongation of the DNA-synthetising phase in a synchronous population of Chinese hamster cells treated during the G_1 phase of the cell cycle (Roberts et al. 1977).

5 Effects of Post-treatment with Caffeine on DNA Synthesis in Mammalian Cells Treated with Genotoxic Agents

One of the first biochemical effects to be observed in cells that had been treated with genotoxic agents and then incubated in medium containing a non-toxic concentration of caffeine was a reversal of the agent-induced depression in the rate of DNA synthesis. Thus caffeine reverses the progressive inhibition in the rate of DNA synthesis in the first few hours after treatment of asynchronous cultures of Chinese hamster cells with MNU and sulphur mustard (Roberts and Ward 1973). This effect has also been observed in synchronised populations of hamster cells treated in the G_1 phase of the cell cycle with both MNU (Roberts and Ward 1973) and cisplatin (Fraval and Roberts 1978 a). The more rapid completion of DNA synthesis in treated cells that were then incubated in the presence of caffeine leads to their earlier entry into mitosis.

The above reversal in the rate of DNA synthesis in treated cells was subsequently shown by Painter (1980) to be due to a reversal of the specific depression of replicon initiation in X-irradiated cells. Similar effects of caffeine were observed in HeLa cells treated with novobiocin, an agent that inhibits initiation but does not apparently directly damage DNA (Painter 1980), and with aflatoxin (Cramer and Painter 1981) and in human colon carcinoma cells treated with nitrogen mustard, 2-chloro-N-(2'-chloroethyl)-N-methyl-ethanamine (HN2) (Murnane et al. 1980). It was proposed that caffeine alters the conformation of intracellular chromatin in such a way that the conformation usually induced by DNA-damaging agents is reversed (Painter 1980).

A limited number of studies have determined the effect of non-toxic concentrations of caffeine on DNA elongation in cells treated with both physical and chemi-

242

cal agents. Caffeine can inhibit elongation of newly-synthesised DNA in Chinese hamster cells previously treated with N-acetoxy-AAF (Trosko et al. 1973), MNU (Roberts 1975; Fujiwara 1975), cisplatin (van den Berg and Roberts 1976), 7-bromo-methylbenz[a]-anthracene (7-BMBA) (Roberts et al. 1977) and the anti-diolepoxide of benzo[a]pyrene (Roberts et al. 1978; Bowden et al. 1979). As a consequence of this inhibition, low-molecular-weight DNA can accumulate during post-treatment incubation in the presence of caffeine over several hours. Support for the concept that caffeine blocks a process that circumvents lesions in the template DNA by some as yet undefined process came from measurements of the size of DNA synthe-sised in the presence of caffeine following treatment of cells with agents for which the extent of reaction with cellular DNA is known. In the case of cisplatin, 7-bromo-methylbenz[a]anthracene, and benzo[a]pyrene diolepoxide-treated Chinese ham-ster cells, the DNA newly synthesised during a 3-h post-treatment period approxi-mated to the distance between lesions on one strand of the DNA. Hence for these compounds it would appear that all lesions are circumvented by a caffeine-sensitive process.

6 Caffeine-Induced DNA Template Breakage in Treated Cells: Double-Strand Break Formation

The molecular weight of template DNA of Chinese hamster cells treated with 7-BMBA and incubated for either 4 h or 24 h is indistinguishable from that of con-trol cells. Hence the excision repair process known to operate in these cells (Dipple and Roberts 1977) is not associated with the formation of persistent breaks or gaps in template DNA. If, however, similarly treated cells are incubated in the presence of caffeine, then a time-dependent decrease in the size of template DNA is observed (Friedlos and Roberts 1978). Similar effects have been observed in benzo[a]pyrene diolepoxide-treated (Roberts et al. 1978) and, more recently, in sulphur mustard-treated hamster cells (J.J. Roberts, F. Friedlos, unpublished results).

A likely mechanism for the formation of breaks in the template DNA of cells treated with DNA-damaging agents and then incubated in the presence of caffeine is illustrated in Fig. 1. The reduced size of nascent DNA synthesised in the presence of caffeine suggests that gaps are left opposite lesions on the template strand, giving rise to single-stranded regions of DNA. These single-stranded regions of template DNA, which still contain lesions, could therefore act as substrates, either for specif-ic endonucleases which are still able to recognize specific lesions on the DNA or for non-specific single-stranded endonucleases. As a consequence of such incisions, double-strand breaks would be introduced into DNA which, if persistent into mito-sis, would result in the observed chromosomal damage. The presumptive endonu-clease(s) involved in the incision of template DNA could be either constitutive en-zymes or be induced by this newly-formed damage in DNA, as possibly implied by the delayed formation of breaks. This model would predict that following the initial incision step of excision repair, an inability to carry out exonucleolytic degradation and repair replication (in the absence of a suitable template) would be expected to lead to a decrease in the rate or extent of removal of DNA-bound adducts from the template strand. Post-treatment incubation in the presence of caffeine does indeed

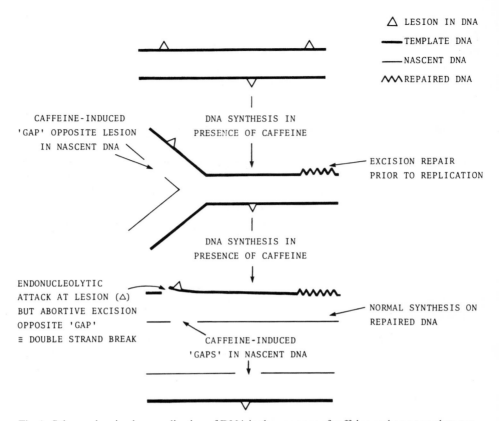

Fig. 1. Scheme showing how replication of DNA in the presence of caffeine and on a template containing excisable damage could lead to DNA template degradation and DNA double-strand breaks. *Above:* template DNA is substituted with 7-BMBA. *Middle:* both excision repair and replication occur on the damaged template. Excision repair in a nonreplicating region proceeds successfully, although possibly slowed by the presence of caffeine, while in the replication region, the influence of caffeine is to disrupt replication repair, leading to gaps in the nascent DNA. *Below:* replication proceeds, but before the caffeine-induced gaps in the nascent DNA are sealed incision of the template strand at the site of the adduct occurs, producing a double-strand break, which, if persistent into the mitosis, could lead to the observed chromosomal effects

result in a small but definite inhibition of excision of 7-BMBA adducts from the DNA of Chinese hamster cells, and the effect is more marked at late times after treatment (Friedlos and Roberts 1979).

7 Caffeine-Induced Premature Mitosis

Recent studies (Lau and Pardee 1982) have suggested that caffeine can potentiate cell killing of HN2-treated BHK cells by a process which is different from those that have been considered so far and apparently does not involve effects either on the initiation of DNA synthesis or on DNA elongation. A dose of HN2 which was only minimally toxic to BHK cells apparently did not produce any significant effect on DNA synthesis but did, nevertheless, cause a mitotic delay for up to 6 h. Unscheduled DNA synthesis could be detected during this G_2 delay period, and when it was completed, cells proceeded into mitosis. Post-treatment with caffeine ($2\,mM$) increased the lethality of HN2 five- to tenfold and allowed the HN2-treated cells to traverse the S and G_2 phases at a normal rate. Importantly, Lau and Pardee found that at the low concentration of HN2 used ($0.5\,\mu M$ for 1 h), not only was there no significant effect on DNA synthesis, but also the rate of DNA synthesis was not further modified by caffeine.

Lau and Pardee (1982) made the further interesting observation that caffeine did not act directly to potentiate the lethality of HN2, but rather by means of some newly-synthesised protein. Thus HN2-treated cells were protected from the lethal and chromosome-damaging effects of caffeine by low doses of cycloheximide. Moreover, even after HN2-treated cells had entered the G_2 phase they could still be protected by cycloheximide. It was presumed, therefore, that proteins might be required for normal mitosis and that these could be induced by caffeine.

The various effects produced by caffeine in cells treated with DNA-damaging agents can be summarised as follows:

1. Reversal of agent-induced depression of DNA synthesis
2. Reversal of agent-induced inhibition of replicon initiation
3. Decrease in size of replicons (also in absence of DNA damage)
4. Inhibition of elongation of nascent DNA (to high-molecular-weight, template-sized DNA)
5. Time-dependent incision of template DNA
6. Time-dependent formation of DNA double-strand breaks
7. Inhibition of excision of base damage
8. Induction of protein synthesis (caffeine effect nullified by cycloheximide)
9. Prevention of S phase delay and G_2 arrest

A feature of many reports is the ability of caffeine to reverse the inhibiting effect of agents on DNA synthesis and on cell division, effects that may reduce the time required for the operation of certain cellular repair processes. However, the time-dependent formation of double-strand breaks in DNA by the action of a single-stranded endonuclease at the site of caffeine-induced gaps in nascent DNA emerges as the most appealing mechanism for the formation of the gross chromosomal damage and chromosome fragmentation frequently observed in cells that have been treated with genotoxic agents and then exposed to caffeine. The further possibility that the endonuclease(s) are not constitutive but are induced following the formation of damage to nascent DNA remains to be established.

8 Modifying Effects of Caffeine on Tumour Induction by Chemical and Physical Agents: Possible Role of DNA Repair

An interest in the possibility that caffeine would influence tumour induction has clearly been stimulated by the known effects of caffeine on the lethal and clastogenic effects of genotoxic chemicals in mammalian cells. The effects of caffeine on mu-

Table 1. Inhibition of carcinogenesis by caffeine

Inhibition, animal	Reference
Benzo[a]pyrene-induced subcutaneous tumours	Leitner and Shear (1942/3)
Inhibition of DMBA binding to DNA of cultured mouse epidermal cells	Shoyab (1979a)[a]
Stimulation of murine hepatic AHH activity in vitro	Shoyab (1979b)[a]
UV-induced skin cancer in mice	(R) Zajdela and Latarjet (1973)
Cigarette smoke condensate-induced skin cancer in mice	(R) Rothwell (1974)
4NQO-induced lung tumours in mice	(R) Nomura (1977)
Urethan-induced lung tumours in mice	(R) Theiss and Shimkin (1978)
Spontaneous melanotic tumours in *Dorsophila*	Ghelelovitch (1975)
Spontaneous pulmonary adenomas in mice	Theiss and Shimkin (1978)
LELO-virus-transformed cell-induced tumours in hamsters (by theophylline)	Reddi and Constantinides (1972)
4NQO-induced transformation of BALB/3T3 cells	(R) Kakunaga (1975)
4HAQO-induced pancreatic tumours in partially pancreatectomised rats	(R) Dendi et al. (1979)

(R), protocols that could implicate early effects on DNA repair
[a] These studies were not directly measuring carcinogenesis, but provide an explanation for the findings of Leitner and Shear (1942/3).

Table 2. Inability of caffeine to effect carcinogenesis

Tumour	Reference
MNU-induced lymphocytic leukemia	(R) Nomura (1980)
MNU-induced lung tumours	(R) Nomura (1980)
N-hydroxyurethane-induced lung tumours	(R) Nomura (1980)
N-ethyl-N-nitrosourethane-induced lung tumours	(R) Nomura (1980)
MNU-induced thymic lymphoma	(R) J.J.Roberts, (unpublished results 1982)
N-butyl-N-(4-hydroxybutyl)nitrosamine-induced bladder carcinogenesis	Nakanishi (1978, 1980)

tagenesis is however less clear since both potentiating and inhibiting effects have been reported (see Roberts 1978 for references) often depending on such factors as the concentration of caffeine employed, the time after treatment when present, and on the precise methodology for determining mutation induction. It is not surprising, therefore, that there should be similar contradictory reports of its effect on carcinogenesis. Thus both inhibitory and synergistic effects have been reported as well as a lack of effect (Tables 1–3). As discussed earlier, for caffeine to potentiate cell killing of UV-irradiated or chemically treated cells it generally needs to be present for one S phase after treatment. In certain special instances, when, for example, some cells were treated with methylating agents, cell killing could be potentiated for up to 48 h after treatment by caffeine. Therefore only in those carcinogenesis experiments in which caffeine is present for such a defined period of time after administration of a potential carcinogen can it be presumed that caffeine is acting so as to modify the immediate effects of the genotoxic damage. Under these conditions it could be acting in a way that might alter the initiating effect of a carcinogen. When caffeine is

246

Table 3. Potentiation of carcinogenesis by caffeine

Action potentiated	Reference
Enhancement of UV- or 4NQO-induced skin cancer	Hoshino and Tanooka (1979)
Benzo[a]pyrene potentiation of FLV-induced leukemogenesis	(R) Raikow et al. (1981)
Dimethylbenz[a]anthracene-induced breast cancer (with fat)	Minton et al. (1982)
Chemically induced morphological transformation of Syrian hamster cells	Donovan and DiPaulo (1974)
Enhancement of induction of SV40 from transformed hamster kidney cells by UV	Zamansky et al. (1976)

given during a subsequent, and possibly prolonged, period after the carcinogen it might be considered to be acting on possible promotional factors in carcinogenesis.

The earliest reports of an effect of caffeine on carcinogenesis came from Leitner and Shear (1942/3) who found that when applied with benzo[a]pyrene it could inhibit the formation of subcutaneous tumours in mice. It now seems possible that caffeine may inhibit the binding of the hydrocarbon to cellular DNA, since the binding of dimethylbenz[a]anthracene to the DNA of cultured murine epidermal cells in culture was shown to be inhibited by caffeine (Shoyab 1979 a). A possible mechanism for such inhibition of hydrocarbon binding to DNA is indicated by the subsequent finding that caffeine stimulates the activity of murine liver aryl hydrocarbon hydroxylase (Shoyab 1979 b), which could result in the more rapid metabolic inactivation of the hydrocarbon. The reported suppression of the carcinogenic effect of cigarette smoke condensate by caffeine (Rothwell 1974) could also be due to the altered metabolism of polycyclic hydrocarbons present in the mixture.

The proposal that caffeine might inhibit an error-prone postreplication repair process in *Escherichia coli* (Witkin and Farquharson 1969) prompted a search for an anticarcinogenic effect of caffeine. Zajdela and Latarjet (1973) observed a decreased yield of skin tumours following application of caffeine to the UV-irradiated ears of mice which they thought accorded with this proposal.

The decrease in the number of 4NQO-induced lung tumours, accompanied by an increased mortality, on post-treatment of mice with caffeine, was likewise thought by Nomura (1976, 1977) to be due to the inhibition of an error-prone DNA repair process. However, the lungs of young adult mice remained sensitive to the antineoplastic action of caffeine for at least 5 days after 4NQO treatment, while the caffeine-sensitive period is confined to the first round of DNA replication after 4NQO for both mutation in *E. coli* (Kondo 1977) and the killing and transformation of cultured mouse cells (Kakunaga 1975). A more detailed analysis of the timing of the antineoplastic action of caffeine coupled to an estimation of the generation time of "target" cells that are converted to neoplastic cells resolved this apparent paradox (Nomura 1980). The final yields of lung tumours produced when either young adult mice or mouse fetuses are treated with 4NQO or urethan are markedly reduced by post-treatment with caffeine. However the lungs of day 15 fetuses were sensitive to the antineoplastic action of caffeine for only 1.5 days, in contrast to the lungs of adult mice, which remained sensitive to the antineoplastic action of caffeine for

21 days after 4NQO treatment and for at least 10 days after urethan treatment. The difference in the caffeine-sensitive period between young adults and fetuses is compatible with the difference in the generation time of the stem cells in the lung between young adults (2–25 days) and day 15 fetuses (1.5 days). The results were therefore considered to support the above-mentioned proposal that caffeine acts during the first postcarcinogen DNA replication period.

Caffeine could therefore be inhibiting carcinogenesis either by inhibiting an inducible error-prone postreplication repair process, or by potentiating the lethal effects of chemical carcinogens, which could lead to the death of cells that would have produced a tumour had they survived. The latter possibility was discounted by Nomura on the grounds that caffeine did not similarly reduce the yield of tumours produced by a number of other agents, such as N-hydroxyurethan, *N*-methyl-*N*-nitrosourea, and *N*-ethyl-*N*-nitrosourea. These latter agents induce mutations by base mispairing (which would presumably not be modified by caffeine), rather than by an inducible error-prone postreplication repair process, as in the case of UV- or 4NQO-induced damage. Inhibition of such an error-prone process by caffeine would therefore be expected to reduce the number of mutagenic events.

Theiss and Shimkin (1978) observed an inhibition of urethan-induced lung tumours in mice by post-treatment with caffeine and the effect was again markedly dependent on the time of administration of caffeine. The most pronounced suppression occurred when caffeine was given as only two injections 3 h before and 3 h after urethan administration. Of considerable interest was the ability of caffeine to suppress the inhibition of DNA synthesis induced by urethan, an effect reminiscent of the effects described above on the reversal of either the suppression of DNA synthesis or the inhibition of replicon initiation in cells in culture treated with a variety of chemical agents. These findings would indicate that rather than antagonizing the lethal effects of urethan (as suggested by Theiss and Shimkin 1978), caffeine is likely to be potentiating the lethal effects of urethan in lung tissue by inhibiting a postreplication repair process. Hence in these experiments, as in those by Nomura (1980), caffeine could be acting in a manner that increases lethal damage while inhibiting the induction of mutations.

Dendi et al. (1979) found that caffeine reduced the number of acinar cell adenomas in the pancreas induced by 4-hydroxyaminoquinoline-1-oxide (4HAQO) in rats that have previously been subjected to partial pancreatectomy. Similar levels of reduction in tumour induction were obtained when the caffeine was given for 6 consecutive days starting either immediately after or 6 days after administration of 4HAQO. The 4HAQO was in both instances given 3 days after partial pancreatectomy, which corresponds to the time of maximum DNA synthesis in the regenerating pancreas. Again, these findings were therefore thought to indicate that caffeine was, as in the above examples, likely to be interfering with the error-prone repair of damage induced in DNA by the 4HAQO, rather than affecting the level to which it interacts with cellular DNA.

Consistent with the reasoning that damage induced by some agents such as UV-irradiation and 4NQO, but not by others such as MNU, is repaired by an error-prone mechanism that can be inhibited by caffeine so as to reduce their mutagenic potential, was the finding that caffeine also failed to potentiate the thymic lymphoma-inducing effect of MNU in C57BL mice when given in four consecutive

248

Table 4. Effect of immediate post-treatment with caffeine on MNU-induced thymic lymphoma in C57BL female mice

MNU dose (mg/kg)	Thymic lymphoma (%)	
	− caffeine	+ caffeine[a]
20	5.3 (1/19)	7.7 (1/13)
30	17.0 (5/30)	15.0 (3/20)
40	19.0 (5/26)	43.0 (9/21)
	28.0 (7/28)	21.0 (5/24)
	27.0 (8/30)[b]	24.0 (7/29)[b]
	28.0 (6/21)	
50	40.0 (8/20)	
80	60.0 (12/20)	
	85.0 (17/20)	
	100.0 (20/20)	

[a] Caffeine (0.75 mmol/kg) was given 1 h after MNU and three times thereafter at 12-h intervals
[b] Male mice

Table 5. Effect of caffeine on MNU-induced thymic lymphoma in C57BL mice

MNU (mg/kg)	Thymic lymphoma (%)			
	− caffeine	+ caffeine[a]	+ caffeine after MNU[b]	− caffeine before MNU[c]
40	19 (5/26)	43 (9/21)	23 (7/30)	
	28 (7/28)	21 (5/24)	19 (4/19)	18 (4/22)

[a] Caffeine (0.75 mmol/kg) was given immediately after MNU and three times thereafter at 12-h intervals
[b] Caffeine treatment (as above) was started 5 days after MNU
[c] Caffeine treatment (as above) was started 5 days prior to MNU

intraperitoneal doses of 0.75 mmol/kg every 12 h for 48 h after the nitroso compounds (Tables 4, 5) (J. J. Roberts, unpublished results 1982). Caffeine administered under the above conditions was, however, able to potentiate the lethal effects of MNU on bone marrow stem cells.

Caffeine has been shown not to enhance N-butyl-N-(hydroxybutyl)nitrosamine (BBN)-induced bladder carcinogenesis in Wistar rats when both agents were administered in the drinking water for 40 weeks (Nakanishi et al. 1978, 1980). It is not known whether the dose of caffeine used in these experiments (0.1% in drinking water) would be sufficient to potentiate the lethal effects of BBN and hence whether the experimental protocol examined the action of caffeine as a possible modifier of initiating damage to DNA or simply its action as a possible promoter of bladder carcinogenesis. The principal metabolite of BBN is N-butyl-N-(3-carboxypropyl)nitrosamine (BCPN). Injection of BCPN by urethral catheter at a dose of 25 mg/kg produced considerable damage to the DNA of bladder epithelium within 2 h as indicated by its more rapid sedimentation in alkaline sucrose than control DNA. However, there were no changes in the DNA of bladder epithelium of rats given

0.05% BCPN solution to drink for 4 weeks, nor in that of animals subsequently given caffeine (8 mg/kg body weight) and killed 2, 24 or 48 h later (Miyata et al. 1980).

There appears to be only one report of the ability of caffeine alone to potentiate the carcinogenic effects of physical, chemical or viral agents (Hoshino and Tanooka 1979). However, the protocol of the experiment was such that it was not apparent whether caffeine was potentiating event in carcinogenesis or having an effect on the subsequent promotional process. Thus it was found that caffeine increased the incidence of malignant tumours in mouse skin from 26% to 49% when the skin, given a single exposure to beta rays and 20 subsequent paintings with 4NQO, was further treated by additional painting with caffeine on alternate days of the 4NQO painting.

On the other hand, it has been shown that caffeine can enhance the ability of a chemical to potentiate viral carcinogenesis. Thus the incidence of leukemia development in STL/J mice given very small amounts of Friend leukemia virus (FLV) can be increased if the animals are first exposed to chemical carcinogens such as methyl methanesulphonate (Raikow et al. 1979) or benzo[a]pyrene (O'Kunewick et al. 1980; Raikow et al. 1981). Post-treatment with caffeine can further enhance this chemical potentiation of viral carcinogenesis. In the absence of benzo[a]pyrene caffeine has no carcinogenic effect, either when given alone or in conjunction with FLV. These results were considered to be consistent with the possibility that the potentiation of virus-induced leukemia may be linked to the damage to the DNA induced by the hydrocarbon. Moreover, if the repair of hydrocarbon-induced damage to DNA is inhibited by the addition of caffeine, this further enhances the potentiating effect of benzo[a]pyrene on leukemia induction. Presumably the persistence of gaps in either nascent or template DNA (see above) could facilitate the integration of viral DNA into host cells.

The induction of infectious virus from some SV40-transformed cells after treatment with chemical or physical agents is well documented (Rothschild and Black 1970). This induction is probably a consequence of the common ability of such agents to produce breaks or gaps in DNA, either directly or during the operation of DNA repair processes. Exposure to caffeine can significantly increase the level of induction of virus by ultraviolet irradiation, presumably by increasing gap formation during the inhibition of a DNA repair process(es) (Zamansky et al. 1976).

Conflicting reports exist with regard to the effects of caffeine on the chemically-induced transformation of cells in vitro. Caffeine has been reported to enhance the morphological transformation of Syrian hamster cells treated with diverse chemicals (Donovan and DiPaulo 1974), but to inhibit 4NQO-induced morphological transformation of mouse BALB/3T3-A-31 clone cells (Kakunaga 1975). The enhancement of transformation depended on a number of factors, including concentration of caffeine, the timing and length of exposure, and type of carcinogen used. However, until the relationship between transformation in vitro in these various systems and carcinogenesis in vivo is better understood, the relevance of these observations to the possible effect of caffeine on cancer induction cannot readily be assessed.

9 Conclusions

The considerable number of studies in which the carcinogenic effects of caffeine either alone or in combination with a variety of chemical agents have been investigated do not suggest that caffeine can, in general, potentiate the carcinogenic effects of chemical carcinogens. In fact a majority of the observations seem to indicate that caffeine can often have an inhibitory effect on tumour induction. The precise mechanism of such inhibition is not known, but it has been suggested that it could result from the inhibition of an error-prone repair pathway analogous to that operating in prokaryotic cells. Certainly there is some evidence that caffeine can potentiate chemically induced cell killing in vivo and that this could be due to an increase in DNA damage following inhibition of cellular DNA repair processes. However, it should be stressed that the concentrations of caffeine required to produce marked potentiation of cell killing and chromosomal damage induced by toxic agents in vitro are far in excess of those which could be tolerated in vivo. Moreover, for such potentiation to occur caffeine needs to be present for a precise period of time immediately following the initial insult to DNA. These factors make it unlikely that the levels of caffeine consumed in the normal course of events are able to modify damage induced in DNA as a result of exposure to genotoxic chemicals.

References

Bowden GT, Hsu IC, Harris CC (1979) The effect of caffeine on cytotoxicity, mutagenesis, and sister-chromatid exchanges in Chinese hamster cells treated with dihydrodiol epoxide derivatives of benzo(*a*)pyrene. Mutat Res 63: 361–370

Boyd JB, Presley JM (1974) Repair replication and photorepair of DNA in larvae of *Drosophila melanogaster*. Genetics 77: 687–700

Cleaver JE (1969) Repair replication of mammalian cell DNA: effects of compounds that inhibit DNA synthesis or dark repair. Radiat Res 37: 334–348

Cramer P, Painter RB (1981) Effects of aflatoxin B1 and caffeine on DNA replicon initiation in Hela cells. Carcinogenesis 2: 379–384

Dendi A, Inui S, Takahashi S, Yoshimura H, Miyagi N, Konishi Y (1979) Inhibitory effect of caffeine on pancreatic tumors induced by 4-hydroxyaminoquinolien-1-oxide after partial pancreatectomy in rats (in Japanese). Isako No Ayumi 108: 224

Dipple A, Roberts JJ (1977) Excision of 7-bromomethylbenz(*a*)-anthracene DNA adducts in replicating mammalian cells. Biochemistry 16: 1499–1503

Donovan PJ, DiPaulo JA (1974) Caffeine enhancement of chemical carcinogen-induced transformation of cultured Syrian hamster cells. Cancer Res 34: 2720–2727

Fraval HNA, Roberts JJ (1978a) Effects of *cis* platinum(II) diammine dichloride on the survival and rate of synthesis in synchronously growing Chinese hamster V79-379A cells in the presence and absence of caffeine-inhibited repair: evidence for an inducible repair system. Chem Biol Interact 23: 99–110

Fraval HNA, Roberts JJ (1978b) The effects of *cis*-platinum(II)diammine dichloride on survival and rate of DNA synthesis in synchronously growing Hela Cells in the absence and presence of caffeine. Chem Biol Interact 23: 111–119

Friedlos F, Roberts JJ (1978) Caffeine-inhibited DNA repair in 7-bromobenz(*a*)anthracene-treated Chinese hamster cells: formation of breaks in parental DNA and inhibition of ligation of nascent DNA as a mechanism for the enhancement of lethality and chromosome damage. Mutat Res 50: 263–275

Friedlos F, Roberts JJ (1979) Caffeine inhibits excision of 7-bromomethylbenz(*a*)anthracene-DNA adducts from exponentially growing but not from stationary phase Chinese hamster cells. Nucleic Acids Res 5: 4795–4803

Fujiwara Y (1975) Post replication of alkylation damage to DNA of mammalian cells in culture. Cancer Res 35: 2780–2790

Ghelelovitch S (1975) Effet de la caféine sure le developpement des tumeurs mélaniques chez la drosophile. Mutat Res 28: 221–226

Hoshino H, Tanooka H (1979) Caffeine enhances skin tumour induction in mice. Toxicol Lett 4: 83–85

Hsu IC, Bowden GT, Harris CC (1979) A comparison of cytotoxicity, ouabain-resistant mutation, sister-chromatid exchanges, and nascent DNA synthesis in Chinese hamster cells treated with dihydrodiol epoxide derivatives of benzo(a)pyrene. Mutat Res 63: 351–359

Kakunaga T (1975) Caffeine inhibits cell transformation by 4-nitroquinoline-1-oxide. Nature 258: 248–250

Kihlman BA (1977) Caffeine and chromosomes. Elsevier, Amsterdam New York Oxford

Kondo S (1977) A test for mutation theory of cancer: carcinogenesis by misrepair of 4-nitroquinoline-1-oxide DNA damage. Br J Cancer 35: 395–601

Lau CC, Pardee AB (1982) Mechanism by which caffeine potentiates lethality of nitrogen mustard. Proc Natl Acad Sci USA 79: 2942–2946

Lehmann AR (1972) Effects of caffeine on DNA synthesis in mammalian cells. Biophys J 12: 1316–1325

Lehmann AR, Kirk-Bell S (1974) Effects of caffeine and theophylline on DNA synthesis in unirradiated and UV-irradiated mammalian cells. Mutat Res 26: 73–82

Leitner J, Shear MJ (1942/3) Quantitative experiments on the production of subcutaneous tumours in strain A mice with marginal doses of 3,4-benzpyrene. J Natl Cancer Inst 3: 455–477

Minton JP, Foecking MK, Abou-Issa H (1982) Enhancement of DMBA-induced breast cancer by caffeine and fat diet. Am Assoc Cancer Res Abstr 272: 70

Miyata Y, Hagiwara A, Nakatsuka T, Murasaki G, Arai M, Ito N (1980) Effects of caffeine and saccharin on DNA in the bladder epithelium of rats treated with N-butyl-N-(3-carboxyproypl)-nitrosamine. Chem Biol Interact 29: 291–302

Murnane JP, Byfield JE, Ward JF, Calabro-Jones P (1980) Effects of methylated xanthines on mammalian cells treated with bifunctional alkylating agents. Nature 285: 326–329

Nakanishi K, Fukushima S, Shibata M, Shirai T, Ogiso T, Ito N (1978) Effect of phenacetin and caffeine on the urinary bladder of rats treated with N-butyl-N-(4-hydroxybutyl)nitrosamine. Gan 69: 395–400

Nakanishi K, Hirose M, Ogiso T, Hasegawa R, Arai M, Ito N (1980) Effects of sodium saccharin and caffeine on the urinary bladder of rats treated with N-butyl-N-(4-hydroxybutyl)nitrosamine. Gan 71: 490–500

Nomura T (1976) Diminution of tumorogenesis initiated by 4-nitroquinolino-1-oxide by post treatment with caffeine in mice. Nature 260: 547–549

Nomura T (1977) Inhibitory effect of caffeine on chemical mutagenesis in mice. Proc Natl Assoc Cancer Res 18: 244

Nomura T (1980) Timing of chemically-induced neoplasia in mice revealed by the antineoplastic action of caffeine. Cancer Res 40: 1332–1340

O'Kunewick JP, Raikow RB, Meredith RF, Brozovich BJ, Seeman PR, Magliere KC (1980) Suppression of stem cells and immune responses and enhancement of viral leukemogenesis by chemical carcinogens. In: Baum SJ, Ledney GD, van Bekkum DW (eds) Experimental hematology today. Springer, Berlin Heidelberg New York, pp 127–136

Painter RB (1978) Inhibition of DNA replicon initiation by 4-nitroquinoline-1-oxide, adriamycin, and ethylenemine. Cancer Res 38: 4445–4449

Painter RB (1980) Effect of caffeine on DNA synthesis in irradiated and unirradiated mammalian cells. J Mol Biol 143: 289–301

Painter RB, Young BR (1976) Formation of nascent DNA molecules during inhibition of replicon initiation in mammalian cells. Biochim Biophys Acta 418: 146–153

Plant JE, Roberts JJ (1971a) A novel mechanism for the inhibition of DNA synthesis following methylation: the effect of N-methyl-N-nitrosourea on Hela cells. Chem Biol Interact 3: 337–342

Plant JE, Roberts JJ (1971b) Extension of the pre-DNA synthetic phase of the cell cycle as a consequence of DNA alkylation in Chinese hamster cells: a possible mechanism of DNA repair. Chem Biol Interact 3: 343–351

Raikow RB, Meridith RF, Brozovich BJ, Seeman PR, Livingston AE, O'Kunewick JP (1979) Potentiating effect of methyl methanesulphonate on Friend virus leukemogenesis. Proc Soc Exp Biol Med 161: 210–215

Raikow RB, O'Kunewick JP, Buffo MJ, Jones DL, Brozovich BJ, Seeman PR, Koval TM (1981) Potentiating effect of benzo(a)pyrene and caffeine on Friend viral leukemogenesis. Carcinogenesis 2: 1–6

Reddi PK, Constantinides SM (1972) Partial suppression of tumour production by dibutyryl cyclic AMP and theophylline. Nature 238: 286–287

Roberts JJ (1975) Repair of acetylated DNA in mammalian cells. In: Hanawalt PC, Setlow RB (eds) Molecular mechanisms of DNA repair. Plenum, New York, p 611

Roberts JJ (1978) The repair of DNA modified by cytotoxic mutagenic and carcinogenic chemicals. Adv Radiat Biol 7: 212–436

Roberts JJ, Ward KN (1973) Inhibition of post-replication repair of alkylated DNA by caffeine in Chinese hamster cells but not Hela cells. Chem Biol Interact 7: 241–264

Roberts JJ, Brent TP, Crathorn AR (1971) Evidence for the inactivation and repair of the mammalian DNA template after alkylation by mustard gas and half mustard gas. Eur J Cancer 7: 515–524

Roberts JJ, Friedlos F, van den Berg HW, Kirkland DJ (1977) Inhibition by caffeine of post replication repair in Chinese hamster cells treated with 7-bromomethylbenz(a)-anthracene: enhancement of toxicity, chromosome damage and inhibition of ligation of newly-synthesized DNA. Chem Biol Interact 17: 265–290

Roberts JJ, Friedlos F, Belka ES (1978) DNA template breakage and decreased excision of hydrocarbon-derived adducts from Chinese hamster cell DNA following caffeine-induced inhibition of post replication repair. In: Hanawalt PC, Friedberg EC, Fox CF (eds) DNA repair mechanisms. Academic, New York, pp 527–530

Rothschild H, Black PH (1970) Analysis of SV40 induced transformation of hamster kidney tissue in vitro. VII. Induction of SV40 from transformed hamster cell clones by various agents. Virology 42: 251–256

Rothwell K (1974) Dose-related inhibition of chemical carcinogenesis in mouse skin by caffeine. Nature 252: 69–70

Shoyab M (1979a) Caffeine inhibits the binding of dimethylbenz(a)anthracene to murine epidermal cells DNA in culture. Arch Biochem Biophys 196: 307–310

Shoyab M (1979b) The stimulation of murine hepatic aryl hydrocarbon hydroxylase activity in vitro by caffeine. Cancer Lett 8: 43–49

Tatsumi K, Strauss BS (1979) Accumulation of DNA growing points in caffeine-treated human lymphoblastoid cells. J Mol Biol 135: 435–449

Theiss JC, Shimkin MB (1978) Inhibiting effect of caffeine on spontaneous and urethan-induced lung tumors in strain A mice. Cancer Res 38: 1759–1761

Trosko JE, Frank P, Chu EHY, Becker JE (1973) Caffeine inhibition of post-replication repair of N-acetoxy-2-acetylaminofluorene damaged DNA in Chinese hamster cells. Cancer Res 33: 2444–2449

van den Berg HW, Roberts JJ (1976) Inhibition by caffeine of post-replication repair in Chinese hamster cells treated with cis platinum(II)diammine dichloride: the extent of platinum binding to template DNA in relation to the size of low molecular weight nascent DNA. Chem Biol Interact 12: 375–390

Witkin EM, Farquharson EL (1969) Enhancement and diminution of ultraviolet light initiated mutagenesis by post treatment with caffeine in Escherichia coli. In: Wolstenholme GEW, O'Connor M (eds) Ciba Foundation symposium on mutation as cellular process. Churchill, London, pp 36–49

Zajdela F, Latarjet R (1973) Effet inhibiteur de la caféine sur l'induction de cancers cutanés par les rayons ultraviolet chez la souris. C R Seances Acad Sci [III] 277: 1073–1076

Zamansky GB, Kleinman LF, Little JB, Black PH, Kaplan JC (1976) The effect of caffeine on the ultraviolet light induction of SV40 from transformed hamster kidney cells. Virology 73: 468–475

Subject Index

258